Copyright Information

Cover art: Martin Mailloux

Copyright © 2011 by Frédéric Patenaude

All rights reserved

First Edition, January 2011

Published by:

Raw Vegan

Montreal, Canada

www.fredericpatenaude.com

Customer support: **www.replytofred.com**

To get the DVD "Raw Food Nutrition Explained" that completes the information in this book, go to:
www.rawcontroversies.com/dvds

Important Medical Disclaimer

The information in this book does not constitute medical or health advice, but is presented simply with the intention of sharing the personal experiences of Frederic Patenaude with healthful living.

Frederic Patenaude does not provide any medical opinions or health advice. If you have questions regarding specific medical or healthcare matters, you should speak directly with your doctor or licensed healthcare provider.

The information contained in this book is not intended to replace the advice of a licensed healthcare provider.

Raw Food Controversies

Acknowledgements

It never ceases to amaze me how certain seemingly insignificant moments have the potential to define our existence. In writing this book, I realized how my thinking has been shaped by all the experiences that I have had, and all the people I have met.

Several people contributed to this book, including all the characters you will meet in it. They are all real people, who were part of this "raw" journey along with me. I'd like to thank all of them, because they all had something to contribute to this book.

I have changed some of the names and sometimes altered the chronology of some of the events I relate, only to make the story easier to tell and to protect the privacy of certain people who would prefer not to be recognized.

I'd like to thank all the raw food "gurus" that I have featured in this book. I know some of my writings will appear as harsh criticism of their philosophies, but in reality, I have no one to blame but myself for some of the mistakes I have made. I wanted to tell my raw food story without hiding behind obscure references to "some well-known people in the raw-food movement," and so I have chosen to name all the people I feature, who have themselves decided to be public personalities by writing their own books.

I'd like to thank my wonderful wife Veronica, who gave me the idea for this book. I thought I had already written my "raw story" in my book *The Raw Secrets*, but she knew I had much more to say. Our conversation in downtown Vancouver sparked the idea for *Raw Food Controversies*, and she contributed key parts to this book.

Table of Contents

CHAPTER 19

CHAPTER 20

CHAPTER 21

CHAPTER 22

CHAPTER 23

CHAPTER 24

CHAPTER 25

CHAPTER 26

CHAPTER 27

CHAPTER 28

Introduction

The Proof is in the Raw Pudding

"To a great extent, when you take up the raw food diet, you become a new and different person. You don't just stay the old person, only a little healthier...You become a person who is more a part of the one great life of Nature and less of the confused human world."

Joe Alexander,
Blatant Raw Foodist Propaganda

This is my raw food story.

Again, I find myself writing a book about the raw food diet, meant for raw food newbies and rookies or simply anyone who wants to avoid common mistakes most raw foodists make.

Amazon.com is filled with books on the raw food diet, many of which are meant to introduce the concept to a broad audience. Those books have already done the job of explaining what exactly a raw food diet is. So why in the world would someone pick up another book with the unlikely title *Raw Food Controversies?*

I've been asked by my graphic artist Martin (my old high-school friend, who has done the cover design for all of my books, and has followed my raw food experiments of the past 14 years as an outsider), "What exactly is a raw food controversy?

"I get it. Raw foodists like to eat raw foods. They're vegetarians who prefer not to cook their food. That part is clear."

"But what controversies could there be within this bunch of health-food enthusiasts?"

When Martin asked me what kind of controversies I was talking about, so that he could get an idea for what to put on the cover of this book, he envisioned that perhaps some raw foodists said we should eat more apples, while others preferred pineapple.

I explained to him that it's a little bit more complicated than that.

"For example, in the raw food movement, there's the fat camp and the fruit camp. Some people think we should eat mostly fruit, while the rest think fruit is bad.

"There are also people who believe we should take supplements and superfoods, while others say that we can get everything we need from bananas and lettuce."

"Let's keep it simple," Martin said. "How about we feature a banana and an avocado on the cover? That should be a symbolic representation of those mysterious raw food controversies."

It would be so much easier if one raw food guru thought we should eat mango, and another said that no, oranges are the way to go!

The controversies are everywhere. We ask a hundred raw food "experts" what a raw foodist should eat, and get a hundred different answers.

The raw food diet itself can be divided into different factions, such as the fruitarians, low-fat raw vegans, instinctive eaters, paleo eaters, living-foodists, nutritarians, liquidarians, sunfoodists... We even have the "breatharians," who believe they can live on nothing but air, who are often raw foodists who decided to take their diet to the "next level."

Should you follow the green juice approach? What about the ideas of Dr. Robert O. Young that all sugar, including fruit sugar, is bad for you? Then, of course, we have Ann Wigmore and her diet of sprouts and living foods, and on the other end of the spectrum, people who live on fruit alone, with no vegetables.

When some raw gurus don't want to recommend a specific diet, they become "just-do-what-works-for-you foodists"; that is, they don't want to commit to any one approach, so just suggest to their readers to try all of them and decide for themselves which one works. I have found out through personal experience that this can be a long and painful process.

Looking for Love in All the Wrong Places

After 14 years, I still haven't tried all the different raw food approaches, and I was disappointed to find that most of them didn't work for me. So what works in the end? Do I have to try out everything to find out?

There's value in learning from other people's experiences. Over the years, one of the things I've found to be the most fascinating is to hear other people's stories with the raw food diet, whether they are positive or negative.

Usually, these experiences are recorded in a short article or a quick rant posted on a discussion board on the Internet. Most newbies read these articles and then decide whether or not to try the diet on that basis.

It would be easier if we had hundreds of scientific studies comparing the merits of various raw food diet approaches. Unfortunately, the scientific community has little interest in the tribulations of health food nuts "who obviously have an eating disorder," they think.

By putting together this book, I'm trying to do more than simply tell my story. The raw food diet has been this dysfunctional love affair that's been part of my life for almost 15 years. She was the love of my life, but after a few years, my life and my health fell apart because of her. I tried to get rid of her many times, but realized I could not live without her. Each time I went back running towards her, it was with a renewed promise to try to do things differently this time! Sound familiar?

If it doesn't, then you're new to this diet. The longer you've been doing this, the more you know exactly what I'm talking about.

The strange thing I realized when writing this book is that almost everybody that I met who was doing raw foods 12 years ago has either stopped eating raw or has changed their diet tremendously to the point of being unrecognizable from what they were eating back in those days.

Raw foodists are suffering from the fact that there is no unified theory of the raw food diet. The raw diet is a niche of alternative nutrition, within which there are dozens of sub-niches and theories.

If you decide to go vegan, you might get a variety of opinions on what you should eat. Surprisingly, the vast majority of influential authors who promote a plant-based (vegan) diet all go in the same direction. You might get a little bit lost when you first get started, but eventually, you will find your way.

Decide to go raw, and you'll be confronted with a circus of gurus with conflicting advice. The newbie is left wondering who is right and who is wrong, and ultimately, most people accumulate a conglomerate of information that they try to put together in practice, often unsuccessfully.

An Inexact Science

There is no consensus in the raw food movement because there is no real raw food science to speak of. In this book, I will debunk many common raw food myths that are often used to claim the superiority of this approach to others.

The reason this book is called *Raw Food Controversies* and not *The Raw Food Diet Myth* is that this is not an anti-raw book. Although the case against the raw food diet would be easy to make (after all, there's little scientific evidence to prove that eating 100% raw has any significant health benefits), the proof is in the raw pudding.

The reason we go back to the raw food diet after having seen it fail so many times, like poor souls lost in toxic relationships, is that *most other diets don't work either!*

You will read this book and wonder many times, "If Frederic had so many problems trying to find the best way to eat raw, why didn't he just give up the diet completely and never look back?"

I eventually went back to the warm embrace of the goddess of RAW and asked for forgiveness every time, because eating cooked foods burned me too, in the end.

Eat raw the wrong way, and you might not experience all the signs of health you were expecting, but unless you do it terribly wrong, you will still feel a certain vitality you never quite experienced in your life before.

Start eating cooked the wrong way, and that feeling will be gone, replaced by a cloud of negative energy that will get worse and worse as time goes by.

In the end, we all just want to be healthy.

The question I ask and try to answer in this book is this: *what is the healthiest diet we can eat that can bring us health now and in the long term?*

I will not answer that question with a set of strict rules that imply: *this is the way it has to be.*

The reason so many people fail on the raw food diet is precisely because of this dogmatic approach that only sees what it wants to see and excludes all other possibilities.

At the same time, I will not leave you hanging with the vague advice to *simply find out what works for you.* I believe you can learn a great deal from my experience, but can also draw some conclusions for yourself.

As the book progresses, I will expose some raw food controversies and try to answer them using what I believe is the most up-to-date and accurate information.

In the end, I am clear on *how not to eat raw,* but I believe that there's still room to learn *what's the best way to eat.*

To the latter end, I can give you a series of suggestions that I believe to be accurate, as well as the consolidated experience of the thousands of raw foodists that I have been in touch with over the last 14 years.

I believe there are a few ways to eat a healthy diet and be happy, and not just one dogmatic and limited approach. Yet, I don't agree with the position that each human being is *completely unique* and there's no one diet that works for everybody.

There is room for personal preferences and addressing individual weaknesses, but we are more alike than we are different. What works for me will probably work for you too, although you might not choose to eat exactly the way I eat to get the same results. My experience with raw foodists over the years is that most of us have had the same experiences; it's only their severity that tends to vary from one person to the next.

I happen to be very sensitive and react promptly to certain influences that might not affect most people immediately. I'm also abnormally prone to self-observation, and therefore, writing an entire book about my obsession with diet and nutrition seems like a normal thing to do.

In the end, it's not about who is wrong and who is right, but rather, *what can we do to achieve our goals of perfect health?*

My goal with this book is to help you make the right choices. I want to tell my story, and I hope that you can learn from my experience and avoid the mistakes that I have made. However, I also want to avoid the wishy-washy vague talk that avoids answering real questions that demand some answers.

The more confusion there is in the raw food world, the more people are likely to make the wrong choices. As one study found in 2000 in Washington State, the more people are confused about nutrition, the more they're likely to eat the wrong foods and neglect taking action to improve their health.

While I may not have all the answers, I know this book holds part of the solution and can help you to avoid common mistakes that may sabotage your health.

To make my point, I'll take you on a journey spanning over 15 years, from the moment I discovered the vegetarian diet, through my discovery of raw foods, across all the various experiments, trials and errors that I made along the way, to where I am now.

The story I'm about to tell is a true story. Every event that I relate actually happened, and every person I have met is a real person. I have sometimes changed some names to protect the privacy of some people who would rather remain anonymous, but the stories are true.

Let the journey begin...

Saturday December 30, 2000
Press Release

SOURCE: Fred Hutchinson Cancer Research Center

Some Americans, Fed Up With Conflicting Diet and Nutrition Messages, Respond With Less Healthful Eating Habits

Some people appear to be responding by tuning out the conflicting advice and eating less healthful diets, according to a study by researchers at the Fred Hutchinson Cancer Research Center in Seattle, Wash.

The results of this National Cancer Institute-funded study, led by Ruth E. Patterson, Ph.D., R.D., an associate member of the Hutchinson Center's Public Health Sciences Division, appear in the January issue of the Journal of the American Dietetic Association.

"The more negative and confused people feel about dietary recommendations, the more likely they are to eat a fat-laden diet that skimps on fruits and vegetables," Patterson said.

(...)

Patterson and collaborators from the Hutchinson Center and the University of Washington conducted a cancer-risk behavior survey that included questions regarding attitudes toward dietary recommendations. The random survey, which involved 1,751 adults in the state of Washington (60 percent women; 90 percent white; mean age 44), asked also about consumption of fat, fruits and vegetables.

The results found evidence both for and against nutrition backlash, defined as negative feelings about dietary recommendations, such as anger, skepticism, helplessness, worry and cynicism.

SOURCE: Fred Hutchinson Cancer Research Center

CHAPTER 1

From Poutine to Tofu Hot Dogs

"You put a baby in a crib with an apple and a rabbit. If it eats the rabbit and plays with the apple, I'll buy you a new car."

Harvey Diamond,
Fit For Life

The Story of How I Became Vegetarian

I was born in 1976 and grew up in North America, in my native province of Quebec, speaking French almost exclusively until the age of 20.

The French Canadian diet in those days was not too different from that of the rest of Canada and the United States. Traditional French Canadian food is a very heavy and fatty cuisine of meat, lard and root vegetables: a diet suitable for lumberjacks who burn an excess of 5000 calories a day!

Like every French Canadian, I ate these traditional foods on special occasions. Things such as beans with lard, pea soup, eggs with maple syrup, pork pâté ("cretons" in French), sugar pie, meat pie, Poor Man's Pudding[1], were not everyday fare, but they were served on special occasions.

The infamous poutine is the official French-Canadian junk food, mixing French fries, gravy, and fresh cheese curd. It sounds gross, but it's the most satisfying and addictive junk food you'll ever taste. As for all teenagers in Quebec, it contributed to at least half of my acne.

Everyday food in Quebec, in those days, is comparable to what most people refer to as "food" in North America today.

These are foods such as pasta with meat sauce, boxed cereals with milk, sandwiches, eggs and toast, occasional "treat" food, like pizza; meat and potatoes, boiled vegetables, some fruits, such as watermelon and oranges, bananas and apples, and a limited amount of salad and vegetables.

The diet wasn't the greatest, but in those days, not so long ago, there weren't any kids in my school that ever got labeled as ADD or ADHD or were treated with drugs. Some kids were smarter than others, but

---

1   "Pudding Chômeur", more accurately translated as the "Unemployed" pudding, is made with maple syrup, sugar, butter, milk and bread.

it seems like we were not as messed up as the new generation growing up today.

I had never tasted a mango or an avocado until I was about 16, and "vegetarian cuisine" was not something that was part of my family's vocabulary.

Between 1980 and 1995, the variety of foods available at the supermarket expanded exponentially. Suddenly, we were getting fruits and vegetables from all over the world, and vegetarianism and healthy eating became more popular.

I never met anyone who was vegetarian until I met Mario, a smart and funny man in his late thirties that my mother had befriended after her divorce.

Like about half of Generation X-ers in North America, I grew up in a divorced family. I was about 10 when my parents split up.

When my parents got divorced, I didn't realize it, but I was missing a father figure in my everyday life.

Although my mom dated a few guys, I felt that none of them had a memorable personality like my dad, who always made me laugh.

Like many women with teenage kids, my mom's favorite activity (besides painting) was to take classes on random topics, ranging from new age divination and palm reading to macramé.

One day, she decided to improve her diet, so she took a class in vegetarian cuisine. That's how she met Mario.

Mario was unlike any other man I had ever met. He was fun. He had a twisted sense of humor. He was intelligent. He looked super healthy, buff, and young for his age. Even more shocking, he was completely independent financially and officially "retired" at the young age of 38! His time was spent working out, hanging out with friends, traveling, and living humbly on his investments.

I thought my mom was "dating" Mario, and I so wanted him to be part of our lives.

I discovered that it was no accident that Mario looked better and healthier than other men of his age. Mario was a vegetarian and had studied Natural Hygiene and natural health.

His kitchen was unlike any other kitchen I had seen so far. It was filled with various jars containing bulk grains, beans, herbs, nuts, and seeds, most of which I had never seen before (with names such as "quinoa" and "amaranth;") everything looked so exotic.

His bookshelf was filled with titles such as *The Natural Hygiene Way* and *The Power of Live Juices.*

He explained to me that he generally skipped breakfast and ate only twice a day. He drank freshly squeezed juices, ate fruits and vegetables in unusual amounts, and got the bulk of his calories from whole grains and plant foods.

He worked out every day, alternating one hour of running with weight lifting sessions.

On top of that, he had become financially independent by working two jobs at once, living frugally and carefully investing every penny he had. For over a decade, he had had the plan to retire before he was 40, and he finally succeeded at the ripe age of 37 (which was one year before we met him).

Mario was an example of what I could accomplish in my life if I set my mind to it. It seemed that nothing in Mario's life was an accident or happened by luck, from his great health and appearance to his financial success.

Without his inspirational example, I probably would have viewed my mom's interest in vegetarianism as another fad, an attempt to make our lives miserable. Instead, I saw that there was definitely something to it.

I had two options: I could turn out like other men in their early forties that I had met—sick, old-looking and unhappy—or I could become healthy, happy, successful and independent, like Mario.

At the time, I did not suspect Mario to be gay and did not know that quite often, if a man is well-informed, dresses fashionably, is wealthy, independent and child-free, then there's a good chance he's homosexual!

When I learned the truth, I was not shocked, but I was disappointed that he couldn't be my mom's boyfriend.

However, I was so impressed by his alternative lifestyle that he became somewhat of a mentor at this critical point in my life.

At that point, our little household (me, my mom and my younger brother) was transformed. Gone were the ground beef and white bread. Now the cupboards were filled with whole grains and beans. Veggie-dogs and other meat alternatives replaced the animal foods in the fridge, together with fruits and vegetables in larger quantities.

Without too much of a fuss, I went mostly vegetarian at the age of 16, although I still ate dairy products and couldn't resist a good hamburger when I could get my hands on one.

We didn't know many vegetarian recipes, so we ate mostly the same foods but in vegetarian versions. The meat in tomato sauce was replaced with lentils, and hamburger patties with Yves' meatless patties.[2]

All my friends were making fun of our kitchen ("all the good stuff is gone!"), but somehow I knew that this change in diet was going to last.

The vegetarian diet had gotten my full attention, but I still had a lot to learn, and hadn't yet been convinced to go all the way. Until by chance, a random meeting with a piano tuner turned me from a casual vegetarian to a militant vegan.

---

2   Yves is a common brand of vegetarian fake-meat products that started in Quebec, now popular all over the world

A year or two after I met Mario and right before I got accepted to music school to complete a two-year curriculum in classical guitar, I went mostly vegan and 100% vegetarian.

I enjoyed eating these newly discovered vegetarian foods, but I was not aware of all the implications of eating animal products and what it really meant to be a vegetarian.

Mario was the only vegetarian person I knew, and he wasn't even 100% strict. Occasionally, he would indulge and eat chocolate or even meat, but he would quickly get back on track. He was more of a "health-foodist" than a strict ethical vegan.

I did not think I would take this vegetarian lifestyle any further, but as I started reading the dozens of books on vegetarian cuisine and health that my mom had purchased, I became more and more interested in the health aspects of this lifestyle.

Most of these books were classical vegetarian books, with recipes containing eggs, butter and cheese. Compared to the wonderful vegan ethnic food that I now know of, most of the vegetarian recipes I tried at the time were terrible, but I did not know any better.

One of the first books about health that I read was called *The Guide to Healthy and Natural Nutrition* by a French-Canadian author, Renée Frappier, who had done a great job of outlining a relatively healthy way of eating, and of describing all the foods that are now common in health food stores, but that were novelties at the time.

What is quinoa? What can you do with it? How do you cook beans? What should you do with mustard greens? How do you cut an avocado? How can you make healthy guacamole? What do you do with seaweed? What is tempeh, and what can you do with it? What nutrients do all of these foods contain?

This book, which I read several times, answered all of these questions and provided a framework for healthy eating.

In Quebec, the slang word in French for someone who eats this way is a *grano* (from the word "granola"). Vegetarian people were *grano*, but so was anyone else who shopped at a health food store, which were almost non-existent at the time, and were very small.

A *grano* is the type of person that would eat tofu, use Tamari sauce instead of regular soy sauce, or make veggie burgers instead of regular burgers. They were people to make fun of and not take too seriously, although many meat-eaters confessed they were a little *grano* themselves, at times, replacing some of their junk foods with healthier items.

The problem with vegetarian diets at the time was that they were often based on antiquated ideas about nutrition, such as protein combining. Protein combining is the concept that plant proteins do not contain all of the necessary amino acids in the right proportions, like meat does. When this theory was "en vogue," it was recommended to combine different kinds of food together in order to get all of the essential amino acids at any one meal.

For example, grains are generally rich in some types of amino acids, while lacking in others. On the other hand, beans seem to be low in the amino acids in which grains are abundant, while being rich in the ones they lack.

Therefore, the recommendation was to always combine two kinds of complementary proteins at each meal. It was also noted that this is what most cultures in the world naturally did, by eating together rice and beans, squash and corn, or tofu and rice.

Any vegetarian at the time was strongly encouraged to follow this principle...or else!

Nowadays, most nutrition experts will agree that it is not necessary for vegetarians to combine their proteins, because amino acids are recycled in the body. What may be lacking in one meal is compensated by what's in the next meal. As long as you get enough calories from a variety of foods, protein deficiency is not to be feared.[3]

At the time, most vegetarians did not know this and, more importantly, the vegetarian recipes in the recipe books were a little too *grano*, even for today's tastes.

So I had to assuage my cravings for heavier and tastier foods by occasionally visiting a fast food joint or buying junk foods, such as potato chips. I would also snack on cheese, because I thought just being vegetarian was enough of a big deal.

But at the time, I did not view myself as a "vegetarian."

Not until I met a piano tuner who told me to read a book that would change my life.

How a Piano Tuner Got Me to Go (Mostly) Vegan

When my grandmother died, we inherited the family piano, which needed to be tuned. So we called a company to get it done, and I was the one at home to wait for the piano guy.

The piano was located in the room where my mom kept all of her books about health and vegetarian cuisine. So when the guy came over, he saw that we had all of these books and asked if I was a vegetarian.

I told him what I was eating, and he said that he, himself, was a vegan, and told me that there was a book that I had to read.

"It's called *Diet for a New America*, by John Robbins, and it's a bomb!"

So the next day, I went to the bookstore and bought the book, since it was not available at the public library. In the French translation, the title was rendered as *Eating Without Causing Suffering*, but I later found out that the original title was completely different and could not

---

3   http://en.wikipedia.org/wiki/Protein_combining

understand why the translators had chosen such a lame and off-putting title in French.But nonetheless, even in a French translation, the book blew me away.

John Robbins was the former heir of the Baskin-Robbins ice cream empire, and he "saw the light" at an early age after researching the evils of our animal-food-based culture.

I thought that eating vegetarian was just a healthy way to go because meat was bad for you, but I did not fully understand the reasoning behind it until I read this book.

From the mistreatment of animals and the cruelty of slaughterhouses to the destruction of our environment and our health—with arguments fully supported by science—this was the ultimate vegetarian manifesto that convinced me to go all the way.

After reading 100 pages, I was shocked.

After 200 pages, I was *angry!*

After finishing the book, I was motivated to change the world!

But even after reading such a convincing book as *Diet for a New America,* I had some doubts. Could the world really be that bad?

After all, if the habit of consuming animal products was really destroying the world and our health, wouldn't we have heard about it before?

I decided to do some research on my own.

As it turned out, I studied music in the little town of Joliette in Quebec, which was also one of the main college centers for agricultural studies in the province.

The college library had all the trade publications that farmers subscribed to, with archives.

I spent a few days at the library browsing all these publications, with titles such as "Pork Today" and "Poultry Insiders."

By reading the magazines those farmers subscribed to and used to discuss industry practices, I made a shocking discovery. *Everything that John Robbins described in his book was true!*

There were articles on how to use certain hormones to make cows produce more milk, how to pack more chickens into a closed space and what to do when they started killing each other, how to change the public's perception that eggs are full of cholesterol to "eggs are nature's food," and ads on how to turn your chickens into "cash machines!"

The farmers were not shy about discussing their practices with each other, and it didn't take a visit to a slaughterhouse or an egg farm to know what was going on, just by reading these publications.

I discovered that the insanity of modern meat production was not something that vegetarians had hyped up or that only happened in the United States. This was how the entire industry was run.

My research persuaded me to go vegan all the way, and from that point forward, I did not eat any meat for many, many years.

I then convinced my brother to read the book, and he, too, decided to become a vegan.

My brother is a little less than two years younger than me. In my teenage years and onward, I was a huge influence on him. Now that he's fully found his own personality, whatever I say or do has little influence on how he's going to live his life.

At the time, I would start to listen to AC/DC, and he would do the same. I would start playing a game, and he'd start to play it too. So when I became vegetarian and then vegan, he naturally followed, but not blindly. He also read *Diet for a New America* and was shocked by what he learned.

Someone once said, "There's nothing like the zeal of the newly converted." It's completely true.

Together, we not only became strict about our way of eating: we became militant about it. We went looking for trouble!

At first, it created some tension in the family. My dad, whom we would visit a couple times a month, every other weekend, was very proud of his limited cooking skills. He had a few recipes in his arsenal, clipped from ancient cooking magazines, and he would keep making them to impress his sons and dates.

One of his famous recipes was the "Italian Crêpe" which was a thin French crêpe filled with a mixture of Italian sausage and vegetables in creamy sauce.

It was delicious, but of course, it was not vegan.

When we told him we wouldn't eat meat anymore, his first reaction was "So you won't be able to have my Italian Crêpes again?"

Perhaps it didn't help that we didn't call in advance ahead of our weekend together to tell him about our new dietary changes and that he had purchased the ingredients to make his famous recipe, just for us!

At that moment, I realized for the first time how so much of our social lives are based on food. I had never given a thought to the fact that my becoming a vegetarian would cause some friction in the family. After a while, though, my dad accepted the changes and didn't make too much fuss about it. He never even asked us about protein at all!

Everybody else we told about our new diet asked us where we would get our protein. They might also tell us that vegetarians have to be "very careful" about what they eat or else they could run into deficiencies.

Whenever someone brings up these objections nowadays, I smile and answer politely, without turning the question into a big argument.

But at the time, we were not even twenty, we were very passionate, and we had memorized all the arguments from the "Bible" of vegetarianism, John Robbins' book. Whenever someone brought up any objection against vegetarianism, we would start an argument.

Common objections were:

If everybody became a vegetarian, what would happen to all the farm animals?

My answer today: ethical issues aside, why bring up an issue that will NEVER in a thousand years happen? No one is going to transform the planet into a vegetarian planet overnight by voting on it, and there will probably never be a time when the entire planet is vegetarian. So, we don't have to worry about those excess farm animals.

I know someone who was a vegetarian, and they became so weak on the diet that they had to go back to meat. Vegetarianism is not for everybody.

My answer today: There is junk vegetarianism, and there's a properly balanced vegetarian diet. The main issue is that vegans generally don't eat enough food to get the calories and nutrients they need. By following some simple principles, everybody can become vegan without running into those problems.

Vegetarians have to be "very careful" about what they eat.

My answer today: So do meat-eaters! We live in a society where diseases are primarily caused by excess, not by lack. Diseases that vegetarians experience are also generally caused by excess of the same macronutrients meat-eaters eat too much of—fat and protein.

On average, vegetarians still live two years longer than the average population, and vegans live another two years longer than regular vegetarians[4].

I couldn't do that. I love meat too much.

My answer today: No one is forcing you. It's much easier than you think to get used to different foods. I love the foods I eat now at least as much as the foods I used to eat, and I don't suffer the negative consequences.

Nowadays, I don't bring up statistics or logical arguments. If someone wants to challenge you, it's because they feel threatened by your choice. Turn that energy around by acknowledging their argument while holding your ground.

If someone tells me, "I tried to go vegetarian, but I got weak because I wasn't getting enough protein," I might say, "That's too bad. I found out that as long as I eat enough calories, I'm okay. By the way, did you see that latest action movie?"

When I first went vegan, the year was 1995. The Internet was barely getting started and our family, like most families, did not own a computer. I had never even been "on" the Internet.

So I gathered information the old fashioned way. I looked up all the addresses that were listed in John Robbins' book as organizations that he recommended, and I wrote letters to all of them requesting more information.

Before I knew it, my mailbox was filled with a ton of magazines, catalogs and pamphlets of vegetarian, vegan, and animal rights associations from all over the world.

---

4 A study done on the Seven Day Adventists showed that vegetarianism added 2 years to life expectancy. The overall healthy lifestyle of the Seven Day Adventists made this group live almost 10 years longer than the general population of California. REFERENCE: Arch Intern Med. 2001; 161:1645-1652.

I discovered that there was even a small vegan movement in Quebec. There was a lady in Quebec who was publishing a small magazine called *Ahimsa,* with articles on animal rights and vegetarian recipes. I even wrote a letter to the editor that was published.

Most of the organizations promoting vegetarianism that I found were coming from an ethical or animal rights standpoint. They wanted the world to know about the horrors of factory farms, slaughterhouses, and the treatment of animals. There was certainly a concern for health, but it was not their primary focus.

The vegetarians I met were converted because they didn't want to participate in the killing of animals. They were not motivated by health, but rather, by the love of animals. Some of them felt repulsed at the sight of meat and decided to stop eating it for that reason.

I was still in music school at the time, working on my classical guitar curriculum that ballooned from a two-year program into three years of study.

I was no longer visiting my local *Harvey's*[5] to pacify my cravings with a hamburger. Instead, I found a completely vegetarian restaurant nearby.

The first time I walked into that place, I knew I was not in a typical restaurant. It smelled like a combination of incense and vegetables cooking with spices. The music played was soothing Indian tunes. The walls were filled with flyers advocating vegetarianism and quotes from Gandhi.

I remember the first time I walked in. The place was deserted, and after taking my order, the owner/chef told me, *"You're not a vegetarian, are you?"* Perhaps I did not fit in, with my long wild hair and guitar!

My visits to this restaurant also exposed me to a new aspect of the vegetarian movement: the unhealthy vegetarian.

---

5   Harvey's is a Canadian chain of fast food restaurants, where you get to build your burger by choosing your own toppings.

The owner complained about his liver problems, and he blamed it on the large amounts of butter he was consuming. He was still overweight and did not look healthy. He was a vegetarian for ethical reasons, and he did not seem to care about being the best example possible for this lifestyle.

Although the book *Diet for a New America* convinced me to become a vegetarian, I had a hard time being completely vegan because most vegetarian restaurants still used dairy products. I kept eating standard vegetarian food, keeping in the back of my mind that I would one day become a pure vegan.

In school, I kept my diet to myself; but sometimes, I shared my progress with a friend. One day, it was corn season, so my friend and I bought a bunch of corn on the cob to cook. Instead of boiling it, I had read in a magazine that you could leave the corn in its husk and bake it in the oven instead, to preserve more nutrients.

That is what being *grano* meant at the time: always trying to seek healthier choices, even when the changes are oftentimes generally insignificant.

I read all the books I could find in my public library and local bookstore about vegetarianism, including the animal rights classics, such as Peter Singer's *Animal Liberation*.

What was great at the time was that if you wanted information on a particular topic, you had to read books. Nowadays, people only skim-read websites that give them only part of the picture.

The selection of books was quite limited, and the public libraries I subscribed to only had books in French. If I wanted books in English, I had to order them from companies in the United States, which meant filling out a form in their catalog, sending a mail order in US dollars, paying ridiculous shipping fees, and waiting weeks for the book to arrive.

Nowadays, we have Amazon and other amazing online bookstores with an incredible selection, and eBooks are widely available for instant download. Today, a great proportion of vegan organizations are primarily concerned with the health aspects of this lifestyle, which is a great plus.

At the time, most vegetarians were tree-hugging environmentalists and animal rights activists that survived on a diet of French fries and tofu. They were not the greatest poster boys and girls for a healthy lifestyle.

I remember in a catalog I saw the *McDougall Program* book by John McDougall, and it had a friendly cover. However, I didn't order it, because I thought it was mostly about weight loss, which was not my concern.

If I had ordered it, I would have learned about the importance of the low-fat diet and how to properly go vegan, and that would have saved me much trouble down the road, as we will later see.

However, without the mistakes that I have made, I also wouldn't have had the experience that I have today.

CHAPTER 2

From Dog Food to Live Food

"Live with passion!"

Tony Robbins

In the summer of 1996, I was on vacation, having only one year left of my music and guitar curriculum. I tried to practice a lot (but not as much as usual), enjoy some sun, and try a few new vegetarian recipes.

One day, out of the blue, I got a mysterious call.

I picked up the phone and said, "Hello...?"

An excited voice on the other end of the line answered, "Frederic? Just the man I wanted to talk to!"

"Huh...."

"This is Dominic! I'm your brother's friend. We're in the same year of high school. I met you once."

"Oh yeah, right..."

"Is this a good time to talk?"

"Sure... what's up?"

"Listen... do you have any plans for the summer?"

"Well, not exactly. I'm practicing guitar."

"How would you like to earn some extra money? I have a great opportunity for you that I think you should check out!"

"Huh...?"

"Listen. Let me come over to your place right now, I'll explain everything."

"Huh... oooohkay."

When I hung up the line, I had no idea what Dominic had just said. Opportunity? What was I doing this summer? What the hell was he talking about? Plus, I only vaguely remembered him anyway.

At that point, I had no idea that Dominic was going to become one of my best friends and that meeting him that day was going to set in motion a string of events that would change the course of my existence and define what I would do with my life in the future.

When Dominic showed up, he had a VHS cassette tape in his hands and asked where the TV was. Then he went on to explain to me that he was going to show me a 15-minute video and that all I needed to do was to keep my mind open and watch.

I suspected that Dominic was going to pull a joke on me, but instead, I ended up watching a sales presentation about a company called "Viva" that was doing something called "network marketing" to sell premium dog food.

The video showed testimonials from people who were now living their dreams because of Viva, apparently earning money on the side by selling this dog food.

I was not necessarily captivated by the cheesy video, but then Dominic had a folder of information with him and explained to me that he got into Viva a few months ago and was now recruiting people and building his business.

"This would be perfect for you! You can do it this summer, earn some extra money, and then have a side job that brings you passive income as you continue your music studies!"

"So, how does it work?" I asked.

"I just have to sign you up. There's a presentation next Tuesday in downtown Montreal where you can meet the company and hear more about how it works. I can come pick you up. So what do you say?"

"All right..." I mumbled reluctantly.

Next Tuesday came, and we showed up at this small conference center in Montreal. Older people in their thirties greeted me enthusiastically and ask me what attracted me to this meeting.

"Uh... my friend Dominic just dragged me here!"

"You won't regret it," they answered, with a million-dollar, Tony Robbins smile.

A charismatic, bilingual, lean guy named Michel Piette, who was the picture of success, led the presentation. He wore a nice suit, sported a great haircut and a perfect tan, and dazzled everyone with his excellent public speaking skills.

First, he made the audience feel at ease by pointing out the obvious fact that someone probably dragged us to this meeting.

"How many of you are here for the first time? And how many of you have no idea what this is about?"

After a few jokes, he explained to us the importance of timing.

"Let's say you could go back in time and buy shares of McDonald's when the company was just starting, would you say that it would be good timing?"

The audience naturally agreed.

"What we call "timing" is the most important thing in business. Being at the right place at the right moment," he continued, placing strong emphasis on certain words.

After a while, he shifted his attention to explain to us the booming pet industry in America.

"Did you know that the pet industry is bigger than Hollywood in terms of total sales and revenues?"

After convincing us that the pet industry is really gigantic and underestimated, he started talking about a new way of distributing products and services called "Network Marketing."

"According to the Popcorn report, by *Faith Popcorn*; in 10 years, 30% of all products and services will be distributed through network marketing."

We had no idea who that "Faith Popcorn" person was, but apparently, it was her real name and she had written best-selling books about investing.

He added a few slides to make his statements convincing.

In the last part of the presentation, he described the business model for Viva. Viva was selling a premium dog food product called "Compagnon Plus." It was so much better than any other dog food out there that animals became healthier, and owners were raving about it.

"Even the police squad of Montreal is adopting Compagnon Plus for all of its police dogs."

It was more expensive than your average dog food, but it ended up costing less because animals needed to eat less of it.

It was easy to sell because animals naturally preferred it, and owners loved it, because their pets became healthier and stopped shedding so much. Additionally, it saved them money.

"All you need to do is find three dogs—*big* dogs preferably!"

The audience laughed.

"Then we have this system where you can put the clients on this automatic delivery system with UPS. You don't even have to bring them the product anymore, it happens automatically."

Then, with the income distribution program of Viva, which worked according to network marketing, you just had to recruit other people to do the same. After just a few "generations", you'd make enough money to basically stop working.

"How easy is it to find someone who has a dog or a cat? How many of you know at least one person who owns a cat or a dog?"

Almost everybody raised their hands.

"Some of our members even walk around with a little tag on their jacket that says, *Do you have a cat or a dog? Talk to me!* And people show up and talk to them, and they make sales automatically!"

Then a few people went up on stage and gave amazing testimonials about how much Viva had changed their lives, how much they were loving their new jobs, and how they were working with a great team.

I ended up being pretty convinced by the presentation and decided to sign up. What did I have to lose after all? The cost of enrollment was only 60 bucks.

For the rest of the summer, I worked with Dominic on the Viva business. We recruited my brother. Then we recruited many of our high school friends and built a team of motivated sellers.

We called everyone we knew who had a dog or a cat and even got a few to try the food.

Every week, we attended the seminar and brought people to try to recruit them. It got to the point where we almost knew Michel's entire presentation word-for-word.

But as it turned out, the reality was a little different from the theory.

Even though most dogs initially preferred the dog food, it was significantly more expensive than other products, and although we could sell a case to an individual, they would rarely buy another one after that.

We discovered that most people don't love their animals enough to buy a $50 bag of dog food when they can go to Wal-Mart and get one for $12.

The suggested savings that Michel had talked about didn't seem to make sense in practice, and no one ever opted for the automatic UPS delivery system.

Furthermore, although it was easy to recruit people to Viva and pay the $60, the people you recruited almost never actually made any sales that earned you commissions, and they were even less likely to recruit other members themselves that would also make sales.

As we would discover farther down the road, Viva was based on a structure of sketchy investments, and almost no one in the company actually made money except the ones at the very top. This was probably only from the $60 charge for everyone signing up!

In spite of this, there was one great thing that came out of it. Every month, Michel Piette would host seminars on a variety of topics in order to motivate his team.

One of the seminars was called "Health and Energy." He looked pretty healthy and energetic himself, so I was intrigued.

At the time, I thought I knew what I needed to know about health. *Just go 100% vegetarian and, eventually, vegan, and that's pretty much what you needed to know.*

When I attended Michel's seminar, my convictions were shattered once again.

Michel's program was copied almost word-for-word from Tony Robbins, who himself copied it from a book called *Fit for Life*. It involved the following elements:

- Only eat fruits for breakfast because fruits are the easiest foods to digest, and they must be eaten alone.

- Eat according to the principles of food combining: so don't mix a protein and a starch together. For example, a dish of rice and beans was to be avoided.

- Don't eat meat and dairy products (I already knew that).

- Don't drink water with your meals, because it dilutes stomach acid and makes digestion more difficult.

- Eat 75% of your diet as living foods, meaning raw fruits, vegetables, nuts and seeds.

After hearing this information, I experienced for the first time a "comfort zone threat."

I had found a health philosophy that I liked and I thought I was doing pretty well. I was learning new recipes. Yet someone was telling me that it was still not good enough and that I needed to change my diet yet again!

Just like when I first read about the horrors of factory farming, I thought to myself, *I have to investigate this on my own.*

So I went to the public library again and got a few books about food combining, which led me to discover other books by authors I had never heard about.

The first book I read was called *Food Combining Made Easy,* by Dr. Herbert Shelton. It was a very thin book, but it was full of new ideas.

The concept of food combining presented in the book was similar to the one Michel had presented in his seminar. It led to a very simple diet of fruit in the morning, vegetables with a complex carb for lunch, and vegetables with a protein for dinner.

Although Shelton's book provided menus where he showed how to properly combine foods like meat and bread, I later found out that Shelton never promoted these foods or served them at his health retreat. He included them in his book as an example of how to make a bad diet better. His book was meant for the masses, and that's why it sold so many copies.

Somewhere in the book, Shelton had a line that caught my attention. He mentioned that the ideal diet for man was one of raw fruits, vegetables, nuts and seeds. This was a revolutionary idea for me, and one that certainly unsettled my status quo.

Food Combining Simplified

Shelton's book on food combining is the foundation of all rules for food combining that many health authors have adopted throughout the years.

It led to many complicated and unnecessary rules such as:

- Don't eat melons with other types of fruit.

- Don't eat more than two types of starchy vegetable together.

- Don't combine acidic fruits with sweet, non-acidic fruits (for example: figs and oranges).

Many people who read Shelton's book also misinterpreted it. Although Shelton said that melons are best eaten alone, he also said that you could combine them with other fruits. Yet some people have only retained the first part.

For half the rules that Shelton gave in his book, no reason or explanation was provided except that he found that his patients did better when these combinations were avoided.

Shelton dealt with extremely sick and weak people at his fasting center, and without a doubt, a simple, easy to digest menu was advisable.

The big advantage of food combining is that it forces you to eat simply and to eat less.

That can be a positive or a negative thing, depending on the circumstances

Food combining theories have been criticized because it led to a diet that often made people weak. The reason is simple: by avoiding most combinations, people following this diet simply didn't get enough calories!

They were having a small breakfast of fruit, but not consuming enough calories from fruit (maybe only a few hundred calories). For lunch, they had a complex starch and a salad, but not enough to sustain them for very long (another 400 calories), and for dinner, they had vegetables with a protein food. We know that protein foods are generally lower in calories, so again, they were running into a deficit.

It was great for weight loss, but not for long-term health.

Food combining forced people to eat less and avoid complicated mixtures. However, I learned over the years that the body could handle almost every combination of food as long as it is in small enough quantities.

There is a lot of wisdom in avoiding certain combinations, such as fat and sugar (for example: nuts and raisins). However, even this combination, which otherwise often leads to fermentation and gas, can be properly digested in small amounts (such as 5 almonds and a small handful of dried fruit).

My main recommendation for food combining is eliminating high-fat and high-protein foods or only consuming them in small quantities. This, in itself, is enough to improve overall health and digestion, and it's not necessary to follow the complicated food combining rules that, for the most part, have no scientific basis.

I was really intrigued by Shelton's ideas, so I got other books he had written. One was called *Superior Nutrition*.

In this book, Shelton laid out simple, but clear, rules for achieving optimal health through proper diet.

His diet was completely different from the "healthy" vegetarian diet I had been following. It was very simple: avoid almost ALL recipes. This kind of simplified cooking, but it made the menu very boring and relied primarily on fruits, vegetables, and nuts.

Shelton championed a fruit-based diet, and he thought it was the ideal food for mankind. His menu plans generally featured one or two fruit meals per day.

Breakfast was always a fruit meal, but sometimes lunch was, too. Later, I found out that in his more advanced book, he recommended skipping breakfast entirely and eating only two meals a day — one of them being a fruit meal.

The other meals generally featured a giant salad or steamed vegetables, with one more concentrated food like a baked potato or a big handful of nuts.

Shelton loved nuts, and he thought that they were one of Nature's most perfect foods. He recommended a generous amount of nuts every day — about 4 ounces — which is a very large handful.

His salads were gigantic, and they did not feature any dressing. A typical *Shelton Salad* would be an entire head of lettuce, with several tomatoes, some celery, and a giant serving of nuts, or an avocado. He also felt that items were best presented simply, instead of all chopped and mixed together in one bowl. So the ideal Shelton "Salad" would not be a salad at all, but a plate of raw vegetables.

Superior Nutrition was also a book meant for the masses, and I did not know at the time that Shelton recommended a raw diet. In *Superior Nutrition*, although Shelton heavily promoted uncooked foods, he also included some cooked foods, such as steamed vegetables or baked potatoes.

Again, those foods were prepared and presented very simply. For example, a cooked meal, according to his guidelines, might feature one baked potato with an entire head of steamed broccoli or some steamed carrots served with a salad.

Shelton thought all spices and herbs were toxic, as was salt. All of the foods he recommended were to be presented as close to their natural state as possible with no addition of condiments or sauces.

In spite of recommending a very austere diet, Shelton had the talent of making this quasi-ascetic life almost sound good and appealing. He said that our palates were so desensitized with the use of condiments that we couldn't taste and enjoy natural foods anymore. He claimed that after eating these foods in their natural state, we would come to crave them just like that.

I was quite inspired by Shelton's book, so I decided to try the diet. At first, I felt extremely hungry with these Spartan meals, but since Shelton had given his seal of approval to nuts, I ended up eating a large serving of walnuts every night.

I did not feel that much better on this diet, but I felt okay. I treated it like an experiment, and I followed it for a few days until I found another book by Shelton that inspired me to try something else.

About Shelton's Diet

As with food combining, many of Shelton's concepts about nutrition were flawed. Although I would commend him for recommending such a simple and wholesome diet, there are some serious problems with his diet that must be addressed:

Without the use of nuts and seeds, Shelton's diet is extremely energy-deficient. A meal consisting of only a few pieces of fruit might contain a few hundred calories, maybe 500 at the most. A meal of a baked potato and a salad might be 400 calories, but only if the baked potato is very big or you eat two. The average person needs about 2000 calories a day, so already; we can see how someone might feel on this diet.

Without realizing it, Shelton created a diet where most of the calories came from fat. Four to five ounces of walnuts is about 740 to 920 calories, 82% of which come from fat! Balanced out with the rest of the meals, we have a diet that is at least 50 to 60% fat, which is far higher than what is healthy by almost any standard recommendation.

Although he had good intentions and a lot of practical knowledge about health, Shelton's concepts about nutrition were seriously lacking in some areas, and they were a bit naive too. That is why, over the years, I have found that almost nobody could follow Shelton's diet as it was described in his books. The ones that attempted to eventually became sick or start binging and purging.

The next book I picked up from the library was the giant tome on fasting by Shelton, which was translated into French as *Le Jeûne*, meaning *fasting*. The actual title in English was the longer *The Science and Fine Art of Fasting*.

It was a fascinating book on the history of fasting, its use in religion and in the animal kingdom, the physiological changes that occur when someone fasts, and how to use fasting to improve one's health.

Shelton's book made fasting sound cool and fun. Because he wanted to prove that fasting was safe, he went to great lengths giving examples of all these people that fasted for long periods of time and were able to maintain their energy levels.

Although the type of fast Shelton recommended involved absolute rest in bed, he also gave examples of people who fasted up to 40 days on water and kept working throughout. It almost sounded like fasting was something anyone could do, and it would not affect your normal life at all, as if eating food was just an optional choice.

After reading the book, I decided to try fasting for 3 1/2 days on my own. I didn't rest in bed, but instead, I stayed active and continued my life as normal.

I found that fasting was a lot easier than I thought. The first day was really easy, and I had a great amount of energy.

I was biking everywhere with no difficulties. On the second day of my fast, I met my high school friend, Hugo, and I told him that I hadn't eating anything for two days and that I felt amazing.

He said, "Man, you're crazy!"

On the second day, I was very hungry, but energetic. The thought of eating an apple made my mouth salivate. Things got more difficult by the morning of the third day.

On the morning of the third day, I felt less hungry and less energetic. I had discovered that my body was adjusting to the physiological effects of fasting and quickly moving into the state of ketosis, where it was starting to feed on its own fat reserves.

During that stage, hunger disappears, along with energy. I've noticed over the years that the only people who feel amazing and energetic throughout a fast are overweight people. Skinny or thin people feel lethargic as soon as they hit day three. On the third day, the fast didn't feel so great anymore.

However, I stuck with it, and ate a fruit meal on the morning of the fourth day, which didn't taste as amazing as I had expected. I wasn't as hungry as I was on the morning of the second day, but I enjoyed it nonetheless.

What this fasting experience proved to me was that it was definitely possible to live for a while without food without harming the body.

In my high school biology class, I had learned that the human body would die after 3-4 days without water and only 7-8 days without food.

I don't know where my teacher had gotten that information, but when I fasted for 23 days on water in 2005, I certainly disproved it!

CHAPTER 3

How an Old Frenchman Would Transform My Assumptions About Diet and Health

"Almost all men die from their remedies and not from their diseases."

Molière

For the rest of the summer of 1996, I continued experimenting a little bit with Shelton's diet, but without taking the plunge.

Towards the end of the summer, I went back to the library to look for some new books to read on diet and health. Among the various titles, from *Fit for Life* to more of Shelton's books, I found a few curious-looking books by a Frenchman named Albert Mosséri.

Without really thinking about it, I picked up a few of his books to add to my collection.

When I opened and started reading the first book, *La santé par la nourriture* (Health Through Diet), I was blown away. After a few chapters, Mosséri had already introduced the concept of eating 100% raw by translating parts of a book by an Iranian author called Hovanessian.

Even though Shelton had mentioned that man's natural foods should be raw fruits, vegetables, nuts and seeds, he didn't insist on that point. In Mosséri's book, the quotes by Hovanessian were so passionate in advocating a 100% raw diet that somehow I started to share that enthusiasm, and began to feel that this was probably the way to go.

The translation of Hovanessian's book, *Raw Eating,* was only part of Mosséri's work. When I opened Moss'eri's books, time would stop. Without realizing it, I would have spent four or five hours reading.

Mosséri was a student of Shelton, whom he considered his biggest mentor. But Mosséri took a very different standpoint on many crucial aspects of the Natural Hygiene diet where he disagreed with Shelton.

Shelton's books are written in a very old, antiquated style and sound very formal and severe, like having an old, cranky, puritan grandfather lecture you on morality for hours.

On the other hand, Mosséri was from a different generation (born in 1925, Shelton was born in 1895), and he was still alive (Shelton died in 1985).

Mosséri's books were much easier to read, and he combined in them stories, interesting quotes, personal experience, and a kind of dry humor only a native French speaker could appreciate.

When I read Shelton's books, it felt like I was presented with ideals that were impossible to follow. Reading Shelton made you feel he was some kind of superhuman, impervious to the influences of modern society, and you were a low-class, corrupted moron for not being 100% pure and natural like he said everyone should be.

Mosséri had a more down-to-earth approach that made you feel like you were normal for struggling in a society that did not promote health, and he also described his personal experience and struggles with interesting stories, which made you feel connected to him, without having met him in person.

The more I read Mosséri, the more I started to understand what this concept of *Natural Hygiene* was that I had discovered in other books, but never quite understood.

Mosséri was passionate about Natural Hygiene and really bitter about modern medicine (for legitimate personal reasons). He also had a lot of experience with his fasting center to back it up, having worked with some of the sickest people in the world, who came to him as a last resort.

More importantly, Mosséri took a strong stand against naturopathic medicines, and he wrote a lot about it, debunking everything from homeopathy to herbal medicine.

His main concept, which he got from Shelton, was that *healing is a biological process only the body can undergo.* No other outside influences, whether they are drugs or herbal remedies, can heal you. At the most, they will suppress your symptoms and not get at the root of the problem, which he referred to as *the cause.*

One example he gave is that of a cold. We know that there are thousands of remedies to get rid of a cold. For example, some people take a drug. Others prefer herbal teas. Yet others go for a more brutal approach, such as drinking a shot of whisky. There are literally hundreds of folk remedies for getting rid of a cold.

Yet what do all of these remedies have in common? *Everybody who takes them eventually gets better.* But the person who does *not* take a remedy at all, and just stays in bed and fasts, also gets better, but much more quickly than everyone else, while addressing the real cause of the cold.

According to Natural Hygiene and even modern medicine, there is no remedy for a common cold. What these remedies have in common is that they suppress the symptoms to some degree. Natural Hygiene says that the symptoms should not be suppressed, because the *dis-ease* is an effort of the body to restore its homeostasis, or state of health, and it should not be interrupted in any way. Instead, we should provide the body with enough rest and other elements of healthful living so that it can go through the disease naturally and heal itself, without any outside interference.

The reason why Natural Hygienists use fasting is not because fasting itself cures anything, but because it allows the body to get enough rest (from digestion and physical activity) so that all its energies can be directed towards healing.

As I read Mosséri's books, I became fascinated with this idea of Natural Hygiene. My mother was a nurse, so I had had my exposure to modern medicine and knew it was not always the perfect savior people often believed it to be. I realized that even "natural" medicines were often just less dangerous ways to suppress the same symptoms that drugs try to suppress.

On the subject of diet, Mosséri differed from Shelton in a few important areas. He believed strongly that Shelton was wrong in recommending a large amount of nuts and seeds in the diet. According to Mosséri's experience over the years, the quantity of nuts recommended by Shelton on a daily basis led to some severe health problems. (He even claimed that he had known people who had died from those problems.)

The problems he mentioned were: bad digestion and gas, constant hunger caused by malnutrition, skin problems, lack of energy, and even cancer.

However, he said that it was not necessary to eliminate all nuts from the diet, but to limit them to about five almonds a day. In his later books, he increased that amount to about one ounce.

Mosséri was also against grains, like Shelton. He claimed that bread and grains were not meant for human beings because we are not granivores like birds. Grains are acid-forming and are the primary cause of mucus in the body. Therefore, he said that if you stop consuming bread and grains you will never catch a cold again.

He promoted vegetarianism and criticized fish as being worse than meat (because it putrefies faster), so all that was left to eat were fruits and vegetables.

In his books, Mosséri quoted Hovanessian's book on *Raw Eating* extensively, which claimed that a 100% raw food diet was the only way to achieve health. However, after this long exposé against cooked food, he gave his own opinion about it, which was more moderate.

Mosséri first quoted some research about some tribes living in New Guinea that were living almost exclusively on cooked sweet potatoes. He said that if cooked foods were so bad, we wouldn't find a tribe in perfect health living on a mostly cooked diet. However, he said that no tribe had ever been found—*in perfect health*—living on a diet of 90% bread or grains.

He also said that Hovanessian made big salads by grating all of these strong vegetables together, like cabbage and onion, with milder vegetables, like carrots and lettuce, and then adding his own dressing of honey and oil.

Mosséri felt that if you couldn't eat a vegetable raw (like cabbage), in large enough quantities, without mixing it in a big salad and camouflaging the strong flavor with questionable items like honey and oil, then you probably shouldn't be eating that food raw in the first place.

Mosséri claimed to have a very sensitive palate, so he didn't enjoy the vast majority of vegetables in their raw state. If he only ate the ones he enjoyed raw, then there wouldn't be much left on the menu.

So, as a compromise, he cooked some vegetables, just enough to make them more palatable, and he included those vegetables with his dinner meal. This included most vegetables and potatoes.

Mosséri also stressed the importance of eating when genuinely hungry. He said that most people do not wait for hunger to eat, but instead, they wake up in the morning, drink some coffee or other hot beverage that makes their throat dilate unnaturally, and eat something without feeling true hunger. According to Mosséri, eating without hunger leads to overeating, which is the primary cause of disease in our society.

He describes hunger as a pleasant feeling, not pain (which is a sign of *false hunger*), and generally for most people only occurred four or five hours after waking up, unless they were athletes—in which case, they would probably wake up hungry.

He offered a basic menu plan, which was described as the *Ideal Diet:*

Morning:

Don't drink anything. Don't brush your teeth. Wait for true hunger.

When you feel true hunger, calm it with a few pieces of fruit. Repeat a few times during the day.

Evening Meal:

Either have a big salad (with avocado and acceptable condiments), cooked potatoes with lettuce, or steamed vegetables. Alternatively, you can have salad at around 4 or 5 p.m. and follow it an hour or two later with cooked vegetables (including potatoes).

Mosséri's Diet

Albert Mosséri was a student of Herbert Shelton, and wrote over 25 books on Natural Hygiene. Although, fundamentally, he followed the basic principles of Natural Hygiene as taught by Shelton, he had different opinions concerning the practical application, especially the diet. Here's a synthesis of Mosséri's opinion of the optimal diet.

Biologically Appropiate Foods

As humans, we're designed to eat fruits and vegetables. Mosséri rejects all grains (including rice and wheat) and all beans (except when sprouted and cooked). In Mosséri's view, root vegetables are superior to grains, and therefore, they can be consumed (potatoes, sweet potatoes, etc.).

Vegetarianism

Mosséri promotes a vegetarian diet with no meat or fish. He also rejects dairy products and eggs. However, in some cases, when someone is not able to digest nuts and seeds, he will recommend a small quantity of cheese (raw and not fermented) or egg yolk (not egg white) for protein.

Condiments

Mosséri condemns all condiments, such as salt, spices, pepper, garlic and onions. However, to make salads more pleasing to the taste, he allows chopping some onion (through oxidation they lose a great deal of their strong oil) and adding them to the salad.

Cooked Foods

Mosséri says a 100% raw diet is best, as long as one does not go through the extremes of eating all-raw and then cheating with bad foods, such as either unhealthy cooked foods or large quantities of nuts and seeds. He finds that most people find it easier to have a few meals of cooked vegetables per week.

Fruit

Mosséri recommends a fruit-based diet, and he himself eats fruit all day, every other day.

Nuts and Seeds, Fats

Mosséri claims he has seen a lot of people getting very sick and even dying from eating too many nuts and seeds on a regular basis. He went through a period where he didn't recommend any at all, and eventually arrived at the position of recommending about one ounce of nuts and seeds, or some avocado, to most people every day.

Hunger

Mosséri recommends eating when genuinely hungry, and for most people, that means skipping breakfast every day.

Fasting

Mosséri is a proponent of fasting for health, but his experience has shown him that fasts longer than 21 days are not beneficial. After 14 to 21 days of a water fast, he switches people over to what he calls a "half-fast," which consists of eating 100 grams of apples several times a day. The added nutrition in the fruit kick-starts detoxification again, according to him.

I consider Mosséri's work an evolution over Shelton. The main problem with Mosséri's diet is the implementation. Because Mosséri is not concerned with counting calories and often recommended waiting for true hunger before eating, he has created a framework that encourages eating disorders. I know some people who took the "wait for true hunger" advice literally and would wait until 2 p.m. every day before they started eating. To compensate for the lack of calories during the day, they overate all evening, which made them feel bad the next day. Every day, they continued this unhealthy cycle of fasting, followed by overeating. In my opinion, it's better to create a stable schedule of meals and follow it as best you can, even if that means eating without being ravenously hungry every time.

I was really inspired by Mosséri's writing and decided to give his diet a try. Fortunately for me, one of Mosséri's favorite foods was the white potato. He was strongly against grains, but advocated potatoes, which, as a vegetable, are naturally alkaline-forming.

When I experimented with Mosséri's diet, I discovered that by waiting for true hunger, I would really appreciate the fruits I was eating, and I thought it was the best meal on the planet. Many days, I would only start eating at around noon or 1 p.m.

In the evening though, I would get very hungry, and I would often make a massive salad or eat a giant bowl of potatoes with some lettuce.

I found that I really enjoyed the taste of the foods I was eating (even without spices or salt), but I had trouble making the diet work.

Because I would wait for true hunger to eat during the day and only eat a few fruits at a time, I would feel ravenous at night. I would then devour almost two pounds of cooked potatoes, and then I would feel tired and stuffed afterwards.

Because the diet was difficult to maintain, I would often fall off the wagon and eat some junk food. I would then pay for it the next day by feeling terrible, which led me to fast even longer, often all day, before I felt true hunger again.

It was my last year of music school and my interest in classical guitar was waning. My true passion now was diet and nutrition and Natural Hygiene. I could see myself working in that field, perhaps even at Mosséri's fasting retreat, and who knows what the future could hold for me.

Although I was determined to complete my studies successfully, I knew that I was not going to continue in university and have a future in classical guitar. I wanted to do something with health and nutrition.

For that school year, trying to follow Mosséri's diet, I felt extremely isolated. I didn't share my new beliefs with most of my friends because I knew they would think I was crazy (no one can live on fruit and potatoes!)

I spent my spare time hunting for new fruits at different markets, and I would buy exotic items, such as papaya, whenever I could afford them.

I also started corresponding with Mosséri. I wrote him long letters that I would mail to his address in France, and he would always reply with a laconic note that I would ponder for days.

When I told him, in a long letter, that I felt so isolated with this new lifestyle he replied saying: "You have to break the isolation. Find other like-minded people you can share your thoughts with."

Naturally, I wanted to go to France to see if I could land a job working at his fasting center. When I asked him about that, he replied, "I closed down the center so that I can focus on writing my books."

He recommended that I read all of his books and Shelton's books several times, and get a basic training in human physiology. I eventually read everything he and Shelton had written that I could get my hands on.

Towards the end of my school year, around the spring of 1997, I felt my options were running out for what to do the following year. Mosséri had closed down his fasting center and was no longer accepting interns. I did not know any other similar fasting center in the world, and I seriously needed to meet some people in person who shared the same ideas and interests.

One day, I got a call from a French-Canadian of my age. Mosséri had given him my number so that we could connect. The young guy called me from France, where he said he had met Mosséri, but only for a brief moment. He was disappointed that Mosséri was not a believer (meaning in God), and told me he had started eating exclusively fruit (which I found a very strange idea).

Then the line got cut off, and I never heard from him again...

So I truly felt I was alone in the world, trying to eat this way and learn about Natural Hygiene. I did at some point correspond with some people of my age that I found in the magazine published by the American Natural Hygiene Society, in the "Connections" section, but I never met any of them in person.

However, right about that time when the spring flowers were in bloom, I went online for the first time and discovered a book that would give me the answer about what to do next.

CHAPTER 4

Nature's First Law: The Raw Food Diet

"There are some truths which are so obvious and for that very reason are not recognized by ordinary people."

Arlin, Dini, Wolfe;
Natures First Law: The Raw Food Diet

"There are some truths which are so obvious that for this very reason they are not seen or at least not recognized by ordinary people."

Adolf Hitler,
Mein Kampf

Spending the winter in Quebec on a mostly raw diet of fruits and vegetables made me acutely aware of a reality that I had taken for granted all my life: the Canadian winter. My parents had always considered me *frileux*, a French term which affectionately describes someone who is more sensitive to cold weather than average.

After my parents got divorced, the heating broke down in our house, and it took forever for my mom to get it fixed. One winter, the average temperature in the house, day or night, was about 12° Celsius (54° Fahrenheit). When going to school early in the morning, I would often quickly wake up, feel cold, and then immediately go run a bath. Then I would go back to bed and wait for the tub to fill up, and soak in hot water for as long as I could before I left the house.

I ended up spending long periods of time in the bathtub, because it was the warmest place I could be and because I wasn't an active kid playing sports. So I read books in the bathtub, and I literally read hundreds of books during my high school years—all while in the bathtub!

During that winter on Mosséri's diet, I felt even more sensitive to cold weather than usual. I wasn't weighing myself, but I knew my weight had dropped. I would feel even colder, because I was often eating cold fruit right out of the fridge.

There was only one thing that helped combat the cold: I was probably doing more exercise than I ever did in my life, just by walking frequently and bicycling to get all my food.

I became an urban food hunter! I was on a limited budget, so I had to hunt for the best bargains for fruits and vegetables everywhere. I would walk or bike to a supermarket, get what I needed, and then move on to the next one, often covering the entire city before I was done, while carrying my harvest home in my backpack.

Besides my growing aversion to the cold weather and snow — which made everything more difficult — I started to think about what it would be like to be able to pick my own fruit from the tree.

All I knew was fruits from the supermarket. I could not find organic produce easily, and I was longing to try these amazing tropical fruits I had read about in yet more books I got from the library. Fruits like durian, jackfruit, and lychees... they all sounded so delicious, but I had never tried them. Little did I know that I could simply go to Montreal and find all of these fruits and more in Chinatown and specialized fruit stores. At the time, I was not aware that such places existed.

For most of my life, until I discovered vegetarianism, I never paid much attention to the foods I ate. Now, food had become the most important part of my life. I started to build an image of paradise in my mind: how amazing would it be to live in a warm country, escape this ridiculous cold weather and snow, and pick my own oranges from the tree?

What about growing a garden? I did some research and found out that Quebec had a very short growing season. Farmers were preparing the soil when the snow melted, usually in mid-April. The first crop of a few vegetables, like radishes, came in early June. August and September were the big months for harvest, and by October, not much was left in your garden. By November and December, the only thing you could pick was parsley, which resisted cold weather and could literally be dug out of the snow.

I also discovered that not much fruit was grown in Quebec because of the harsh winter. We had some berries and, of course, an abundance of apples, but only select Northern varieties like Cortland and Macintosh. You could also plant pears and plums, but forget about peaches and nectarines. Cherries were not common, unless you planted hardy varieties that could endure the cold winters. However, to this day, I have never seen a cherry tree in Quebec.

Southern Ontario enjoyed a warmer climate and could grow all of these fruits and more, and I read that somewhere in BC there was a place called the Okanagan Valley where a lot of fruit grew. Otherwise, it seemed to me that the rest of Canada was a very cold place for a raw foodist to live.

I started researching the places where I could relocate. France had a much better climate than Quebec, but I did not have any options besides Mosséri's health retreat, which was closed to the public.

I was so jealous because Mosséri often described having a big fruit orchard. He said he cultivated over 15 varieties of apples that he ate year-round, by keeping them in special boxes. He also had persimmon, cherry, plum, peach, fig, and pear trees.

A place like that must cost a fortune, but I told myself that one day I would also grow my own fruit trees.

I looked at where I could go in Canada, but it looked like we had cold weather everywhere, except a few enclaves with distinct, milder climates. One of them was the city of Vancouver and another was Victoria on Vancouver Island, where apparently it only froze a few days a year, and spring flowers came as early as February. Compared to Quebec and our six-month winter, it sounded wonderful! However, I had never been there, did not know anybody, and it sounded a bit out of reach.

I looked at the United States and noticed how Americans could enjoy such a wide variety of warm climates in one big country. From the islands of Hawaii, the states of Florida, California, Arizona, and Texas, to the US territory of Guam — there were plenty of great places south of the border. Again, I had no opportunity there and no one I knew, except a cousin who lived in Los Angeles that I hadn't seen for ages.

So I had to put my dream of fruit-picking on hold.

How to Deal with the Winter on a Raw Food Diet

The winter in cold climates can be a difficult time for those trying to eat a raw food diet. The raw foodist's body temperature may be lower than average (my own body temperature is a couple degrees Fahrenheit lower than the norm), although this can have advantages, such as the ability to improve personal fitness and sustain longer hours of training.

I personally have not noticed that I'm more sensitive to cold weather when eating raw, unless I eat cold fruit. By paying attention to a few principles, I can deal with the cold weather. This does not mean that I like it, and for that reason I now spend several months of the winter in tropical countries. (For more information on this, check out my program "How to Move to a Tropical Paradise" **www.fredericpatenaude.com/tropicalparadise.html**.)

Here are some of my favorite tips to help you to stay warm and healthy during the coldest days of winter:

Tip #1: You don't need more fat during the winter

Most people imagine that they need to eat significantly more fat during the winter to stay warm. Eating more fat will cause body fat gain, which can be useful if someone has a very low body fat. In general, more calories might be required during the winter if you spend a lot of time outside. The energy required to maintain your body temperature will be manifested in an increased caloric need. However, if you are staying inside all the time with artificial heat, you do not need to have a higher body fat percentage in the winter.

Tip #2: Not everything has to be so cold!

Get your vegetables out of the fridge a few hours before dinner. Before going to bed, select the fruits you'll want to eat in the morning and keep them at room temperature.

Tip #3: You can warm up a soup

You can always warm up a raw soup, or make a simple cooked soup by steaming some vegetables and blending them (carefully) in a Vita-Mix or other blender with some of the steaming water, along with seasonings if desired.

Tip #4: You can drink hot drinks

Drinking hot drinks doesn't alter the high-energy feeling you'll get from eating a raw food diet, as long as you take in only the liquid. For example: herbal teas are okay (caffeine free), as is the broth made by boiling vegetables (only drink the broth, don't eat the veggies). I enjoy drinking all kinds of herbal teas (not those sold in bags but bulk dried fruits and flowers, sold at tea shops), including Teeccino (a coffee replacement available in health-food stores or at **www.teeccino.com)** and Rooibos tea.

Tip #5: Stay warm!

You might get colder on a raw food diet because your body is getting used to a lower, more natural and healthy body temperature. To overcome this obstacle, wear additional clothing.

Tip #6: The best way to raise your body temperature is to exercise

But don't just exercise at specific times! Plan exercise "breaks" during the day, to raise your body temperature and avoid afternoon fatigue. Short exercise breaks can last only a few minutes with exercises such as jumping jacks, a short jog or sprint, lifting weights, etc.

Tip #7: Don't skip a day of exercise

According to recent research, when skipping exercise for two days in a row, the body's efficient use of insulin decreases.[6] I suspect there could be other negative health aspects, including lack of resistance to cold weather.

---

6   http://walking.about.com/od/healthbenefits/a/skip2days.htm

Tip #8: If you're looking for an indoor exercise, try rebounding

Want an exercise you can do on a snowy day? Try rebounding. It can be a great cardio-endurance-toning workout if you know what to do with the rebounder. Get a good rebounder, such as the Needak. Rebounding exercise DVDs are available online.

Tip #9: Hydrate and nourish your skin

Take plenty of hot baths, give yourself a footbath or try a facial mask. Be sure to use a heavy moisturizer after you bathe and before you step outside in the cold, and you'll be sure to be ready for the coldest days.

Finding Raw Foods on the Internet

In 1997, the Internet was just getting popular. I thought it was so cool to be able to browse from one website to the next, looking for information, even though there was not a lot available compared to what there is today.

Naturally, one of the first terms I searched for was "raw food diet."

One of the first websites that popped up was *rawfood.com*, which presented a curious book called *Nature's First Law: The Raw Food Diet*. On the home page of the website, I could see the cover of that book, where three young men in their late twenties were naked in an avocado tree, with leaves conveniently covering their private parts.

That was a pretty shocking cover, and I had no idea who these people were. The cover gave the impression they were living in some kind of tropical jungle, foraging fruit, and laughing at the rest of modern civilization. I had no idea these guys were living in San Diego, California—a big modern city—and driving cars, while buying their foods at the grocery store like everybody else!

The book looked interesting, and I decided to order it. To do that, I had to mail them a money order and wait a few weeks for the book to arrive.

When I got the book in my mailbox, I read it in one day. It was probably the most militant, pro-raw food book I had ever seen.

While all of these hygienists that I had read believed in the raw diet, they were shy and rarely advocated a 100% raw diet. Even though they often considered it an ideal, they also considered it to be out of reach due to the corrupted circumstances of modern society.

Nature's First Law said that unless you ate 100% raw foods, you could not possibly be healthy. Even just 1% of cooked food in your diet, such as steamed broccoli, was enough to keep those cooked food cells alive and make you sick. Their diet was to be 100% raw and nothing less.

Having read the translation of Hovanessian's book *Raw Eating* in Mosséri's work, that message sounded quite familiar. In fact, the more I read *Nature's First Law*, the more I became struck at the similarities between their book and *Raw Eating*.

I did not have the original, English version of *Raw Eating*, but from Mosséri's translation I could still see the striking similarities between the two books. In fact, long paragraphs of *Nature's First Law* were almost word for word paragraphs of *Raw Eating* by Hovanessian. I found that strange, but the book fascinated me nonetheless, in a way that an old, Iranian, long-dead author didn't.

These were real guys, maybe 5 or 6 years older than me, who were doing this, right now, in 1997! They were so enthusiastic about the raw food diet that it was hard not to share their excitement.

They did not try to tone down their message. In their opinion, the raw food diet was *the* answer to all of humanity's problems. It had to be done right—100%—no exception. They even ended each chapter with four words that resonated like an ominous warning: *"Cooked food is poison!"*

As long as you ate cooked food, you were going to stay sick, because any cooked foods consumed would feed those *cooked food cells* in your body. These morbid cooked food cells were what caused your cravings, so you had to starve them completely by eating *only* raw food without any exception.

It wasn't very scientific, but for some reason, it sounded exciting and fun. Maybe I had fooled myself all along thinking I could be healthy on Mosséri's diet, eating these big plates of potatoes and steamed vegetables. According to *Nature's First Law*, even a piece of cooked broccoli was a laughable meal and one that would lead to illness.

After reading the book, I became seriously excited about going 100% raw. Summer was coming, and I could really do this. *Nature's First Law* was somehow devoid of any useful menu plans or guidelines on what to eat, but they said that if it's a raw fruit, vegetable, nut, or seed, it's okay. Eat as much as you want, as often as you feel like. That sounded like an easy plan to follow, so I decided to try it.

At the end of the book, there was a page that said that *Nature's First Law* was seeking correspondence with any like-minded people, and that all inquiries would be replied to. They also had a catalog of products you could order.

So I wrote them a long letter, describing all of my story and adventures that led me to raw foods and their book.

To my surprise, a few weeks later, I received a reply from one of the authors, David Wolfe himself. It was a good two-page answer, handwritten, and signed by David "Avocado" Wolfe.

Over the next few months, I exchanged a few letters with David, before we moved on to the more convenient form of communication: email.

I pointed out the fact that their book seemed awfully similar to *Raw Eating* by Hovanessian, to which David responded that they had indeed "gotten some inspiration" from that book to write theirs. That was not such a big deal to me, but also I did not have the entire book *Raw Eating* at my disposal to see how much they had really used as "inspiration" for their book. I could only tell that every part of *Raw Eating* that I had read was included in a modified form in *Nature's First Law*.

A few years later, some people found out about this plagiarism and exposed it on some Internet forums. It turned out that *Nature's First Law* had copied the entire book *Raw Eating*, almost word for word, and used it as part of *Nature's First Law*, without giving any acknowledgement to the author, except for a vague dedication at the start of the book.

Because *Raw Eating* was written in an old-fashioned style with poor English, they had modernized it a bit and added a lot of their own stuff to create their book. Eventually, they changed future editions of the book to include a clear acknowledgement of where the material was from. At the time of the controversy, David told me that I was the first person to point out the similarities.

I told David in a letter that I could probably translate their book into French for them. There was really not much available on the raw food diet in our language, so I offered my services for this task.

David responded with something like, "Lets do it!"

One day, I talked to David on the phone. We had a short conversation, in which he told me he was now following a 100% fruit diet. I said, "Does that mean you're not eating spinach?" At the time, I was eating large quantities of raw spinach. David almost laughed at me for eating greens. He said, "Dude... Spinach? Ha, ha, ha... no way. Just fruit."

When I told him that I felt quite isolated in Quebec and did not know anybody who shared my lifestyle, he said, "Why don't you come to San Diego? You can stay at my place!"

I said, "Really? Ok... that sounds great!"

Going to California? Meeting the authors of *Nature's First Law*? That sounded amazing! I was amazed at David's friendliness. I had never met him in my life. I was just one of his readers, but yet, he treated me like an old friend.

I realized that this dream of going to France and working at a fasting center was just not going to happen, and California and the raw food diet was where things were really happening. Mosséri and Natural Hygiene were old, and the raw food diet was the new wave.

CHAPTER 5

California's Raw Food Superheroes

"I'll say it point blank... Dude, you've got to go nude!"

The Raw Courage Vegetable Man,
aka RC Dini

During my first days 100% raw, my raw food diet was going quite well. Even though I was constantly hungry, I had good energy levels and felt great.

One thing I hadn't figured out yet and none of these raw foodists were insisting on was the importance of calories. Instead, everybody said that you should just eat as much as you wanted. They said that during your first few months raw, you would need to eat more. Over time, you would be able to eat less and less to the point where some raw foodists claimed they only needed to eat very little to feel great.

Every major author was guilty of this magical thinking. Shelton dismissed the calorie theory and provided a menu plan that was seriously lacking in energy and too high in fat. Mosséri, with his program of eating when you're genuinely hungry, promoted undereating followed by large, never-ending evening meals to compensate. Hovanessian claimed he ate only two meals a day: a meal of fruit at noon and a large salad in the evening. Finally, the authors of *Nature's First Law* claimed they only needed a few pieces of fruit a day to thrive.

In practice, the concept rarely worked. I have found over the years that undereating in total calories and overeating certain macronutrients (namely, fat) is the single biggest mistake raw foodists make with their diet.

Calories are just a measure of the energy value of food. Like all animals, we need to eat primarily for energy, not just for vitamins and minerals.

As a young man of 21, active as I was, walking and biking everywhere to get my food, I probably needed about 2500 calories a day, at the very least. In rawfood terms, that would mean about 25 bananas a day (100 calories in each banana).

At the time, I did not understand how to properly balance a raw diet, so I was eating all the time. I was constantly hungry. I relied exclusively on willpower and the desire to thrive on this diet to get me through.

Fortunately, undereating for a few months, when you're still young and capable, is something most people can handle fairly well. They might even feel more energy as they are burning off their fat reserves and getting stimulated by higher levels of stress hormones to get them through the day.

I remember one day, I was walking down the street, feeling this amazing craving for food. At that moment, I would have eaten anything: burgers, French fries, or even a steak. However, I didn't allow these thoughts into my consciousness. I was determined to keep eating 100% raw.

When I got back home, I gulped down 8 bananas in a row. That was the most fruit I had eaten at once, ever! I felt a little guilty about it, because Mosseri condemned raw bananas in his writings and, instead, recommended avoiding them or eating them cooked. Yet, I felt great after eating this much fruit, which is only 800 calories after all, probably what the average teenage boy eats for breakfast.

At some point in his life, Mosséri started to believe that raw bananas were detrimental for health. He made a few observations on his patients and later learned that gorillas did not eat bananas, which strengthened his belief. For some reason, he thought that bananas were not properly digested. He said that if you cooked them briefly, the problems went away. He later revised his theory and admitted that as long as they were perfectly ripe, bananas were okay.

When I was following Mosséri's diet, I often cooked bananas, which helped me get extra calories. Strangely enough, cooked bananas don't taste that bad. They get very sweet and juicy, and I found I could eat more of them that way than when I ate them raw.

I didn't know about making giant smoothies using a blender, so all I was eating was raw fruit and big salads. Because I was still under the influence of Mosséri's writing, I was avoiding nuts and seeds, for the most part, but still ate some avocado.

That summer, I went to Montreal to the world-famous *Jean-Talon Market,* because I was told that it was a great place to find fruit. When I got there in May, the quantity of fruit overwhelmed me. I filled my backpacks with as many mangoes as I could, and I brought them back home.

Those mangoes that I bought were so incredibly delicious. I had never tasted anything quite like it. I thought at that moment that it was great that I could get tropical fruits imported from all over the world, but it would be even better if I could pick them myself from my own trees.

Little did I know that Montreal is one of the best places in the entire world to find fresh fruits and vegetables, if you know where to go. The *Jean-Talon Market* is probably the single best produce market in North America. If I had hung out there a little bit longer, I would probably have met some other raw foodists there, who inevitably would have come to get their weekly groceries.

But I already had my exit strategy: California.

How was I going to get there? I researched prices for airfares, but found out it was quite expensive. So I looked at the Greyhound bus company, and I found out that they had a special for the summer. You paid the fare of around $80 in advance, and you could go anywhere their buses went in North America.

So I booked my ticket for October 29, 1997. The total cost was a little less than $80 for a one-way ticket to San Diego, which was the farthest I could go with this deal, except Alaska!

It was not going to be an easy ride, either. I would have to take a bus to one city, transfer to another city, and so on, until I reached my destination, which would take a total of three days.

I got this huge ticket that unfolded almost to the floor when I opened it. From Montreal, I was going to go to New York City, to Cleveland, to Chicago, to Denver, to Las Vegas, to Los Angeles and, finally, to San Diego. I was going to arrive in San Diego on November 1st.

When I prepared my exit strategy, I analyzed the weather patterns and growing season in different areas of Quebec. I found out that if I ever lived here, the best time to stay would be from May 1st until November 1st. After that, the winter started, and it was probably a good time to leave!

Having the defined goal to leave at the end of October made me extremely motivated to do what was necessary to leave.

First of all, I needed money.

During all my time in music school, I hadn't had a job because I wanted to live at home and focus exclusively on practicing. My thinking was that, since I started playing later than many people, I needed to compensate by practicing more than them. I noticed that most people in music school had a part-time job. I decided that if I stayed with my parents and did not get a part-time job, I could easily get an extra two hours of practice per day, which would give me an edge over everybody else.

The strategy worked, but I was also extremely broke because of it. So my goal for the summer was to save as much money as I could by working every day.

I tried to apply for jobs in the area, but I could not find anything. Then a friend of mine told me about this food preparation company that was hiring, so I showed up and was hired on the spot.

It turned out that there was a reason why it was so easy to get a job there: the work was terrible.

Up until that point, I had been unaware of how little food preparation most restaurants actually do. When restaurants want to save time and not have to cut cabbage for their cabbage salad, or slice bell peppers for their stir-fries, they buy these vegetables from a company that specializes in food preparation for restaurants.

The job that I got was for one of these companies.

It's not that the job was that terrible, but the hours were. Surprisingly, a lot of the cutting was done manually and not with machines. To keep the vegetables fresh, they kept the temperature in the workspace at around 5° C (41° F).

It was the height of summer, so going from a cold temperature to hot weather was quite shocking to my body. But every time we had a break, I went outside to soak up some sun and eat some fruit even so.

When other workers were eating their bologna sandwiches for lunch, I was having fruit or salad. All the male workers were making fun of what I was eating, but in the back of my mind, I was going to have the last laugh, knowing that in October I'd be leaving this place and enjoying another summer, while they were going to freeze their butts off in Quebec!

Every day, the company received orders from different restaurants, and my shift was only over when all of these orders were completed. Usually, I ended up working 12 hours in a row but sometimes, it was even more.

One day, I worked 24 hours in a row (with only a few 10 minute breaks). I was so tired when I got back home, but the raw food diet helped me survive and stay healthy.

At some point, I had enough of this craziness, so I did what any disgruntled worker should do: I left.

We had already worked 16 hours in a row that day, and the manager wanted us to keep working to finish the order. I asked him, "When are we going to be done?"

He answered, "When the order is done! Now, go back to work!"

"You know, I can't do this anymore," I replied.

"What are you talking about? You can't leave!"

"Well, watch me." I replied, and then removed my uniform and left.

I was happy to have left that crappy job, but I still needed to earn some more money to have a reserve good enough to last me for a while in California.

I was lucky enough to get a job at a supermarket that had just recently opened in my area. Again, everybody thought I was crazy, this time for buying so many fruits and vegetables after my shifts. I didn't necessarily enjoy this kind of job, but I didn't care because I had a clear goal in mind. I knew that by the end of October, I would be out of there.

San Diego, Here I Come

The day that I left for San Diego, the snow hadn't yet started, but it was cold enough to make me long for warmer climates. I had my passport ready, enough money saved to last me who knew how long, and I had said goodbye to all my friends and family.

All of my friends were convinced that I would run out of opportunities within a few months and quickly come back home. However, I saw this trip as something more. I was leaving Quebec, and I didn't intend on coming back. I had no idea where in the world I would end up, but I knew going to San Diego was the first step.

I didn't bring many belongings with me— just a few clothes, a blank journal and a pen to write with, a few books, and some basic items. I knew that while traveling on the Greyhound network, there would probably be nothing for me to eat anywhere, so I also brought with me a 12-pound bag of apples and two pounds of medjool dates.

Once on the bus, I knew I had a big trip ahead of me. A plane ride would have taken me only 5 or 6 hours, but I was in for a total of 72 hours on the bus and waiting at bus stations.

For a once-in-a-lifetime experience, I actually enjoyed the ride. I had plenty of time to reflect on why I was leaving Quebec and what I was hoping to find once I reached my destination. For the first part of the trip, the landscape was quite similar to Quebec and still familiar. Once we headed to Colorado though, everything changed. Near Denver, people were skiing in the mountains. A day later, I was seeing the deserted landscape of Utah, which reminded me of old Western movies. When I arrived in Las Vegas, I saw my first palm tree and the weather was already much nicer. I started to relax and feel at home.

When you travel on a bus for that long, you don't get to sleep anywhere comfortably. Sometimes the bus was packed, and I was crammed next to a big fat person. Sometimes the bus was nearly empty, and I could have two seats to myself and spread out. I slept on my seat, passing out for a few hours at a time, but often, my sleep was ended abruptly when we arrived at a new city. I had to get out and wait for the next bus to arrive at the station.

It turned out that my idea of bringing my own fruit with me was a good one. There was literally nothing I could eat at those bus stations, except for the occasional unripe banana or orange. So I ate apples and dates for three days, and I felt quite good overall.

When I arrived in San Diego, David Wolfe picked me up at the Greyhound station. I had only seen his picture in a book, so I didn't know what to expect. These guys were almost like cartoon characters to me, so meeting them for the first time was very strange.

It didn't take very long to recognize David once I got out on the street and looked around. He showed up in an old, beaten up Honda Civic, walked up to me bare-chested, sporting the darkest tan I had ever seen on a white guy, with well-defined pectoral muscles that paid testimony to the hours he had obviously spent in the gym. He radiated an overall glow of health, unlike I had ever seen in my life, but similar to how Mario had appeared to me when I first met him.

"Are you Frederic? Hi! I'm David Wolfe!"

We got into his car, which was filled with random papers and fruit peels. David picked up a few ripe bananas and started eating them. He then turned on the radio and started blasting some *Slayer*, a heavy metal band I knew very well, since I had been a heavy metal fan in my teenage years, before I started learning classical music.

"You listen to heavy metal?" I asked, startled.

"Of course, dude! I love this shit!" he replied.

Then David cranked the volume a few notches, and continued, "Listen, dude, I have a bunch of stuff to do today with my school, so I have to drop you off at a friend of mine's, and you can hang out with them for the day. I'll come pick you up later. Ok, dude?"

This was my first introduction to the word "dude," but I quickly realized that Californian guys used it in every sentence.

I was in shock after my first meeting with David Wolfe. I had expected some kind of nature boy, more of the hippie type, cultivating fruits and living peacefully, eating only a few pieces of fruit a day, as he had claimed in the book.

Instead, by the time we reached our destination, David had already consumed the few daily pieces of fruit that one could supposedly live on for an entire day. He was driving a car, listening to heavy metal, and "duding" me all the way. He was the typical Californian, relaxed by the warm weather and enjoying the coolest life in the world.

Speaking of weather, I was quite amazed by my first day in San Diego. It was November 1st, and it was probably only 7°C (45°F) back home in Montreal. In San Diego, it was at least 25°C(78°F), and the sun was shining brightly.

David dropped me off at a typical suburban house, where a friend of his named Don "The Raw Guy," was living. He also told me that his cousin, "Raw Courage," simply called RC, was there too, along with his girlfriend, Heidi.

Then David excused himself to go back to school and drove away with his windows open and the heavy metal music blasting. I went inside the house, and I met Don the Raw Guy, who was expecting me. He had been christened with this name because it sounded cool, and because every raw foodist seemed to have some kind of raw food superhero name.

Don was a thirty-something, friendly and slightly geeky Jewish guy, with whom I immediately felt at ease.

After I said a few words to Don, RC showed up from the kitchen. He was also around thirty or thirty-one, and was walking around shirtless, wearing only old sweat pants, with fruit juice stains all over them. Like David, he was extremely tanned. He had this crazy beard that was totally out of control, and looked like a homeless person, but he smelled like fruit and garlic instead of beer and cigarettes.

Without introducing himself or saying anything to break the ice, he brought out the biggest bowl of guacamole that I had ever seen in my entire life and said, "Have some of this, dude."

The guacamole was in a giant salad bowl and reeked of onions and garlic, and because of my Natural Hygiene background I did not eat those items. I asked, "Is there garlic in this? I don't eat garlic."

RC answered, "You're going to love it." He handed me a leaf of cabbage to use as a bowl, and scooped a generous amount of his guacamole into it with a spoon.

I couldn't really say no, so I smiled and ate the guacamole sandwich. It tasted really good, and I was hungry. Don smiled at me and said, "Dude, you're going to eat so much food while you're in San Diego; it's not even funny."

Don was right.

I also met Heidi, who was RC's girlfriend and was seventeen at the time. RC seemed to be completely in love with her.

RC was a very funny, hyperactive guy, who had lost over 150 pounds on the raw food diet in the last year or two. He had pictures of himself in the book *Nature's First Law* that showed how he looked when he was over 300 pounds and used to work as a manager at the fast-food chain *Jack in the Box*. After David converted to the raw food diet, Fouad Dini (his real name), decided to go raw, and "Raw Courage" Dini was born.

Heidi was more the quiet type. She didn't say much, but she giggled often. She had only been a raw foodist for a few months and didn't have a raw food name yet. I was starting to wonder whether I would also receive a raw food name during my stay in California.

After this quick introduction at Don's house, we headed to the beach. In the car, I was told we were heading to Black's Beach, a nude beach north of San Diego. I had never been to a nudist beach before, and certainly wasn't planning to take my clothes off on my first day in San Diego. However, I didn't really care too much, and I was open to any experience.

RC brought a big bag of fruit with him. He was living with his dad and had dozens of fruit trees that he and David had planted years ago. He gave me the biggest and sweetest pomegranate I had ever had, and I was blown away at how delicious it was. He then started to feed me the most amazing oranges that I had ever tasted too.

As soon as we got to Black's beach, RC took his clothes off. Almost as fast as Clark Kent could remove his suit and fly away in his Superman costume, RC was naked and ready to jump in the ocean.

I also got undressed and enjoyed the glorious San Diego sun.

While we were at the beach, RC showed me some interesting new raw food techniques that he had invented. He liked to bring certain fruits, like tomatoes and avocados, and dip them in the ocean to make them salty. I wasn't sure that it was such a good idea, but RC seemed to love his ocean-dipped tomatoes.

At the time, the El Niño current had warmed the ocean to an unusually high temperature. When I got in the water, it was probably at least 25°C (78°F). As a first introduction to Southern California life, I was quite blown away. I thought to myself, "This is paradise. I can never leave this place. This is too good."

Unfortunately, the ocean never got quite that warm again. But I thought, at that moment, that this is the way it was all the time. I don't think I ever swam in the ocean again in all of my time in California, but this was perfect for my first day there.

It occurred to me that all I had needed to make new friends here was to be a raw foodist. Just eating this way made you immediately part of an exclusive club, where you lived in a completely different reality, in a world where everything seemed possible, and where cooked food eaters were not welcome.

Guac Around the Clock

When I showed up in San Diego, I was a scrawny, pale French Canadian, living on a diet of fruits and vegetables. I ate very little fat, because of Mosséri's influence, and I also avoided all salt, spices, condiments, garlic, and onions. I ate very simply. I knew no raw recipes, and I did not blend my food ever.

Although I was not consuming enough calories for a young guy of my age, I felt pretty good and did not have any health problems.

One year later, I would be spending several months in bed, completely sick, with my health falling apart, in spite of being on what was supposed to be the best diet in the world.

RC's giant guacamole was the starting point of this descent to hell.

When I tell people nowadays that I've seen raw foodists destroy their health because of their almost religious adherence to the raw food ideal, while completely ignoring basic nutritional concepts, I am not kidding.

I was there at a time of renaissance in the modern raw food movement that would fully take off in the 2000's, and I witnessed the drastic difference between the ideal of raw food and the reality of raw food.

The vast majority of people I met at the time, who were so adamant about the ideal of the raw food diet, are no longer eating all raw today. They all quit, because it simply didn't work for them in the end.

The story of how people destroy their health by blindly following an ideal and nutrition misinformation is an interesting one that I intend to reveal in the following pages.

CHAPTER 6

Discovering the Avocado

"Almost every raw foodist I have ever met is an avid fan of the avocado."

David Wolfe,
The Sunfood Diet Success System

After this first day in San Diego, I went back to David's place. At the time, David was still finishing his law degree. He lived with a roommate, spent a good number of hours in school, and worked as much as he could on his business on the side.

After those three days on the bus, I was quite exhausted and slept for 9 to 10 hours the first night. David made fun of me for sleeping so long. I noticed that he himself only slept about 6 to 7 hours a night.

Over the years, I've noticed that most raw foodists claim to need less sleep, in some cases, dramatically less than what is recommended as the "norm." In my own case, especially in my early twenties, I found out that I did not function properly unless I got 8 to 9 hours of sleep. As I got a little older, my need for sleep decreased by an hour, unless I exercised a lot, in which case I needed my 8 to 9 hours, if not 10.

I was kind of jealous of people who were able to sleep only a few hours a night, and I thought that eventually this was going to happen to me if I kept going on a raw diet. However, no matter how many modifications I made to my diet, I still needed my sleep.

I then realized that in most cases, people living on a few hours of sleep a night are not healthier: instead, they are overworking their bodies. Sleep requirements will vary from one person to the next, but for healthy adults, the general amount needed is 7 to 8 hours. The more physical activity one does, the more sleep is necessary to recover as well.

How Much Sleep Do We Really Need?

In 2002, Daniel Kripke from the Scripps Clinic Sleep Center in La Jolla, California, compared death rates among more than one million Americans. He compared it to their reported average amount of sleep.

This study brought interesting results that have been duplicated in other studies as well. It showed that people getting between 6.5 and 7.5 hours of sleep a night live the longest.[7]

People who sleep less than 6.5 hours or more than 8.5 hours have a higher rate of depression, obesity, and heart disease.[8][9]

The biggest surprise in his study was that long sleep starts at 8 hours.

My own theory on that is that the relationship is not necessarily causal. Sick people need to sleep more. Therefore, it is quite normal to discover that people who sleep the longest are the sickest and don't live as long. The amount of sleep they need is a reflection of how sick and depressed they are.

On the other hand, people who don't sleep enough are destroying their health by not giving their body the recovery time it needs. This relationship is probably more causal than the first one.

So how long do we need to sleep? We've been told all our lives that we need to sleep eight hours a night, but there's little evidence that eight hours is the right amount of sleep for the human body.

Your need for sleep will be determined by a few factors, such as:

- Age (young people need more sleep)

- Activity levels (athletic people need more sleep to recover)

---

7   http://www.time.com/time/health/article/0,8599,1812420,00.
    html#ixzz13T5VmlNS

8   Another study to support this: (2006). Amount of sleep affects risk of diabetes, hypertension. *Geriatrics*, *61*(6), 16. Researchers found that men who get fewer than 6 hours or more than 8 hours of sleep each night have a higher risk of developing type 2 diabetes.

9   Kripke, D., Garfinkel, L., Wingard, D., Klauber, M., & Marler, M. (n.d). Mortality Associated With Sleep Duration and Insomnia. *Archives of General Psychiatry*, *59*(2), 131.

- Health (sick people need more sleep)

- Quality of sleep

Some people might need a lot of sleep because they are very sick or because they are very fit! It would be a shame to prevent yourself from getting enough sleep because you think that sleeping more than 8 hours is too much.

However, if you find that you have symptoms of depression and lack of energy, it could be because you're sleeping more than you need to.

How to tell if you're getting too much sleep:

- You have difficulty falling asleep at night.

- You wake up in the morning in a daze.

- You feel depressed.

- You lack energy.

How to tell if you're not getting enough sleep:

- You feel very tired.

- You're falling asleep during the day.

- You're feeling extremely tired at around 2 or 3 p.m.[10]

Most natural hygienists I have studied will say it is not possible to get too much sleep, but scientific literature and personal experience contradict that. Too much sleep can be depressogenic.[11,12]

A more important aspect of proper sleep management has to do with circadian rhythms.

10 Neubauer, D. (2010). "We're not sleeping enough!" *Primary Psychiatry*, *17*(2), 19-21.

11 Foley, D., Vitiello, M., Bliwise, D., Ancoli-Israel, S., Monjan, A., & Walsh, J. (2007). Frequent napping is associated with excessive daytime sleepiness, depression, pain, and nocturia in older adults: findings from the National Sleep Foundation '2003 Sleep in America' Poll. *The American Journal Of Geriatric Psychiatry: Official Journal Of The American Association For Geriatric Psychiatry*, *15*(4), 344-350.

12 Stroe, A., Roth, T., Jefferson, C., Hudgel, D., Roehrs, T., Moss, K., et al. (2010). Comparative levels of excessive daytime sleepiness in common medical disorders. *Sleep Medicine*, *11*(9), 890-896.

Because we live on Planet Earth, a wonderful and unique place in the Universe where days are 24 hours long with 12 hours of darkness and 12 hours of sunshine near the equator, our bodies have adapted to a certain rhythm through evolution.

The circadian rhythms coordinate many metabolic processes, and they are mainly regulated by sunlight, digestion and timing of meals.

That is why as soon as our eyes are exposed to daylight (or even artificial light), our body thinks it is daytime and sets various metabolic processes in motion. Melatonin production is inhibited, and we feel more awake. Even if we are exposed to sunlight at the wrong time (such as when flying to a new time zone by plane) or artificial lights (such as blasting artificial lights in the middle of the night), our body will be confused and respond accordingly.[13,14]

It's also important to understand sleep cycles.

Each night, we go through a series of sleep cycles, where we go from lighter stages of sleep to deeper stages of sleep, finally ending the cycle in REM sleep (rapid eye movement stage), where dreams occur.

If we get woken up during deep sleep or before the completion of a sleep cycle, we will feel sleep inertia. The worst type of sleep inertia occurs when we get woken up from deep sleep, which occurs about 30 minutes after falling asleep.

If you suffer from sleep inertia, you will find yourself very groggy and irritable, and you will suffer from impaired alertness and a decline in motor dexterity, which will make it difficult for you to perform some mental and physical tasks adequately.

I had a friend who told me that she used a technique to get through her sleepless nights of college, when she was studying to become a nutritionist. She said that often she could only get 4 or 5 hours of sleep a night, but would time her sleep so that she would never be woken up in the middle of a sleep cycle.

---

13   Missildine, K. (2008). Sleep and the sleep environment of older adults in acute care settings. *Journal of Gerontological Nursing, 34*(6), 15-21.
14   Burgess, H. (2010). Partial Sleep Deprivation Reduces Phase Advances to Light in Humans *Journal of Biological Rhythms, 25*(6), 460-468.

For example, she figured that her typical sleep cycle was 90 minutes long. So if she was going to fall asleep at 1:30 a.m. and needed to wake up before 8 a.m., she would set her alarm for 7.30a.m. If she set it at 8, she would be woken up in a stage of deep sleep, which would lead to sleep inertia and would be terrible.

That's why if you naturally wake up in the morning at a certain time, but for some reason decide to go back to bed for another 30 minutes, you can end up feeling terrible. Unless you have at least 2 hours to dedicate to more sleep, it's better to just wake up then, even if you feel you haven't had enough sleep.

Nowadays, a more accurate way to time our sleep like this is to use a *Sleep Cycle Clock*. The *Sleep Cycle Clock* works by analyzing your body movements during your sleep. We tend to toss and turn when we are in between sleep cycles, and the clock software takes that into account. It will then chart your sleep cycles and wake you up exactly when you need it! The program works with the iPhone OS (for iPhone and iPod Touch) and can be found here: **http://mdlabs.se/sleepcycle/**. At the time of writing, it only costs 99 cents. If you worry about having a cellphone next to your body while sleeping, make sure you turn off the wireless functions before going to sleep. This is such a useful tool when traveling, and if I had to get up to go to work every morning I would use it regularly as a pleasant way to wake up instead of a stressful blaring alarm clock.

If you suffer from insomnia, you may be giving your body too much sleep. By waking up earlier, you will feel more natural fatigue later in the day and fall asleep easily. The rule of thumb is that if it takes you more than 5 minutes to fall asleep once you close your eyes and lay your head on your pillow, you are probably sleeping too much.

Advice for Sound Sleep

Based on everything we've just said, here are some tips for perfect sleep:

Tip #1: Go to bed at a regular time

Our bodies expect a rhythm. Going to bed at different times every night disturbs that rhythm and messes with our internal clock. Remember that people who live long lives have very established habits concerning their bedtime.

Tip #2: Go to bed before midnight

It's been said that the hours before midnight count for two. While it's not quite accurate, it's fair to say that we'll get better sleep if we go to bed an hour or two before midnight, mainly because we'll respect our body's internal clock, which is regulated by sunlight.[15]

Tip#3: Sleep in complete darkness

Darkness is the most important factor for melatonin and serotonin production. For optimal sleep, make sure you sleep in total darkness. Close all doors and get rid of night lights (except red light, which doesn't disturb sleep). Use blackout shapes or drapes to create total darkness in your room. When traveling, use a sleep mask to recreate total darkness artificially.

Tip #4: Use the sleep cycle alarm clock

The sleep cycle clock I mentioned works great for timing your sleep cycle and waking you up at the appropriate time.

Tip #5: Keep your bedroom cool

A drop in body temperature is necessary for your body to get the signal to go to sleep. Therefore, keep your bedroom cool at night (no more than 21°C/70°F).[16]

Tip#6: Don't eat or drink late at night

Avoid eating or drinking at least 2-4 hours before going to bed so that you aren't woken up at night to use the bathroom too many times.

15   Abe, T., Hagihara, A., &Nobutomo, K. (2010). Sleep patterns and impulse control among Japanese junior high school students. *Journal of Adolescence*, *33*(5), 633.

16   Togo, F., Aizawa, S., Arai, J., Yoshikawa, S., Ishiwata, T., Shephard, R., et al. (2007). Influence on human sleep patterns of lowering and delaying the minimum core body temperature by slow changes in the thermal environment. *Sleep*, *30*(6), 797-802.

Tip #7: Avoid fruit or carbs late in the day

You can have fruit with your evening meal, but this should be about 3 or 4 hours before going to bed. Avoid a late-night sweet fruit snack, especially the very sweet fruits like dates, bananas and mangoes. They will raise your blood sugar and delay sleep.

Because raw food meals are less dense in calories, many people find that they get hungry right before going to bed. In that case, I recommend snacking on low-sugar, low-acid fruits such as apples, pears, ripe starfruit, or dragon fruit (a tropical favorite). This may wake you up once to go to the bathroom, which is manageable.

Tip #8: No computer after 10 pm

A good rule to implement in our modern world is to avoid any computer use after a certain time, such as 9 or 10 p.m. That means no Facebook, no emails, no web-browsing, no watching TV shows, etc. The limitless distractions of the Internet are not conducive to falling asleep.

Tip #9: Use earplugs

That way, you won't get awakened by a noisy, early-bird roommate, family member or neighbor.

Tip #10: Read some fiction

Instead of watching TV or browsing the web, read a good novel before going to sleep. Fiction reading deactivates the analytical part of your brain (left brain) and is relaxing, especially if most of your day is spent in analytical activities.

Tip #11: Avoid caffeine

Caffeine disturbs sleep, even if you just have one cup of coffee per day. This goes for chocolate, too.[17]

---

17   Sin, C., Ho, J., & Chung, J. (2009). Systematic review on the effectiveness of caffeine abstinence on the quality of sleep. *Journal of Clinical Nursing, 18*(1), 13-21.

Tip #12: Avoid alcohol

Drinking alcohol impairs the body's ability to enter the deeper stages of sleep. Even though drinking alcohol may make you feel drowsy, this effect is short-lived, and the overall quality of your sleep will be affected.

Tip #13: Exercise at least 30 minutes every day

Exercising daily will naturally fatigue your body and help you fall asleep. Make sure you don't exercise too close to bedtime, or else the stimulation from exercise may keep you awake.

Tip #14: Get natural sunlight as soon as you get up in the morning

By exposing your eyes to real, natural sunlight first thing in the morning, you help your body curb its melatonin production and time its circadian rhythms to wake you up.[18,19]

Alternatively, you can also use full-spectrum light bulbs to achieve a similar effect, if it's too cold to go outside.

Tip #15: Eat at regular times

Just like sleeping at regular times, eating regularly can help you with your sleep. By eating a meal, you give your body a signal that helps it monitor the circadian rhythms. Eating meals at regular times will help your body time when it should fall asleep and when it should be awake.

I observed how David lived his life, and I admired the kind of discipline he was able to muster on a daily basis. He woke up early, and he immediately jumped on the computer to work on his book. He also worked out at the gym every day for an hour. He spent most of

18 HARADA, T., MORISANE, H., & TAKEUCHI, H. (2002). Effect of daytime light conditions on sleep habits and morningness–eveningness preference of Japanese students aged 12–15 years. *Psychiatry & Clinical Neurosciences*, 56(3), 225-226.

19 Smith, S., &Trinder, J. (2005). Morning sunlight can phase advance the circadian rhythm of young adults. *Sleep & Biological Rhythms*, 3(1), 39-41.

his car-time listening to self-improvement programs by the company Nightingale Conant, who produced titles by Tony Robbins, among others.

We ended up chatting about raw food diet theories, and we ate some more fruit. When I had talked to David on the phone a few months earlier, he had been living on a 100% fruit diet (avocados included). I was wondering how this experiment went.

"Are you still eating just fruit?" I asked.

"No, dude. I lasted three months, but I found out that greens are necessary."

He didn't fully elaborate on the subject, but obviously, he was no longer a strict fruitarian and had changed his mind.[20]

After a few days staying at David's place, I knew I had to move on. David had been kind enough to talk to his cousin RC, who lived on a fruit farm in the town of Encinitas, east of San Diego. He told me I could probably go and stay there for a while on the farm, in exchange for work.

RC had been living with a woman named Barbara, who lived on a few acres of land with lots of fruit trees, in the agricultural area east of San Diego. He was living there with Heidi in a parked RV.

This California trip was a complete adventure for me, and I was willing to go with the flow and do whatever came next. I knew I couldn't stay with David Wolfe forever, and it seemed like the wrong time to talk about me working with them on his business. So I went to Encinitas and stayed with RC and Heidi on Barbara's land for a month.

---

20 Although the definition of a fruitarian diet often includes nuts, seeds, and greens, some people go as far as only eating fruit and vegetable fruits (tomatoes, cucumbers, zucchini, etc.).

During that time, I got to taste the most delicious citrus fruits I ever had in my life. RC had a special recipe that he called "grapefruit soup," which was made only with grapefruit and grapefruit juice. To make the recipe, he made sure he picked only the ripest, sweetest grapefruits that naturally fell from the tree and would normally never have been sold in any market. He then cut the grapefruit in half, scooped out the grapefruit flesh in a bowl, and hand-squeezed some grapefruit juice on top.

This "soup" was delicious, even though it wasn't really a complex recipe, but just another way to eat grapefruit.

RC was full of these one-ingredient "recipes," as he strongly believed in eating "perfect fruit." He said that any fruit could be the best fruit you ever had if you picked it when it was perfectly ripe.

However, RC's diet was far from perfect. His ideal was to eat only perfect fruit, one at a time, when hungry. But, as a former fast food addict, he had carried his overeating habits to the raw world.

RC would eat constantly, but if I could have analyzed his diet, I would probably have found out that it didn't contain many calories, since most of the foods he ate were low-calorie fruits like citrus, pomegranates, or other seasonal fruit.

He often made these giant bowls of guacamole with locally grown avocados. One of his most infamous recipes consisted of guacamole on a cabbage leaf, with some almond butter, honey, crushed garlic, and hot pepper on top.

Before coming to San Diego, I thought I knew what a good avocado was. I would buy these Hass avocados that were only good for part of the year. The rest of the time, they tasted watery and did not ripen properly.

In California, I tasted varieties of avocado I had never had before, such as the *Fuerte, Reed,* and *Pinkerton* avocados. My favorite was the *Fuerte* variety, which tasted so rich and creamy. It reminded me of eating cream cheese, but better.

In the past, I thought that half an avocado was a good amount to have, but I would sometimes allow myself to eat an entire avocado, which felt like a lot. I could have eaten more if I wanted to, but my studies of Natural Hygiene had taught me that too many nuts, seeds, and even avocados was not a good thing.

In California, it seemed like every raw foodist ate avocados in massive quantities. RC probably ate two or three Fuerte avocados a day, which were actually larger and heavier than your typical Hass avocado, so it was probably the equivalent of three to four regular ones.

David Wolfe claimed that avocado was his favorite food, and that he had eaten several avocados every day since going raw. He even told me that his personal record for the most avocados consumed in a day was 17. "They were small," he added after a pause.

I attended a talk that David did later that month where he shared some of his strategies for success on the raw food diet.

"I spent a lot of time talking to hundreds of successful, long-term, 100% raw foodists over the past 3 years, and I noticed some interesting patterns. Every raw foodist I met seemed to eat a lot of avocados. In fact, most successful, long-term raw foodists have eaten 3 to 5 avocados a day. I personally eat 3 to 5 avocados a day, and I'm here to tell you that this is one of the secrets for success on a raw food diet."

Then David delivered his famous line, placing special emphasis on certain words:

"It's *okay* to eat three to five avocados *a day.*"

In spite of my inner voice that told me that it still seemed like too much avocado, I succumbed to social pressures and the fact that these Californian avocados were just too darn delicious to resist.

So I started eating avocados, massively.

I also started eating a lot of raw food in general.

In Montreal, I had sometimes tasted fruit as good as what I was eating in California, but could not find it all the time.

The tree-picked oranges and grapefruit were out of this world. We would often pick the ugliest fruit, but strangely enough, those were the best. If they had ripened on the tree for long enough, they had almost no acidity and were so juicy and fragrant.

The pomegranates that RC brought back from his dad's place were insanely good and really, really big. I did not think that pomegranate was such a great fruit until I tried those. Each kernel was so juicy and sweet, and each fruit contained hundreds of them, so it was very rewarding to eat this fruit!

The avocados were of course extremely good, as were the freshly picked tomatoes (still in season) that we used for guacamole.

The reason why we ate so many avocados was simple: one avocado packs in 300 calories, compared to only 50 for an apple. Eat three avocados a day, and you've already taken care of almost half of your caloric needs. For most people, that was a lot easier than eating 20 apples! Because raw foodists hadn't learned to balance their diets properly and get enough calories from a variety of low-fat foods, the avocado seemed like an easy answer.

Back in Montreal, I needed a lot of willpower to stay on the diet and ate less than my young body needed. Although I felt great, I was pretty skinny.

With all those delicious fruits in San Diego, my "hunger" switch finally got turned on. I started to eat and eat to compensate for months of undereating. After a little while, I had gained some weight and did not look as scrawny as before.

RC even thought he should find me a raw food name. One day it occurred to him to call me *Raw Demolition*, because he said I would demolish and devour any fruit in sight, leaving a path of destruction and mess behind (which my wife can still attest to this day!)

CHAPTER 7

A Wrong Turn Down Raw Meat Street

"When your body needs it, even raw chicken can taste delicious."

Guy-Claude Burger,
Inventor of Instinctotherapy
(and convicted pedophile)

My main goal when going to California was to be part of the raw food movement. It seemed like it was the place where things were really happening.

I left everything behind: my passion for classical guitar and my possible career as a music teacher, my family and friends, and my home province of Quebec, where everybody spoke French, which was what I had been familiar with since birth.

The main thing that compelled me to leave was that I felt I did not have many friends that could understand me anymore. Besides my brother and my friend Dominic, I did not know any other raw foodists. I also did not know any girls who were raw foodists.

Before I left, I had been in touch with a high school girlfriend of mine, Mélanie, and shared with her my whole process with vegetarianism, veganism, Natural Hygiene, and now raw foods.

I wanted her to understand it and even to apply it in her life. I was pushing my new philosophy on her too hard and none of what I was saying made that much sense to her. She kept replying with objections, but she was nonetheless fascinated by my new lifestyle. Besides her and a few close friends, I had not revealed much about my raw food lifestyle to anybody else, for fear of being ostracized by my peers. I thought that nobody could possibly understand me, and I needed to go to California to meet people who finally would.

In the back of my mind, I nurtured the comforting thought that maybe during my trip to California I would meet a girl who was a like-minded spirit that could understand me.

I had felt so alone for so long that suddenly meeting so many people who shared the same lifestyle overwhelmed me. I put aside everything that I had already studied and thought was true about health and nutrition, and I totally invested myself in the experience of being a raw foodist in California.

Towards the end of November, I was still staying at Barbara's ranch. Somewhere around that time, I went back to San Diego for a weekend, because David was throwing a "raw food party" and was inviting everybody.

The last time I had been to a party was during my high school years and before I started my music studies. For most people of my age, a "party" was always synonymous with alcohol and possibly illicit substances, and this was not a scene I wanted to be part of anymore.

David had had an interesting idea for his party. He called it a "juice party," where everybody invited had to bring fruits and vegetables. Then everything would be juiced and served at the party.

I quite liked the idea, and the party turned out to be a success. Many people had shown up, like Stephen Arlin, who was David's friend and business partner; Roe Gallo, another raw foodist I had heard about who had written the book *Perfect Body* and followed a mostly fruitarian diet, and many other now-famous raw foodists.

Among the people at the party was a very cute girl named Claudia, who came all the way from Los Gatos, in the San Francisco Bay Area. She was from Switzerland, but she was in the US on a working visa, as a babysitter for an affluent couple living in Los Gatos. She came with her older friend, Gail, who was also a raw food chef and had written a raw food recipe book.

The first time I saw Claudia, I knew I had to talk to her. She was so pretty to me, and I thought her name was so beautiful and exotic. When she started talking with her Swiss-German accent, I just couldn't resist.

I also thought she was Stephen's girlfriend, because they were hugging. I thought, "Wow, Stephen is a lucky man."

Hugging people for no apparent reason other than just getting a hug was quite popular in the Californian raw food scene, and it didn't necessarily mean these people were going out.

I did not know that at the time, so the perceived unavailability of Claudia made me desire her even more.

After the party, a group of people ended up going to some hot springs, and I was invited to come along. I had never been to a hot spring, so this sounded like a terrific idea. Claudia was coming too, and I was thrilled.

We went to a private club of which one of our party was a member, and he got everybody free passes.

At the club, there was a giant pool fed by natural hot springs, which kept the water temperature very hot.

Because it was December, it was raining outside at night and a little bit chilly, so soaking in the warm springs was just perfect.

I ended up talking to Claudia the whole evening, and we never ran out of things to say. I eventually realized that she wasn't Stephen's girlfriend, and that she was heading back to San Francisco the very next day.

"Why don't you stay in San Diego?" I asked. "I won't have enough time to get to know you..."

"I can't, my dear. I have to go back to work in Los Gatos. But maybe if you come to San Francisco you can come see me?"

Everybody in California in the raw scene talked to each other as if they had known each other for years. By the end of the evening, we were hugging in the car on the way back. This was confusing to me, because I wasn't sure whether she really liked me or this was just another strange Californian custom.

Heading to San Francisco

When I got back to Barbara's ranch, I knew I had to change my plans and do something different.

David had told me about a guy in the San Francisco Bay area named David Klein who had been a raw foodist for a number of years and published a newsletter called *Living Nutrition*.

"Why don't you just go there?" RC asked me.

I got in touch with David Klein, and he was willing to host me for a couple of days. I purchased my bus ticket to San Francisco and got ready to leave just a few days later.

It occurred to me again that without the raw food lifestyle, I would not have been able to travel around the way I did. I had been in San Diego for over 5 weeks and not once did I have to pay for a hotel room or even a hostel. The fact that I was a raw foodist was enough for some generous souls to host me for a few days, and it seemed like common practice among the raw foodists in California.

My friends back in Canada predicted I would be back in a month or two, when my money ran out. The people I knew who headed out West could barely survive by getting a job as a waiter in a restaurant, and they did not know anybody to host them unless they had some family there. Even though I had a cousin who lived full-time in the Los Angeles area, I hadn't seen her for years. It just seemed like I had more in common with raw foodists, who were my "true" family.

I took the bus to San Francisco and then headed to the town of Sebastopol, where Dave Klein met me at the bus stop.

David had been a raw foodist for several years, after suffering from an acute case of IBS (Irritable Bowel Syndrome) and Crohn's disease. He had healed himself by going raw, and he worked full-time as the publisher of *Living Nutrition,* a small newsletter promoting the raw-food lifestyle, helping clients with similar bowel problems.

David Klein was also a Natural Hygienist, and he ate a very simple diet, which at the time was described by David Wolfe as "very good." He described his lifestyle as follows:

"After waking up, I usually go for a 10 to 15 minute jog, and after the jog, I drink some freshly squeezed orange juice, which is my breakfast. Then, I eat several bananas during the day, up to 15 or 20 a day. I'm also very fond of cucumber, which I snack on often. For dinner, I have a salad with more fruit. I try to limit my fat intake to a few avocados a week — max. I avoid strong spices, like garlic and onion, and never eat salt. But I also include some dulse, a type of seaweed. I believe eating some dulse helps me get some extra minerals in my diet."

Dave Klein lived in a house that he rented in Sebastopol, which looked to me like a rustic Canadian house. Northern California didn't look at all like Southern California. It was cooler at night, cooler during the day, and rained more, which made the vegetation much greener and lusher. It reminded me more of Canadian summers in the backcountry, minus the mosquitoes!

Dave had a few fruit trees on his property, which I thought was very cool, and he kept his thumbs green by gardening a little. He was also a bit older than the raw foodists I had met in San Diego.

I showed up as this young, fresh-faced raw foodist from Montreal, full of ideas about the raw diet and eager to meet more people who shared this lifestyle.

After Dave Klein picked me up from the bus stop, we stopped at an organic food store. In Montreal, I had only known of a few of those places, which were very small, and generally the produce selection was limited. In California, organic stores abounded, and they had a lot more organic produce, which was also more expensive than what I was used to at home.

The prices for food in California totally confused me. In Quebec, I was used to never paying more than 99 cents for an avocado, and sometimes getting them two or three for a dollar. In California, they generally sold for $1.99 each. I thought, "But they grow here! How come they are more expensive?" Then I realized that everything was more expensive in California—just because it was California.

We talked a lot about raw foods, how he got into it, what he believed in, etc. Later that day, I met John Kohler, a friend of his who came over for a visit. John was a programmer who had put together probably the first complete website on the raw food diet—**www.living-foods.com** (which is still around today)!

It was the very first website I had discovered in my initial searches, along with *Nature's First Law*, so I was quite impressed to meet the man behind it.

When I came to Dave Klein's place, I brought with me a case of big Fuerte avocados I had picked in the San Diego area. They had had time to ripen on the way and were now perfect.

When John showed up, I offered to share some avocados with everybody. I devoured an entire avocado, while John was savoring his slowly.

"Dude, you have to take your time eating it. *Savor it!*" he told me.

I offered Dave Klein some avocado, but he declined. "I wish I could eat one or two of those a day like you guys, but I can't. If I eat more than one or two a *week*, my energy diminishes."

John struck me as a very balanced person and not the average hippie raw foodist. He took care of his hair, wore trendy clothes, and was smart enough with computers to have built the most popular raw food websites on the net. He also had enough self-control to not eat an entire avocado in just a few bites...but I didn't.

At that point, I was eating one or two big Fuerte avocados a day, which was the equivalent of probably three to four regular Hass avocados.

I tried some dulse that Dave Klein had. Most Natural Hygienists I had been reading were against seaweed, which they qualified as "unnatural" for human consumption. Even some raw foodists I knew had laughed at Dave Klein's dulse-eating habits. After all, who would go get some "fresh," slimy seaweed at the beach and eat it?

But Dave Klein believed that after a few years eating mostly fruits, the enamel on his teeth started to erode. He said that by eating some dulse every day for the minerals, he was able to remineralize his teeth and probably his entire body. It was a compromise, and not necessarily a bad one. "After all," he told me, "even T.C. Fry ate some dulse."

T.C. Fry was another raw foodist I had heard about, who had recently died under mysterious circumstances at the age of 69. He was the force behind the book *Fit for Life*, which had sold millions of copies, and was probably the most well-known Natural Hygienist after Shelton. He had gotten into raw foods and Natural Hygiene in his early forties, after suffering from every proverbial SAD disease in the book. After earning his fortune with a mail-order Baroque music company, he became a powerful workhorse and published countless books, courses and magazines.

T.C. Fry recommended an all-fruit diet, which included oranges, bananas, and every sweet fruit we know of. He also ate non-sweet fruits like tomatoes and peppers and a limited amount of avocados. He claimed that greens were absolutely not necessary for the human body and that humans were biologically designed to eat fruit.

Dave Klein seemed to be a big fan of the man, and at his place, I got to read more of his philosophy.

T.C. Fry was certainly a compelling writer. In every article, the evidence and arguments he presented were so clear and powerful that you had no choice but to say, "If that's true, that makes a lot of sense." He was apparently a great chess player too. "The guy had a brain," Dave said. "I don't know anybody who's smart like he was."

Something inside of me said that maybe the next step in my evolution as a raw foodist was to become a fruitarian. But right now the avocado-dulse-lettuce combo tasted a little too good to give up.

The Death of T.C. Fry

T.C. Fry arguably turned more people on to the raw food diet than anyone else in history. He was the inspiration behind the book *Fit for Life* by Harvey and Marilyn Diamond, a bestseller that promoted Natural Hygiene and raw foods. Many of today's leaders in the raw food movement were inspired by this book.

T.C. Fry had one of the most interesting stories of "before and after" of any writer in this field. He came to Natural Hygiene at the age of 45, being overweight and with a heart condition. He was a very successful businessman with a large mail-order Baroque music company. By applying the principles of Natural Hygiene, T.C. Fry was able to regain his health. In the process, he became so motivated to spread the word about health that he became the most prominent voice in the raw and Natural Hygiene movement.

Then in 1996, the year I first learned about raw, T.C. Fry died. He was just 69. I remember discovering T.C. Fry's writing in a book by Mosséri, and then learning the next week that he had just died. Like many raw foodists, I was left confused by his untimely death.

When T.C. Fry died, he was overweight, had gastric problems, heart and lung condition, and bad teeth.[21]

Since he died, many articles have been written to attempt to explain his death. Ex-vegans claim that he died from lack of B12, while others say that he simply lacked protein in his fruitarian diet. According to Dr. Fuhrman, who saw his blood work, his B12 levels were severely deficient and the lowest he had ever seen.[22]

---

21 *The Life and Times of T.C. Fry*, Health and Beyond, Vol 4. No. 7, **http://chetday.com/v4n7.pdf**

22 DHA Deficiency Linked to Parkinson's, **http://curezone.org/forums/fm.asp?i=1388220**

The strict raw foodists attribute Fry's death to the fact that the man himself was not following the raw food diet strictly enough, and he sometimes ate coleslaw drenched in mayonnaise, or had been seen on a few occasions eating macaroni and cheese.[23]

Others mention that he was a workaholic who only slept a few hours a day, and that's probably what killed him. There were also many questions about some of the treatments he received before his death that went against his philosophy, including a series of ozone therapy treatments that he received in the Caribbean, as a last desperate attempt to restore his health.

Finally, some people were actually impressed that he had lived that long, because at the age of 45 his health was failing dramatically and his doctors had told him that he didn't have much time left to live. Maybe his change to Natural Hygiene gave him an extra 25 years of life, which was still remarkable.[24]

Most likely, all of the above is true to some degree. His death does not necessarily prove anything, other than that our heroes are sometimes more vulnerable than we think. T.C. Fry did some things wrong, but he also did some things right. His idealism and extremism probably led him to make some wrong choices, and combined with an obsessive nature and pre-existing health issues, everything together led to his untimely death.

Dave Klein told me some crazy stories about other raw foodists who had stayed at his house. He told me of a man that everybody called Dr. Bernarr who was a militant natural hygienist who promoted fasting. But in practice, Dr. Bernarr had started eating large amounts of raw meat and fish.

When he had stayed at Dave's house, Dr. Bernarr would wake up in the middle of the night and lift weights. Dave also witnessed his raw meat-eating habits, which were quite disturbing to me. Yet in his writings, Dr. Bernarr pretended he was a raw vegan.

---

23 *The Life and Times of T.C. Fry*, Health and Beyond, Vol 4. No. 7, **http://chetday.com/ v4n7.pdf**

24 Why Did TC Fry Die So Young? **http://debbietookrawforlife.blogspot. com/2009/06/why-did-t-c-fry-die-so-young.html**

For some reason, the image of a middle-aged man waking up in the middle of the night to lift weights compulsively, while bingeing on raw meat, didn't sit well with me. Who were all these crazy raw foodists?

I only stayed with Dave Klein for a few days. Someone once said that "Guests are like fish. After three days, they start to stink."

Dave Klein was a single guy used to his privacy and space. So after three days, he told me politely that his place was too small for an extended stay by guests, and I should probably move on. Luckily, he knew another cool guy in Santa Cruz, just south of San Francisco, that I could probably stay with. David Klein was just going there, so he could drop me off to meet this guy named Bodhi.

Santa Cruz was a lot closer to Los Gatos, where Claudia lived. I was excited by the possibility of meeting her again, so I enthusiastically embraced the idea.

We headed to Santa Cruz, across the iconic Golden Gate Bridge I had seen in so many movies, but never in person, and then showed up at Bodhi's place.

Bodhi was a tall, long-haired guy about my age, who was also a raw foodist. He had a little apartment built on the same small property where his parents had their house and lived. The apartment had a little kitchen, a second floor with just enough room for a bed where Bodhi slept, and was accessible by stairs. It had access to the family backyard, where there was a hot tub. The place was filled with Bob Dylan albums and memorabilia. He had a guitar as well, which I thought was cool.

His legal name was actually "Om Bodhi". His parents were the hippie type when he was born, hence the name.

Just the fact that I was a raw foodist again gave me a free pass to stay with Bodhi, who had an extra couch I could crash on. Bodhi seemed to be cool with the idea, although I did not know exactly how long I could stay there, and if he would throw me out after three days like Dave

Klein. It would probably soon be time to get my own place anyway, I thought.

I hit it off pretty quickly with Bodhi. He was definitely a unique guy with a charming personality, but quite on the eccentric side. He played some guitar, and for the first time in months, I played some too.

We talked about everything except raw foods. I found out quickly that Bodhi was much more interested in talking about his biggest passion: Bob Dylan. He was the biggest Bob Dylan fan I had ever met, and he owned every album. I'm quite certain that by the time I showed up to his place, Bodhi already had the evil secret plan of converting me into a Bob Dylan fan as well. He started slowly by introducing me to his favorite Bob Dylan songs.

Right from the get-go, I knew that Bodhi wasn't the kind of raw foodist I had pictured him and others to be. I found out that every morning, he would go to his hot tub, bring a plate of oranges, and sit there eating them while smoking pot.

At first, he tried to hide his pot-smoking habit from me, but eventually it was too obvious to go unnoticed. He asked me if I smoked too, and I emphatically said "no." He didn't push it on me, but probably felt more comfortable continuing when he saw that I wouldn't chastise him.

I found it very strange that Bodhi thought he could smoke pot and be a raw foodist at the same time. It had been very obvious to me right from the start that the two things were not compatible, so much so that it never even occurred to me that some raw foodists would even think about smoking anything.

Bodhi ate a lot of food he got for free. He worked part-time for a company called Rejuvenative Foods, which made raw sauerkraut and other fermented vegetable dishes, such as Kim Chi. By working there, he got jars and jars of the stuff for free.

Bodhi would eat an entire jar or two of raw sauerkraut a day, which retailed in health food stores for about ten dollars each. His favorite was the red cabbage/beet/garlic combo.

I was skeptical, but when I tried it I became instantly addicted to it. I found out that it tasted exceptionally good with avocados too.

Speaking of avocados, Bodhi would often go on avocado "hunts" on the grounds of UCSC (University of California, Santa Cruz), where there were plenty of avocado trees. He knew the location of most avocado trees in the city, and he would often go at night to "forage" them. Bodhi would literally bring back bags of avocados to his place, so there was an unlimited supply of them in the kitchen.

Besides avocado and Rejuvenative Foods' sauerkraut, Bodhi ate a lot of citrus fruit, some greens, and very few other foods. I continued eating avocado every day and combining it with dulse or sauerkraut whenever possible. I also ate all the fruit I could get my hands on.

Bodhi's girlfriend, Jenny, was a vegan but not a raw foodist. She was a shy girl and quite the opposite of Bodhi in personality. One thing that she told me that stuck in my head was this, "Now that you're a raw foodist, you should watch out for your teeth, Fred. Bodhi's teeth got bad since he started out on raw foods, eating all that citrus fruit every morning."

I pondered that for a moment, and noticed that indeed, Bodhi's teeth didn't look that great. I couldn't imagine exactly why going raw would not be good for your teeth. After all, fruit has natural fiber that washes your teeth as you eat them. A dentist had told me once that when you eat an apple, you crush it with your teeth and that action cleans your teeth, so the sugar doesn't stick on them. I thought that as long as I ate whole foods, I was going to be fine.

Instinctive Eating

After a few days, I also learned something about Bodhi that I didn't know at first. Bodhi was not a vegan. He started out as a vegan, but then had started reading about "Instinctive Eating" and had begun to eat some raw animal products, such as fish and raw egg yolk.

I was quite aware of the Instinctive Eating movement, which was started in France by author and cello player Guy-Claude Burger. I had read his big book in French, called *Manger Vrai* (Eating Real), which was a detailed exposé of his theory.

The book by Burger (pronounced Bur-jay and not like "hamburger"), was one of the most fascinating and convincing books I had ever come across on the topic of raw foods. It was written as an interview with the author, answering questions and explaining the concept of instinctive eating.

In French they called it "instinctothérapie" — instincto therapy, or "instincto" for short. The idea was this: humans never evolved to eat cooked foods. The source of most human diseases was to be found in the kitchen, since cooking altered the molecular structure of food and foreign proteins were getting in the bloodstream.

More importantly, cooking foods messed with our natural instinct, which could tell us exactly what to eat, when to eat it, and how much to eat. According to Burger, all cooked food was toxic, but the worst were dairy and wheat products.

Confusion in nutrition came from the fact that our natural instincts could not work anymore when foods were cooked, seasoned, or even mixed together. In order for instinct to work, we had to eat foods in their natural state, without processing them, cooking them, or even mixing them with one another.

And this instinct was miraculous. According to Burger, people recovered from every disease in the book, simply because they let their bodies decide what to eat.

At his center in France, inside an actual castle they rented out, guests could see and smell an incredible variety of raw foods from all over the world. From the smell, they would then decide what to eat. Then once they picked what to eat, they would continue eating it until their instinct told them to stop. The "stop" was a complete change in taste where what was once pleasant and tasty could become suddenly repulsive or otherwise unpleasant.

For example, if your body gave you the green light to eat pineapple, you might eat an entire pineapple before your mouth and tongue started to feel the acidity. If your body did not require pineapple that day, it would taste acidic immediately.

When you ate the foods your body needed, they tasted amazing. That was the sign that you should be eating it. Then you only stopped when you had enough and the taste changed. Your body was telling you exactly what to do.

At first, Burger was a vegetarian, but then he realized that meat could also be part of the human diet, so he introduced it. He also claimed that some of the biggest miracle recoveries he had witnessed were from people eating large quantities of raw meat.

However, the meat had to be 100% pure. Not only did it have to be organic, but also the animals were not allowed to have eaten cooked foods at all. It had to be 100% perfect.

On a typical instincto table, you might find an incredible selection of tropical fruits (instinctos were very fond of durian), vegetables, nuts, seeds, but also eggs, shellfish, fish, raw meat, and even raw chicken.

Burger had noticed that once he introduced meat into the diet, he had better musculature and his followers didn't look so flimsy either. He emphasized that you wouldn't necessarily eat it every day or in large quantities all the time. You'd only eat it when your instinct told you to do so.

In instincto, you could only eat foods one at a time. Even taking one bite of tomato before taking a bite of lettuce was not allowed. You ate one food until you were done, and then could move on to the next.

Instinctos generally didn't eat breakfast, so they only had two meals a day, at noon and in the evening.

At noon, they ate fruit, and maybe honey for "dessert." In the evening, they ate vegetables, and some protein or fatty foods (avocados, sprouted seeds, nuts, etc.) or meat or fish, or egg yolk.

They had bad results if they mixed protein and fruit together, hence the two separate meals.

At the instincto center in France, guests had access to the most insane variety of foods from all corners of the world. At home, they had to settle for whatever they could get. That's why some instinctos created a company called Orkos, which mail-delivers hard-to-find and exotic items in Europe. The prices were expensive, but most instinctos felt that quality food was the number one priority in their lives.

The Flaws of Instinctotherapy

Although Instinctive Eating sounded great in theory, it often failed in practice. The theories that Burger had about instinct and evolution were flawed. Nowhere in the history of the world did anyone have access to such an incredible variety of high quality food that could be selected according to taste and smell.

Never in history did humans eat two separate meals a day, one of fruit, and one of vegetables and protein, while smelling everything and selecting by their instinct. Humans are opportunists. We ate what we could find, and we have the amazing capability to adapt to almost any diet, and often thrive on it in the short term (often at the expense of our long-term health).

Instinct certainly plays a part in all this, especially when it comes to the body's amazing ability to gauge and evaluate the number of calories consumed, and tell us when and how much to eat next. This instinct, as Burger correctly stated, works best when we eat whole foods, but it is not necessary to go to the extent that Burger and his followers went in trying to separate everything and eat only one food at a time until the taste changes.

Many of these taste changes are related to certain irritating aspects of the plant. For example, figs have a skin that can literally inflict micro cuts and numb your tongue if you eat too many of them. It's not your body magically telling you you've had enough — you are actually hurting yourself (although your body can obviously heal it later) by rubbing all those fig skins on your tongue! You can try eating until that "stop", or simply do like the monkeys and peel your figs, or only eat the inside of them.

The fatal flaw of instinctive eating is that they designed a diet that is nutritionally imbalanced. In a typical instincto lunch, one may eat anywhere from 500 to 1200 calories' worth of fruit on average. That means that if someone needs 2000 or 2500 calories in their day, that is a pretty tough gap to fill with just vegetables and fat for dinner. Over time, the calorie deficit is so massive that instinctos come to think that they crave meat (as it is a denser and richer food), and won't feel satisfied without it. Many instinctos I met ate such large amounts of meat that they felt they could not be satisfied without eating it every day. Again, the Achilles' heel of all nutritional mistakes is the same: designing a deficient plan that just doesn't work in practice, with a lot of fluff talk around it to explain in improper scientific terms why things are the way they are.

When instinctos feel terrible because of that massive meal they had last night, they blame it on detox. They don't eat breakfast because their dinner is so heavy, it takes a long time to digest.

The instinctive diet can also be very dangerous for health. Burger's wife died of cancer, which Guy-Claude himself attributed to eating too much meat. Burger had a cyst that he also attributed to too much meat. As a group, I also noticed that instinctos had the worst teeth of the entire raw food movement, which I attribute to a very acidifying diet (all the animal products), an improper consumption of vegetables (not enough greens), and a large consumption of honey, which fed the decay in their mouth.

Bodhi was reading a book by an American guy who called himself Zephyr and promoted instinctive eating. The book was just called Instinctive Eating. It was an entertaining story of Zephyr's path to raw foods, but also of how he vanquished his cooked food cravings by eating meat, how he became a man (so to speak) by killing a chicken and eating it raw, and how he did not believe in monogamy, but instead polyamory (sleeping with as many men and women as possible).

Bodhi was himself a polyamorist, which was only tolerated by his girlfriend because she accepted his eccentric nature. However, she obviously wished things were different, and she had more stability in the relationship. Bodhi was happy about the polyamory lifestyle, which allowed him to sleep around without too many reprimands from his long-term girlfriend, but it resulted in a lot of tears for Jenny nonetheless.

I noticed that every instincto that I heard of was a polyamorist. I had nothing against polyamory as a choice. In fact, all the evidence is there to show that evolutionarily, the preferred choice for men is to not be polyamorist, but polygamist, a term that is frowned upon by polyamorists, who feel their lifestyle has more glamour. In all of history, the trend has always been that some men control a lot of women, while most men have none. For women, the preferred choice has always been monogamy. Over time, cultures have evolved in their own ways and monogamy became the preferred choice in most societies because of the social stability it provides.

So polyamory as a choice doesn't surprise me, but for some reason, I found that most instinctos who go deep in this lifestyle don't just stop there. Many end up bisexual (even when they didn't start out that way), and Burger himself was condemned in 1997 to 15 years in prison for "rape of an underage 15 year old person." In the French press, Burger was depicted as a "pedophile guru." This final condemnation was just the last in a series of crimes. In 1978, he was sentenced to four years in prison in Switzerland for sexually abusing his son and a 9-year old girl.[25]

What most people don't know is that Burger wrote a book on sexuality after his first one on instinctive eating, in which he proposes his theory called Meta-Psychoanalysis. It says that having sex with children (even your own) is a natural and normal thing for humans to do. Burger even fantasized that this kind of "new sexuality," not bound by society's norms (such as adult-children sexual relationships) would be able to solve many of our problems, such as crime, and even develop extra-sensory abilities such as clairvoyance and telepathy.[26] Most of the English-speaking raw foodists don't know about this because it has only been publicized in the French and German press, both of which, luckily for myself, I can read fluently.

In any case, the question is out there: are instinctos more inclined to experiment with unconventional sexual choices, and if so, why?

As the days went by, Bodhi revealed his modified instincto diet more and more. He wasn't a true instincto, but ate animal products.

One day, I witnessed him eating an entire jar of raw honey. He also loved raw egg yolks, and enjoyed eating raw fish.

---

25 In French: **http://fr.wikipedia.org/wiki/Guy-Claude_Burger**
26 In French: **http://sites.google.com/site/metapsychanalyse/home/ qu-est-ce-que-la-metapsychanalyse**

One night, Bodhi's parents invited a couple of traveling girls and Bodhi and myself for dinner. It was an interesting dinner, since Bodhi's parents were vegan, but not raw. The two girls said they had been vegan before, but they felt something was missing so went back to meat. I was raw and vegan. And Bodhi was raw but not vegan at all.

In order to please everybody, Bodhi's parents cooked some rice and beans. The parents and traveling girls were happy to eat just that. For me, they made a special salad, filled with vegetables, cherry tomatoes and avocados. Bodhi decided he was going to feast on raw egg yolks exclusively, so he sat down with us and ate a meal consisting of 5 or 6 raw egg yolks in a bowl with a spoon, and nothing else.

The girls were obviously grossed out by this ridiculous meal, but Bodhi had this huge smile and thought he was the coolest guy in the world. He obviously did not care how weird his diet looked to others, and I honestly think that he was more interested in shocking people than being a true instincto.

Bodhi's parents were probably the most relaxed, permissive people one could ever imagine. Their philosophy seemed to be to let their son live his life, make his own choices, and come to his own conclusions.

However, they seemed to be a little worried about the quantity of egg yolks that Bodhi was ingesting. "We're worried about the cholesterol and how it might affect his health, but he's young and needs to decide for himself," his mom once told me.

After a couple of weeks in Santa Cruz, I started to feel that my health had taken a turn for the worse—especially my energy levels. I would have the hardest time waking up in the morning, and I would often spend the rest of the day in a daze of brain fog, with low energy. I was craving more and more food, and I ate a record number of avocados to satisfy my cravings.

Everything I was eating was 100% raw. I wasn't even eating the nuts and seeds that Mosséri had condemned, but something was starting to go wrong. I didn't know what to do.

I wrote an email to David Wolfe and asked him what he thought of all this. He replied, "You're going through detox, listen to more heavy metal music!"

I was puzzled by this unhelpful answer, but figured that maybe David was right. I was probably detoxing all the bad cooked foods I had eaten in my life.

The Truth About Detox

For years, people in the raw food movement have been brainwashed into thinking that whatever negative symptoms they were experiencing after going raw were due to "detox" from growing up on cooked food.

They come to believe that they have poisoned themselves since childhood, and it would take years for these "poisons" to exit their bodies on a raw food diet.

Although there is a bit of truth to this, in reality, a lot of what they call "detox" was simply caused by their poorly balanced raw food diet.

For example, if you eat the typical diet promoted almost everywhere in the raw food movement, which consists mostly of fatty foods for calories (avocados, oils, nuts, seeds), salt and spices for flavoring and an insufficient amount of fresh fruits and vegetables, you are inevitably going to experience negative consequences

The most common ones are:

Candida

Lack of energy, drowsiness

Inability to maintain weight

Blood sugar instabilities

Deficiencies

So the "detox" that these people are experiencing actually consists of negative consequences from their current diet.

There Are No Magic Potions or Foods to Take to Detoxify Faster

No special herb, colonic, enema, or any "magic potion" will help you detoxify faster. Your body does the healing, and there are no external agents that can make this healing happen any faster.

The only way I know to accelerate the process is *fasting*. During a fast, the energy that the body would normally spend on digestion and daily activities can now be spent on healing.

Take your time and let your body do its own thing in its own rhythm. If your body's agenda doesn't match yours, keep in mind that you probably know less than it does!

My First Bite of Raw Flesh

As I was reading about instinctive eating and hearing Bodhi talk about it, I started to think that maybe there was something to this instinctive eating theory. The thought started to grow in my head. What if I would actually like raw meat? What if it was the missing key that would transform my health? Maybe the vegan concept was flawed from the start.

The instinctos described eating raw meat and fish with such gusto that it sounded like it might be the most satisfying, delicious food in the world. Many said that after they started eating it, all of their cravings for cooked foods completely vanished.

In my mind, I started to think that maybe eating some fish could solve my current health problems and increase my energy. Even though I felt uneasy about breaking my vegan vows, I wanted to at least try and see if there was any truth behind the claims about instinctive eating.

I told Bodhi that I wanted to try some raw fish. His parents were almost 100% vegan, but sometimes they went out to a Japanese restaurant and ate some fish, so we decided to all go there for dinner.

Bodhi ordered a plate of sashimi, and when I saw the slices of raw tuna in front of me, I hesitated a little bit. Bodhi's step-dad started digging in, dipping generously in soy sauce. "Are you going to have soy sauce?" he asked.

"No," I answered, "It's cooked!"

"What? That's the best part!" he said.

I took a piece of raw fish, and carefully tried to chew a part of it. It tasted awful, and surprisingly not exciting and satisfying like instinctos had said it would. It fact, the taste of raw fish was so revolting to me that after swallowing the first little bit I couldn't eat it anymore. I felt I would probably vomit if I continued.

That's how my raw fish experience went! I was a bit disappointed and felt deceived by the instinctos. How could they think that raw fish tasted good? Maybe their bodies needed it, but not mine.

After a few weeks at Bodhi's place, I had definitely reached the limit of what could be considered an acceptable stay. I decided to go back to San Diego to find a place of my own.

Right before I left, Claudia came from Los Gatos to visit me. We only spent a few hours together, before my bus left to go back to San Diego. Again, this short time together made me feel drunk with love. I knew I had something important to do in San Diego, but I hoped I would see her again soon, if I could.

CHAPTER 8

You Eat Chicken. You Eat Bread. Everything You Eat Is Dead!

"Is the truth so hard to swallow? It shouldn't be. Just take a handful of watermelon and shove it into your face!"

The Raw Courage Vegetable Man

When I got back to San Diego, I was determined to find a place to stay. I knew I could not afford an apartment, so I had to find something more "alternative."

I got back in touch with a guy named Kendon that I had met through David and RC when I first got to San Diego. Kendon's raw name was "Durian," and he was a friend of Nature's First Law. He was called Durian because of his love of the fruit of the same name.

According to David, Durian was a gay guy that went raw, and then "left the dark side" and decided to go for women.

David and Stephen were convinced that homosexuality could be "cured" by the raw food diet. More specifically, they thought that the "hormones" in wheat and bread were causing men to become gay.

However, when I talked to Durian himself, he told me that even though he had tried to date a girl, it had been more out of curiosity. He still preferred men. So much for the theory of "bread makes you gay," as Durian was still a militant raw foodist.

I did not care whether Durian was gay or not. He was a really cool guy and the only person I knew that was willing to help me find a place in San Diego.

Durian knew a man named Morten who had a big garden down in a canyon, in a rough part of town called City Heights. It was truly the weirdest place I had ever seen in a city.

The small house sat on the street and the property extended down a steep hill, where one could walk down many man-made steps and go through several "levels" of this garden, descending towards the edge of the canyon.

Throughout this unleveled garden, Morten had planted many fruit trees, like avocado, orange and olive. He had little waterfalls running, activated by an electric motor. There were bells chiming here and there, struck by the wind. You'd find a random couch on one of these levels, with a bookshelf next to it. At the very bottom of the garden, Morten had built a platform for Durian, literally extending the limits of his property into the air. Durian had planted a tent on this very sturdy platform, and slept there. He paid some money to Morten for the "rent," while being able to use the facilities of the house to prepare food and to shower.

It looked like a very peaceful place, and when I talked to Morten I found out that he was also Canadian, originally from British Columbia, but now a naturalized American. He had come to California years earlier, to work with a spiritual community called "Yogananda," which I knew nothing about.

He had bought the place in City Heights a few years earlier and had worked hard to make it a haven of peace in a bad part of town.

I told him I was looking for a place to live, and he was quite flexible with the most unusual arrangements. He had a guy who parked his tiny RV in the parking lot and lived there, also using the house for the bathroom, kitchen and shower. He rented one room inside the house for more money, but I wasn't willing to pay that much yet.

For me, he suggested an area of the garden where I could "build a hut." Well, not a hut but more like a tent. Morten put a large wooden platform on the grass, and I bought a futon at a nearby store to sleep on. The futon covered almost the entire surface of the platform, leaving enough space to have a small bedside table and a few plastic boxes where I could store my stuff. We brought electricity in using extension cables, so I could have light. To make this more private, we stuck several long and thick pieces of bamboo on each corner of the platform, which would be our "pillars." For a roof, we put up a large piece of corrugated plastic that Morten had, which would work to protect me from the rain. For my "walls," I simply hung up some bedsheets all around, which provided absolutely no insulation, but some visual privacy.

Like everyone else living there, I could take showers in the house, use the kitchen to prepare my food, and I would even have a small section of the fridge that would be designated for me.

My "rent" cost me $25 a week, or $100 a month. Eventually, Morten raised it to $35 a week. It was like camping, but with some amenities, and the privilege of living in San Diego on the cheap.

Living in City Heights was quite an adventure in itself. The entire neighborhood was Mexican and quite poor. Whenever I would tell people I lived in this part of town, they would say, "City Heights, isn't that dangerous?" Even taxi-drivers advised their clients not to go there.

I never felt threatened even once, but the shabbiness of the area was quite noticeable. The thing that bothered me the most was the noise at night. There were local dogs that would literally bark all night, and their owners did not make any attempt to stop them. It was so annoying that I eventually started wearing earplugs, after having dreamed (while the dogs were barking) that I was kicking the culprit dog as hard as I could, sending it flying in the air! I loved animals and did not want to hurt them, so I got some earplugs instead.

It wasn't just the dogs. Frequently, helicopters would hover loudly over the neighborhood. I had no idea if it was the army or the cops chasing bad guys, but they were close and really loud!

Sometimes, you'd hear people screaming. One night, the guy living on the other side of the canyon got so loud, screaming at his wife and verbally abusing her, that Morten got out and started shouting at him too, threatening to call the cops.

Morten's house was like an oasis of peace in all of this madness. You'd hear his little waterfalls, the sounds of the bells and the tree leaves moving in the wind. I would pick fruit straight from the tree, and supplement my diet with cheap fruits and vegetables from the Mexican and Asian markets nearby.

I was living in San Diego. I had made my dream a reality, on a shoestring, and I was still there after a few months, even though all of my friends had told me I'd be running back home faster than I could say "Red Delicious Apple."

It was now time to do what I had originally come here to do, which was to get involved with the growing raw food movement of California.

Behind The Scenes at *Nature's First Law*

When I came back to San Diego after my adventures in Northern California, I called up David Wolfe and asked him if I could somehow help him with his business *Nature's First Law*. He didn't really have anything for me when I first arrived in San Diego back in November, but now it seemed like things had picked up a little bit with their business and they might need some help.

One day, David picked me up at Morten's place in his old, beat-up car to go meet his business partner Stephen Arlin and see what I could do to help.

David didn't really have to knock on the door. I was expecting him, and all I needed to hear was the loud, symphonic heavy metal music blasting from his car to know that he had arrived.

We drove to a posh neighborhood in the hills of San Diego, where they had established headquarters at Stephen's mom's place. It was the neighborhood where Stephen and David, both from affluent families, had grown up.

Stephen's mom's place was a typical, large, two-story California-style house, with a beautiful view overlooking a canyon and the city. Stephen lived there on the second floor, where he had his room as well as an extra bedroom they used to store all the books they shipped and prepare the orders that came in. On top on the stairs, there was a large hallway that had been converted into a computer room, where Stephen was to be found most of the time, typing away or updating his website. From this hallway-office, we could see the rest of the house downstairs and access the extra bedroom where the books were stored.

In the house lived two large dogs, one of which was named Fenris and looked like a beautiful, giant white wolf. Whenever I came in, Fenris would run away. After a while, I realized he would only trust the few people he knew, and any women, but never men he did not know!

David officially introduced me to Stephen, who seemed like the complete opposite of him in terms of personality. While David was exuberant, extroverted and loud, Stephen was more the quiet, introverted type. But because he was tall and physically imposing, he still radiated a certain "quiet power."

At first, Stephen wasn't too enthusiastic about bringing someone else on board. David seemed to be very motivated to start growing their *Nature's First Law* as fast as possible, while Stephen was more conservative and wanted to do as much as he could himself, while spending as little money as possible. In spite of the initial resistance, Stephen quickly adopted me as a member of the *Nature's First Law* team.

They had started their business a few years earlier when they decided to publish the book *Nature's First Law*. When I met them, their business essentially consisted of selling their book through their website, and sending their customers a thin, photocopied catalog of other products they carried.

They had a limited selection of books on the raw food diet, such as Joe Alexander's *Blatant Raw Foodist Propaganda*, as well as a few special reports such as *How to Gain Weight and Muscle on the Raw Food Diet* that they sold for $10 each. It wasn't a big operation, but you could feel that something big was about to happen. They were motivated to become the biggest names the world had ever known in the field of health and raw foods.

Often, they would make fun of the rest of the raw food movement by saying "There's no raw food movement! This *is* the raw food movement, Fred," pointing at the office where we were sitting.

On my first day, I helped them put together some orders they had received. Stephen would print out the orders from the web and collect the mail orders (that David had picked up in the morning at their P.O. Box) and deposit them in a shoebox. I would look at the order and gather the necessary books and put them in an envelope or find the appropriate package to send the order. I would wrap the order, write down the addresses, and, of course, remember to add the catalog. If it was an international order, I would fill out the appropriate declaration forms. Then I'd put all of the orders in a pile, and at the end of the day, David and I would go to the post office to mail everything. I also took care of photocopying and putting together their catalogs and special reports.

On my first day, I helped out for a few hours. David would come in the afternoon or morning only, because he was still going to university to finish his law degree.

There wasn't much to do at first, but Stephen seemed to be happy to have someone around to help out a little bit, even though he was reluctant at first to hire any help. After my first day, Stephen asked me if I could come back the next day. "Sure!" I said.

Working with David and Stephen was a unique experience. First, they were completely different than what I had imagined from reading the books. Although I expected them to live in the jungle and cultivate their own fruits, they were the urban people you would expect any Southern Californians to be.

They had a particular sense of humor and constantly cracked jokes about the raw food lifestyle. For them, it wasn't just a diet choice — it was a mission. The jokes essentially revolved around the theme that the rest of the world was "cooked" and pathetic, and that they were raw and cooler than everybody else.

Sometimes, David or Stephen would walk around and scream loudly for no reason, "You're a f*-ing cooked food moron, a f*-ing cooked food moron!" and apparently that was an inside joke I did not know, but somehow it was funny anyway.

They might also sing a song they made up, "You eat chicken, you eat bread, everything you eat is dead!" or make fun of someone they knew by calling them the worst insult they had, "totally cooked." Although all of this may sound harsh and "cult-like," it was all a joke and a way to have fun with the raw food lifestyle and not be so uptight like the older raw foodists who were our mentors.

As an example of the kind of humor that was going on in the office, David and Stephen loved to tease me by trying to make me admit that I ate cooked foods. "Fred, I heard you ate an entire roll of bread last night!" Stephen would say out of nowhere. Then David would continue, "Fred totally binged on bread!"

Eventually, we found a raw name for me. Instead of the strange "Raw Demolition" that RC had given me, they preferred *Pineapple Fred*.

Stephen liked it, so he would often scream out of nowhere, in a loud high pitched heavy metal scream: "Piiiiinneaaapple Freeeed!"

Essentially, every high-testosterone day at *Nature's First Law* was spent listening to heavy metal music, making fun of cooked food eaters, talking about girls, Stephen and David exchanging inside jokes that I could never fully understand, and going crazy about what's cooked and what's raw.

At first, I could barely understand what they were saying because of all the slang they were using. My English came from books and not from actual conversations, so I did not know that "rad" meant "radical" and was another way to say "cool," among hundreds of other slang terms. I was surprised at how fast I picked it up, and eventually started using those words myself.

The raw food diet became my life. I would go to *Nature's First Law* every day, and stay there for a few hours. We would talk all day about the raw food world and other raw-related stuff. Then I would come home, sit in my "garden," and enjoy the San Diego sun. During this time period, I also regularly went "urban foraging."

Durian was a master at "Urban Foraging." It seemed like he knew every single fruit tree planted in all of San Diego, and would bring back huge quantities of fruit from his "harvesting" trips.

The fruit trees he foraged belonged to private owners who had them on their properties. In some areas of San Diego, many people had fruit trees, but they didn't necessarily pick or eat their own fruits. That's where Durian came to the rescue. He would go in an alley and help himself to fruits that were hanging over the property line and "liberate" them. When the fruit trees were inaccessible, he would knock on the owner's door and simply ask them if they would mind letting him pick some of their fruit. Nine times out of ten, people would say "Sure! No problem. You're going to help us anyway... otherwise, these fruits are all going to rot and ruin the lawn!"

One fruit Durian particularly liked was the white sapote. It's an apple-sized green fruit that gets a yellow tint when ripe and becomes extremely soft. Inside, the flesh is white and comparable in taste to vanilla pudding. Whenever the fruit is picked hard and green, it will ripen but the flavor will be lost. When it ripens on the tree, it becomes too soft to ship. The fruits become so soft that they bruise at the slightest touch, and when they drop from the tree they can make a terrible mess. People who had white sapote trees saw it more as a curse than a blessing, since they didn't care for the fruit themselves.

We picked so many white sapotes, we didn't know what to do with them. For a while, along with other "foraged" fruits, I ate a diet composed mostly of sapotes! Durian also worked at a health food store called "People's Market," where he would get an employee discount, so I would take advantage of that and get a few items from the store as well. I then complemented these two sources of food with cheap fruit from the Mexican produce markets in the neighborhood, and that's how I managed to be a raw foodist in San Diego on a budget.

In spite of my large intake of fruits, the fat content in my diet kept creeping up. In addition to eating my beloved avocados (at least one or two a day, if not three or four), I started eating nuts and seeds.

When I first went raw, I rarely ate nuts and seeds because Mosséri had written so passionately against them. In his experience, eating nuts and seeds on a regular basis caused a wide range of health problems – everything from skin disorders to cancer. He never blamed the fat content per se, but instead referred to nuts as "acid-forming" and "not human food." I was actually so scared of eating nuts that I didn't consume any for the entire first year I was raw! I didn't realize that Mosséri, in his later books, came to realize that quantity was more the problem, and admitted that eating a maximum of one ounce of nuts a day with no other fat was okay.

When I first talked to David Wolfe on the phone, he also told me that he never ate nuts. When David went fruitarian for three months, he didn't have any nuts or fat, besides avocados. When I finally met David in person, and started spending time with him, I noticed he was often eating some Macadamia nuts he got from the store Trader Joe's. I asked him why he changed his mind, and he told me, "When I first went raw, for the first few years, I didn't eat any nuts at all. I didn't even think they were raw! I never had raw recipes either because I didn't think those were raw... so I just stuck with fruits and vegetables."

Stephen Arlin did the same at first, but because he was a bodybuilder, he felt he needed something more than fruits and vegetables. He then discovered that many nuts could be purchased raw, so he started eating them. That influenced David to do the same, so when I met them, both of them were eating nuts and seeds on a regular basis.

I asked David if he felt any different eating nuts. "My sex drive is up," he replied, and laughed. David told me that in his first few years on the raw food diet, eating only fruits and vegetables and no nuts, he felt much less sexual desire. Since introducing the nuts, his "mojo" was apparently back.

I had also felt that on this raw food diet, I was not bothered with as many sexual thoughts, even at my age. I even started to think that maybe sexuality was something different than we had been led to believe. Some authors said that the constant desire to "reproduce" was unnatural, and was only brought about by sick bodies, which could sense that they were "dying," and, therefore, were boosting up the sex drive so that they could reproduce and pass their genes along before it was too late!

Stephen also believed that nuts and seeds contained some important minerals and proteins that would be difficult to get from just fruits and vegetables. The author of *Raw Eating*, Hovanessian, was also a big fan of nuts.

I had never tried macadamia nuts before, so I started eating some once I discovered how delicious they were. There was even a macadamia nut tree in Morten's backyard, but those were not ready to be harvested yet.

Over the next few months, my diet started to change again, through the influence of the raw food movement in California. When I first started, I didn't even know a single raw food recipe. I didn't blend anything, I didn't dehydrate anything, and I didn't eat nuts or seeds, or oil, or garlic, or onion, or salt. I was a purist.

One day, Don the Raw Guy took me to a raw food restaurant just north of San Diego. I was really excited because I had never even known that raw food restaurants existed! I wasn't sure what to order, so I just got the same thing Don got, which was a carrot soup followed by a "Nori Roll."

The carrot soup was delicious. It tasted sweet, savory and creamy, and had finely grated pieces of vegetables in it, so it was also chewy. It was served with two flax crackers, which you could eat like regular saltine crackers.

The Nori Roll looked like sushi, but was made with a nut pâté, grated vegetables and raw, marinated ginger. Again, it tasted amazing, and even though I had not had any food like this in over a year, I realized what I had been missing the moment I tasted those recipes! There was no salt in it, but for the savory taste they used something called "Braggs" which they described as a raw soy sauce.

As I was experimenting with new raw foods, David and Stephen were also slowly changing their diets and influencing the rest of us.

At first, David was a purist like I was. He only ate fruits and vegetables, never had any recipes, or salt, or even seaweed, which he considered gross. One day he even made fun of David Klein, the publisher of *Living Nutrition*, because he was eating some dulse.

However, over the months I worked with David, he did some experiments of his own and started incorporating new foods into his diet.

One day, after he picked me up to go work at *Nature's First Law*, he told me that he had made an "incredible discovery" about olives. He had finally figured out how to eat olives *raw*. He was so excited about it, as if he had just invented cold fusion or the perpetual motion machine.

"For years, I just couldn't figure out how to eat olives raw! I thought you had to marinate them in brine, and process them. I have so many olive trees where I live, and I tried and tried to eat them raw, but they just tasted awful. But the other day I decided to try those dried, shriveled up olives that stayed on the tree, and fell on the ground. And dude, those are amazing!"

He had a little bag of those olives that looked like large raisins. So he handed me a few, and even though they were quite bitter, they were indeed edible.

David didn't stop there. He got really excited about olives and started researching them, and then got to the point where he believed that olives were one of the most nutritious foods *on the planet*. He was eating them constantly with avocado and dulse (yes, he also started eating seaweed).

At some point, he was even telling people that if he had to live on *one food only, it would be olives*.

This experiment with olives led him to try olive oil. Again, for his first few years of raw foods, David didn't think oils could be raw. Then he discovered a family-owned company in California called Bariani that made truly raw olive oil, using an old system of crushing olives instead of using heat for extraction.

One day, David and I went to the gym to work out, and I was surprised to see him pull out a giant bottle of Bariani olive oil from the back seat, open it, and drink a generous amount straight from the bottle before heading to the gym. My jaw dropped when I saw him do that, but he told me that he had been experimenting with olive oil as a fuel source and that it was *amazing*.

David liked to use a lot of superlatives.

Although I never drank pure olive oil straight from the bottle, I also started using some of the Bariani olive oil on my salads. And yes, it did taste amazing! But I didn't realize that I had just instantly doubled the fat content of my meals.

Then *Nature's First Law* started to carry some food products. When I first met them, they were just doing the books and special reports. Now they started selling the Bariani olive oil, and eventually, they added a wide range of raw food items to their catalog. This kept me busy, since those items took a lot more time to package and ship.

My Diet Came Full Circle

Most people who discover the raw food diet go through some kind of evolutionary steps. They may first discover vegetarianism, then veganism, then regular gourmet, high-fat raw food, and then maybe find their way to the low-fat approach.

I went through a full circle, by discovering Natural Hygiene first and then going to 100% (high-fat) raw. That may seem curious to some, but my progression seems completely normal to me when I look at what happened.

I'm 34 now, but I was only 20 when I discovered Natural Hygiene and the raw food diet. My mentors were a few dead guys who had written some books, and an old Egyptian living in France. Although I tried my best to apply the principles in my own life, I failed to find role models that I could relate to. At the time, I honestly thought I was the only raw foodist in the entire province of Quebec. I knew of a raw food family who had appeared in a popular magazine, talking about their experience, but I had learned that they had decided to move abroad.

When I discovered the Californian raw food movement, I finally found people of my own age that I could relate to. I saw the 100% raw food lifestyle as a better way than the antiquated ideas of Natural Hygiene. It was cool, fun, and trendy.

Little by little, my energy levels were dropping, but I was still attributing it to detox. The theory was that detox was this long and complicated process that the body went through once you became a raw foodist. You had to "pay for your sins" for all the cooked foods you had eaten in your life, by eliminating old toxins. Some raw foodists believed that this "detox" could last several months--several years, even. Whenever someone wasn't feeling too well on the raw food diet, it was blamed on the detox.

Stimulants & Detox

When someone switches from a regular diet to a raw diet, the biggest "detox" will come from the elimination of stimulants – mainly caffeine. During that time, one can experience headaches, depression, low energy, sleepiness, and a general feeling of "spaciness." It usually takes a month or two for things to be back to normal and for the person to feel even better than when they started.

Besides stimulants, another "detox" comes from eliminating junk foods, fatty foods, chemicals and preservatives, animal products and other processed foods from the diet. However, this process usually leaves you energized rather than depressed. I always tell people to expect to feel a little "off" for a few weeks when they first go raw, but if the feeling lasts more than a month or two, they're usually doing something wrong. I also recommend progressively reducing caffeine rather than going "cold turkey." The best approach is to use an herbal coffee replacement such as *Teeccino*, and brew your coffee as usual but cut it with some *Teeccino* as well.

Progressively increase the ratio of *Teeccino* to regular coffee over two weeks until at the end of the two weeks you are drinking only the caffeine-free product.

CHAPTER 9

Just Eat an Apple, What's So Hard About That?

"I was actually a fruitarian at that point in time. I ate only fruit. Now I'm a garbage can like everyone else. And we were about three months late in filing a fictitious business name, so I threatened to call the company Apple Computer unless someone suggested a more interesting name by five o'clock that day, hoping to stimulate creativity. And it stuck. And that's why we're called Apple."

Steve Jobs,
CEO of Apple Inc.

I always loved the idea of a specialized magazine or newsletter. When I was in high school, I started writing horror and fantasy short stories, and decided to put them together in a sort of gory newsletter. I asked my mom to draw the cover (which was not that scary), and put together a newsletter, which I photocopied and distributed in school. However, the project was quickly stopped by the school principal, who thought that this "frivolous" project was taking precious time away from my other studies.

Ever since that time, I always felt resentful of that principal, who sought to curb and destroy my desire to be creative and produce a project on my own, outside of the context of the established guidelines. I knew that one day I would get back at her by succeeding with my own projects, and I would prove that whatever they attempted to teach me in school, I could learn better on my own.

When I arrived in California, I noticed that although the raw food movement was getting bigger every day, there was almost no magazine or publication on the topic. I asked David Wolfe if they had a magazine, and he responded by saying, "Sure, we have one! It's published by David Klein and called *Living Nutrition*."

I already knew about *Living Nutrition*, the short newsletter published by Klein. Although *Nature's First Law* was selling it, it certainly wasn't *their* magazine. I asked David, "What if you had your own magazine? I'd love to put it together for you!"

David loved the idea, but he didn't have time to be involved in the creation process.

He told me, "Look, you have the green light to do it. Just put it together, and we'll sell it!"

I was super excited at the possibility of creating *Nature's First Law*'s magazine, but I had no idea where to start.

I had no idea how to put together a newsletter. I did not own a computer. I didn't even know how to touch-type! On top of that, English wasn't my first language.

I didn't let any of that stop me, and somehow, I managed to find the answers to those problems.

I realized that to put together the newsletter, I only needed to have some articles ready. If I had access to a computer, I could then type in the articles and organize them in a basic layout. Those pages could then be printed and photocopied to produce the final copies. It wasn't going to be perfect, but it would work.

So I started writing some articles and getting some guest writers to contribute some of their own. As for the computer problem, I quickly found a temporary solution: because David still studied at UC San Diego, he would drop me off at the campus, and there I would sneak into the computer lab, take a seat at one of the computers, and start using it, saving my files on a disk. No one ever even asked me for a student ID!

I wanted the newsletter to be different. In fact, I wanted it to be downright funny, shocking and provocative.

For example, the very first issues contained titles such as:

- "Interview with a Breatharian!"

- "Urban Foraging: How to Get Free Food from the Urban Jungle"

- "How to Increase Penis Size on a Raw Food Diet"

- "Street Fighting on the Raw Food Diet!"

...and other improper and irreverent articles.

I was still stuck on the name of the publication, though. I thought of a few titles, such as *The Raw World*, *The Raw Times*, and even *Raw Demolition*. Nothing seemed good enough.

Then it came to me: there was this running joke at the *Nature's First Law* office, started by David's cousin, RC Dini. He used to say, "Just eat an apple, what's so hard about that?" That would be his only answer to everyone's question on the raw diet. People would ask him, "What should I eat for protein?" He would answer: "Just eat an apple." If the question was "What is good for Candida?" he would say, "Just eat an apple!" and so on. When he was really exasperated, he would say: "Just eat an apple, what's so hard about that?"

One day, I was in David's car, and I told him what I thought the new magazine should be called. I said, "It's going to be called *Just Eat an Apple!*"

He looked at me, laughed, and said, "Dude, that's it! That's the name!" I then thought of my first trip to California, bringing along only a big bag of apples, and everything made sense to me. That name was the best name ever, and the one that totally represented what I wanted to do with this magazine.

After a few issues of the "magazine" came out, we started getting a flood of letters from our customers. Many thought it was the best thing ever, while others were completely (and rightly) insulted by the juvenile humor in the articles.

When people would ask David if we could make the magazine a little bit less provocative and a little more mature instead, he would reply, "We did a lot of market research and discovered that this is what people want!" (Obviously he was just pulling this answer out of thin air.)

Eventually, though, after the first four or five issues, the tone of the magazine changed a bit and became more professional, and more like something you wouldn't be completely embarrassed to lend to your 75-year old grandmother.

One day, we got an order from Steve Jobs, the now newly appointed CEO of Apple Computer, and one of the richest and most successful businessmen on the planet.

We already knew that Steve Jobs had had an early interest in the raw diet. According to the story, at the time when the company Apple was founded, he was on an all-fruit diet. He threatened to call the company "Apple Computers" unless someone suggested a more interesting name by five o' clock that day. It seems the name stuck, and that's why they called it Apple.[27]

When we got the order from Steve Jobs, it simply said: "One subscription please. Thank you. Steve." This was followed by his address in Palo Alto and his credit card number.

We were absolutely blown away by that order. Obviously, it couldn't be a fake. It was the exact address where Jobs was known to live.

After that day, Stephen looked at me and said, "We can't mess around anymore with this magazine. Steve Jobs is reading it."

I don't think that Steve Jobs was too impressed by *Just Eat an Apple,* especially in those early stages. But his invisible presence forced me to write better and more mature content. It was almost like I felt this presence peeking over my shoulder as I put the magazine together. "What would Steve Jobs think?" was a question I asked myself often, as I imagined him opening his mail and discovering my publication.

In spite of that, I could not completely contain my impulse to write some crazy, completely out-of-hand raw food propaganda. Writing *Just Eat an Apple* was like having all of my creative impulses on overdrive: I could be funny. I could be provocative, and I could also promote meaningful discussions and connections within the raw food movement.

---

27 Don't believe this story? Watch some of the documentaries made on the history of Apple Computers. In one video I've seen, one of the early investors in Apple tells his version of the story and describes how he was shocked to learn that Steve was living on fruit only!

Quite often, though, the "crazy" part took over.

For example, every month we featured a section called "What's Raw, What's Cooked;" the equivalent of the "What's Hot, What's Not" in popular magazines. What was "raw" was über-cool, and what was "cooked" was, well...cooked!

I published a new issue of Just Eat an Apple every other month. In total, 22 magazines were published. Those old magazines can now be found as part of a compilation available at **www.fredericpatenaude. com/enchilada.html**

CHAPTER 10

Raw Cuisine Gone Mad!

"The concept of raw food is the ability to eat junk food and not wind up in the hospital. We have found a way to make junk food out of non-toxic ingredients. It's pretty amazing."

Juliano,
Raw Food Chef

In early summer 1998, I went back to San Francisco to attend a big raw food expo with *Nature's First Law*. It was the first time I had gone to a raw food event of that size, where all the raw food speakers had been invited.

I had decided to volunteer that week at San Francisco's greatest raw food restaurant, *Raw*, in exchange for room and board.

Raw was the creation of raw food chef Juliano, a Las Vegas native who had proclaimed himself not only as the greatest raw food chef in existence, but also as having literally "invented a new cuisine." He was working on a book that had been accepted by a major publisher (also simply called "Raw"), which he hoped would propel him to new heights of wealth and celebrity.

Juliano's food was by far the most addictive, gourmet raw food I had ever tasted. It made the simple "combo-abombos" (Combo-Abombo stands for *combination-abomination)* of RC Dini look like preschooler lunches.

Juliano had figured out how to make raw foods taste even more authentic and decadent than the cooked foods they were supposed to replace. He had also made raw food equivalents of cooked recipes that no one had ever dared to try to substitute before.

The most obvious one was his infamous "Raw Cheeseburger," where he would put a patty made with various nuts and vegetables in between two pieces of "raw bread," along with an almost melted type of cashew cheese, with all the toppings and condiments you would expect in an American cheeseburger.

There were raw pizzas, raw vegan sushi, all kinds of raw nut pâtés and cheeses, pasta alfredo, and the most decadent desserts you had ever tasted.

Juliano specialized in indulgence. His philosophy was to add as much salt, as much fat, as many spices and as much garlic as the palate could tolerate, to the point where it was "almost too much," but instead, in his own words, "just perfect."

He took the philosophy of "as long as it's raw, it's okay" to an extreme, promoting alcohol and wine consumption (it's raw and vegan!), as much olive oil as you want, and liberal quantities of sea salt (as long as it's raw salt, of course).

In person, Juliano was as much of an eccentric as his cuisine would suggest. I found him extremely friendly most of the time. In his restaurant, he sometimes turned into a complete despot, screaming at his employees and often scolding his patrons if he caught them with bad posture. Juliano was obsessed with proper posture, and if he saw anyone in his restaurant slouching on their chairs, he would angrily put them in their place by shouting: "You! Yeah, you, green shirt! Your posture is bad! Lift up your chest! Straighten your back!"

It was almost unreal to see that happening, and the customers seemed so intimidated that they didn't say anything back. Maybe they didn't even realize that the person shouting at them was the owner of the restaurant.

On my first night there, Juliano smoked pot and offered me some, which I politely declined. He didn't force my hand, and admitted that I was doing the right thing by not smoking. I was a little shocked to see him smoke marijuana on the side and at the same time promote the benefits of "natural living," but at that point, I was no longer too surprised at the incongruence of some raw foodists.

His staff members told me that Juliano would often stay up all night, sleeping only a couple of hours, and partied constantly.. He would maintain that routine for a few days, and then be so exhausted that he would need to sleep an entire day to recover. Curiously enough, he did not even eat his own gourmet food, preferring to live on a diet of peaches and "pot."

Over the period of 7 to 10 days that I spent working and sleeping in the basement of Juliano's restaurant, I started feeling extremely sick. San Francisco was rainy, and I developed a cold and sore throat that did not go away, but got worse and worse with every day I spent at *Raw*.

The food served at *Raw* went beyond traditional raw recipes. Juliano would not hesitate to use half a cup of olive oil in just *one* serving of his pasta primavera, or an entire cup of cashew butter would go into one slice of one of his desserts.

Ever since I arrived in California, I had lost the feeling of purity, lightness, and health I had first experienced on the raw food diet. Instead, I started to feel worse and worse as each month passed. I was attributing it to detox, when in fact I was just getting sick from what I was eating. At the same time, I was living the greatest adventure of my life, and the excitement of my travels shifted my focus so that I was not as aware of what was really happening as I might have been.

That week at Juliano's *Raw*, I got *sick* for the first time on raw food. My sore throat didn't go away. It was like having a cold, but without sneezing all the time. I felt tired, my body ached, and I wasn't hungry. In spite of my lack of appetite, I could not resist eating more of the food served at *Raw*, and each day spent at the restaurant, I felt progressively worse. Even after I left, it took me over a month just to recover from my cold symptoms.

The Legendary Appetite of Mad Mango Seb

After my week-long stop at the expo, I came back to San Diego, where I was about to experience one of the most memorable, yet deplorable, summers of my life.

I was still living at Morten's place, where my rent for my tent/room was only $35 a week.

It was about time summer arrived, because I had been so cold at night during the previous winter. I had not known this, but San Diego can get chilly at night. Although days are sunny and beautiful, nights can be downright cold in the winter, especially if one is camping outside year-round.

With the arrival of the summer came longer days, summer fruits, and the excitement of new possibilities. What was the next step in my journey? Would I see Claudia again? I had been in touch with her by email ever since I had left San Francisco, but I had yet to see her again. She was still in Los Gatos, and I did not know when she would come back to San Diego.

In the meantime, my brother was coming to San Diego to visit me, but also to accomplish a sort of raw food pilgrimage of his own, while traveling throughout California for a month.

Even since I had left Canada, Sebastien had remained a raw foodist, and he had not tried to stray from the diet even once. Being on a limited budget too, he decided to follow my lead and take the Greyhound bus all the way from Montreal, which took him three days.

He arrived in San Diego as a taller, scrawnier version of myself (he's the tall one in the family), and seemingly, he was not too exhausted from the long trip. He stayed at Morten's place for a few days, where I showed him the unusual life I had created for myself there. I took him to all the spots I had discovered, went fruit foraging with him, brought him to *Nature's First Law* to meet David, Stephen, and Fenris the dog, introduced him to all my friends, and got him to try the local raw food delights.

"Man, it's so cool to discover your little universe, after imagining it in my head since you've been gone!" he told me.

After his initial stay in San Diego, Sebastien went off for his own adventure in California, where he stayed with different raw foodists that he had been in touch with by email, as well as some contacts I had given him.

As my brother traveled in California during that month, I had the strange experience of running into people who had just seen him a few days earlier. In every instance, they commented on my brother's prodigious appetite. Coming to California had apparently unleashed a monster!

One guy, who worked at the *Living Light House* in Los Angeles, had just seen my brother there and commented to me, "He's a great kid...but boy can that guy eat!" Later during the same month, I ran into Juliano, who was traveling in San Diego as well, and he reported to me: "Your brother is a cool guy. But, my God, can he eat!"

As reports of Sebastien's legendary appetite were reaching me, I figured he was having a pretty good time. I was eager to hear some of his own travel stories. I didn't have to wait too long: a few weeks later, he was back in San Diego, on the last leg of his trip before heading back to Montreal by bus.

"So, what happened?" I asked him. I wanted the juiciest stories of his trip.

My brother had first gone to the *Living Light House* in Los Angeles, a sort of house turned into raw food center where potlucks and events would take place regularly. There, he had met Juliano, who was giving some recipe classes and partying. Sebastien had offered his help in exchange for free room and board, which was probably an exchange all to his advantage, since he was helping himself to massive quantities of Juliano's gourmet raw food.

Sebastien was just as surprised as I had been at the difference between the image he had had in his mind of raw foodists and the reality. Juliano stood out as the most eccentric, unlikely character he had ever met.

At the time, he told me Juliano would stay up all night, and then pass out on the kitchen table, while extremely loud, *death metal* music was blasting from the speakers. My brother would wake up and see him passed out on the table, totally oblivious to the absolute discomfort of his improvised bed and the insanely loud music he had been playing before he had fallen asleep.

The most troublesome part was when my brother told me that Juliano had tried to convince him to do LSD. "Don't believe what you've been told about LSD, Sebastien. It's all a lie. It's actually good for you."

My brother was not quite convinced by this argument, as he did not see Juliano as someone qualified to give any life coaching advice. But the food he made seduced him, and like me, he had not tasted raw foods before that were as delicious and addictive. He did not have anything bad to say about Juliano, though. Sebastien was grateful for the hospitality, and he found Juliano to be quite a friendly guy, but definitely eccentric.

At the *Living Light House*, a controversy was raging between the raw vegans and the raw meat-eaters. One of the raw foodists living there also ate raw meat, which was not well received by the raw food community, especially Denis, the manager of the house. My brother spent some good times with the raw meat-eater and had no problem with his diet. The man was in his fifties and looked pretty healthy. He took my brother on hiking trips in the area. During his stay, my brother Sebastien witnessed some pretty harsh arguments between Denis and the raw meat-eater. At some point, they almost physically fought together. At the end of the week, the meat-eater was kicked out and ostracized, and then my brother continued on his journey.

During his trip, Sebastien did some hitch-hiking. He told me a strange story. He was at a gas station, heading to a national park, Montagna De Oro, having missed the only daily bus; he was trying to hitch-hike. My brother is not religious, but at that moment, he was really desperate because if nobody came, he would have to spend the night outside. He decided to pray, asking God to send him someone.

About ten minutes later, a guy arrived in a car at the gas station. He saw my brother and asked him if he was "the one" he had to pick up. Sebastien was confused, thinking that maybe the guy was supposed to meet someone else, but he told my brother that he had been at the beach, when suddenly he had heard a voice, telling him he had to pick someone up at the gas station.

The guy was not heading to a particular place. In fact, the car was rented. He was supposed to have returned the car days ago, but he had just kept it. So he brought my brother to the national park. The guy was rather weird, and at some point, my brother got scared, thinking he could be some kind of psychopath. He asked my brother to withdraw some money from his own debit card, give it to him, and then tell the bank he had lost his card. My brother refused, but he realized that he might not be quite safe with this weirdo. Fortunately, he left and arrived safely at Montagna De Oro and lived to tell the tale!

The Truth About Raw Food Recipes

Raw foodists try to be trendy by creating a cuisine that imitates cooked foods using only raw ingredients. Their main mistake is that they start off with a false premise, which is the idea that eating cooked food is the main cause of human disease.

Raw foodists believe that raw foods are superior to cooked foods because they have not been denatured, contain more "life energy," or might have all of their enzymes intact. Although some of these ideas are true, the major mistake is to think that eating raw is some sort of miracle cure by itself.

There's nothing magical or mystical, or even healing, in raw foods by themselves. When people experience extraordinary recoveries on the raw food diet, it is simply because they have abandoned most of the foods that made them sick and given their bodies a chance to heal. The improved nutrition in raw foods, with their intact vitamins and minerals, is also beneficial, but only secondary to the main benefit of the diet: avoidance of rich and concentrated foods, such as bread, meat, and dairy products.

The enzyme theory has long been the main argument for a raw food diet. The reference work is a book by Dr. Edward Howell called *Enzyme Nutrition*. In his book, Howell proposes the theory that enzymes in raw foods (called "food enzymes") are an important help in digesting the foods themselves.

Since cooking destroys all food enzymes, Howell theorized that the body has to produce more of its own digestive enzymes than it would to digest those foods consumed raw.

Howell also claimed that the body has a finite lifetime supply of enzymes, and that by eating a cooked diet year after year, we eventually exhaust that supply and end up being sick and tired.

More than being just catalysts, enzymes are supposed to carry the "life force" of the food, which is transferred to the body and reputed to cure human diseases and enhance our vitality.

Howell's work has never been validated by a significant number of scientists, and his theories have never been proven.[28] Most of the references he provides in his book are at least 70 years old and extremely outdated.

Howell claimed that his book *Enzyme Nutrition* was just an abridged version of a longer, 700-page work — which, unfortunately, has never been published or found anywhere by anyone that I have ever known. In other words, it only exists in theory, not in reality. Nowhere in the book is there definite proof of any of the claims proposed by Howell, other than references to his mysterious, unpublished book, and outdated scientific research.

We now know that enzymes are catalysts. They are responsible for millions of chemical operations in the natural world. For example, the enzymes in a banana are responsible for converting the raw starch of a green banana into the sweet sugar of a ripe banana.

In our own bodies, enzymes are also responsible for digesting food. For that purpose, we do not require the enzymes present in foods, which are made for the purposes of the plant itself. The enzymes in a banana are for ripening the banana, not for you to digest the banana once you eat it.

As for the life force in foods, I find that it's a nice metaphor but an unlikely reality. Often, Kirlian photography (a particular type of photography that shows the "aura" of a living thing) is used as an argument for raw foods. In some books, you can even see beautiful pictures of the "aura" of a kiwi or another raw food versus the dead aspect of a cooked food.

28 (2003). Enzymes -- the spark plugs of life: what exactly are enzymes and why do we need them?. *Alive: Canadian Journal of Health & Nutrition*, (253), 160-161.

Tom Billings says this about Kirlian photography:

The logical, plausible explanation for Kirlian photos is that they show the effects of a type of corona discharge (the same phenomenon that produces lightning). The power of such a discharge will depend on moisture content (which in humans may vary with stress, e.g., sweating) and other relevant physical factors.

A corona discharge effect depends on ionized gases that result when a small electric current is applied to the object being photographed. Cooked foods have been heated, and heating can cause a loss of ions via steam and compounds dissolving into the water used in cooking (and the cooking water is usually discarded). Hence, one would expect Kirlian photos of raw foods to have a stronger corona discharge than similar cooked foods.

Even more telling, is if Kirlian photos were actually the "life force" instead of a corona discharge effect, one would expect there to be no difference between Kirlian photos taken in a vacuum (where there are no ionized gases to create the corona discharge effect), and photos taken in normal atmospheric conditions.

However, Kirlian photos taken of an object in a vacuum show no "aura." Thus, we conclude that Kirlian photos do not show the "life force" or "aura," and are not credible evidence in comparing raw and cooked foods.

Readers interested in Kirlian photos should check out the links **http://www.dcn. davis.ca.us/go/btcarrol/skeptic/kirlian.html and http:// www.theness.com/pseudo.html. (Note that the information on Kirlian photography in the second link occurs about halfway down on the page linked to.)**

FROM: http://www.beyondveg.com/tu-j-l/raw-cooked/ raw-cooked-2b.shtml

So, if raw foods are not better for us because of their enzymes and their life force, then why is it that so many people feel better on a raw food diet? Again, the answer is pretty straightforward: Raw foods are not denatured. Therefore, they are unlikely to contain toxins that could be created as by-products of the cooking process.

Raw foods are more intact, and likely to contain more vitamins, minerals and anti-oxidants than cooked foods. (There are some exceptions.)[29,30,31,32]

It is my belief that raw fruits and vegetables are superior to other foods because we are biologically adapted to eat them as a species. They are the foods that we can most thrive on, as long as we eat them in sufficient quantities to meet our energy needs.

Raw foodists avoid most of the foods that are the causes of human disease: animal products, bread, pastries, cakes, refined sugar, etc.

The mistake that raw foodists make is to think that cooking, in and of itself, is the main cause of human disease and that eating raw is enough to create perfect health.

With this mistaken philosophy in mind, and the obsession with preserving the "life force" of enzymes in foods, raw food chefs have created some of the worst cuisine on the planet, nutritionally speaking.

Thinking that anything goes, as long as it's raw, they have created substitutes for cooked dishes using raw ingredients. The trade-off is that by doing so, they have been forced to use excessive quantities of nuts, seeds, oils, avocados, and other fatty foods to bulk up these sparse vegetable dishes.

They dehydrate, blend, chop, and do everything to the food except cook it, and to achieve the flavor they desire, they use unhealthy quantities of fat in everything, to the point where their cuisine is much fattier than even a typical American diet.

Nowadays, whenever I enter a raw food restaurant, the smell of their dehydrated breads and nut pâté almost makes me nauseous. Because of my early experiences with the raw food diet, I have absolutely no desire to taste

29   Graff, J. (2006). The Benefits of Raw Food. *New Life Journal: Carolina Edition*, 7(5), 13-16.
30   Watanabe, F., Hiemori, M., Nakano, Y., Goto, M., Abe, K., & Fujita, T. (1998). Effects of microwave heating on the loss of vitamin B12 in foods. *Journal of agricultural and food chemistry*, 46(1), 206-210.
31   OckKyoung, C., Smith, N., Sakagawa, A., & Chang Yong, L. (2004). Antioxidant properties of raw and processed cabbages. *International Journal of Food Sciences & Nutrition*, 55(3), 191-199.
32   Sungpuag, P., Wasantwisut, E., Chittchang, U., &Tangchitpianvit, S. (1999). Retinol and beta carotene content of indigenous raw and home-prepared foods in Northeast Thailand. *Food chemistry*, 64(2), 163-167.

or try any more "gourmet raw cuisine," and I avoid raw food restaurants at all costs. I would much rather eat in almost any vegetarian restaurant than a raw food restaurant (unless I can order a fruit smoothie or a simple low-fat salad).

CHAPTER 11

Raw Love is in the Air

"When I get the question, "Will eating raw food improve my sex life or make me sexy?" My answer is a definite "maybe.""

Roe Gallo,
author of The Perfect Body

In the middle of the summer, 1998, I got an unexpected call from Claudia.

"My visa is expiring in a few months, and I haven't been able to renew it. I need to go back to Switzerland in just two months, but in the meantime, I need a place to stay. Do you think I could stay with you?"

I was quite excited to get this news, yet nervous at the same time. It was clear that I had been pursuing Claudia ever since I had met her at David's "juice party" back in December. Circumstances had prevented me from spending more time with her. We had already kissed, but I felt that there were obstacles in the way of taking our relationship any further. I wasn't even sure she liked me that much, perhaps preferring an older man to a young, inexperienced pup like me.

What did I really have to offer her?

I didn't have a place of my own. I lived in a shack. Not even a shack, it was a more like a tent, except a little more comfortable. I was living in the middle of a garden in a canyon, in the worst part of San Diego. The house was owned by an aging spiritualist, who paid at least part of his bills by letting young people rent rooms, park RVs, and if necessary, plant a tent like I did.

The scene at Morten's place was quite unique.

In the house, he had a proper room available, which was currently rented by a 20-something guy who studied classical guitar at the local university.

In the parking lot, there was the small RV of Scott, another raw foodist in his thirties who had moved all the way from Chicago on a whim, just to be in the sun and eat raw. He had a past of addiction and excess, and for him, the raw diet was the path to salvation.

Like most of us at the time, he had trouble with cravings and would tend to overeat in the evening, stuffing himself with nuts or dried fruits. To attempt to control his cravings, Scott told me he had started to frequent the local San Diego group of *Overeaters Anonymous*.

In the backyard, as one went down the garden path toward the canyon, the first tent encountered was mine. It was just a platform with a futon on it, with a tin roof and some sheets surrounding it.

At the very edge of the canyon, on a platform that extended above the open air, was Durian's residence: he had actually pitched a tent there.

Durian had been my first true friend in San Diego. After all, without him I wouldn't have had any place to stay, and I might have been forced to go back to Montreal. The fact that he was gay did not bother me at all. I had met plenty of gay people ever since my mom had befriended Mario (who would often introduce us to his boyfriends), but I had never met gay people of my age before.

I had the feeling that he would have liked to be more than just "friends," which put me in a very awkward position, since I had absolutely no attraction for him or for men in general. However, I still felt grateful for his friendship and his help. I felt like some women must feel when they have male friends to whom they feel no attraction, but know that these men secretly desire them and hope for more.

I told Claudia that she could come stay with me, and I was forced to admit to myself that I was not sure what kind of impression this place, or I, would make on her.

On top of the eccentricity of the place itself and its residents, there was the neighborhood, where police helicopters still did surveillance at night and dogs kept barking like crazy. I did not feel unsafe here (probably because I had no material possessions I feared could be stolen), but it was claimed to be the roughest part of town.

I told her in advance about the place. I warned her about the humbleness of my dwelling. "I don't care. I just want to spend some time with you," she said.

All of my concerns went away when Claudia finally arrived. She did not seem to mind anything at all, and in fact, she loved just to be able to be in San Diego, surrounded by fruit trees.

I was barely 21, while Claudia was 29. I did not feel any concern over this difference in age for some reason. To me, she was just a person, and I was falling for her.

I actually don't even remember much of what we did during those two months, except that I was drunk with love.

We took the bus to go everywhere in the city, and we kissed so much in public during that time that once she left, some random stranger even asked me what had happened to my girlfriend.

I kept writing my newsletter *Just Eat an Apple,* and going to *Nature's First Law* every day of the week, but I could not wait to get back home to see her again.

I loved listening to her cute Swiss-German accent, as she was talking about what her life was like in Switzerland or countries she wanted to visit in the future.

During that time, her cousin was also traveling in California, and she also spent some time with us at Morten's place in a different room.

As the weeks passed, her return to Switzerland drew inexorably closer. Claudia had exhausted all possible legal ways to remain in the USA, and she had to go back home. Although she could have tried something else, she decided that she had to go back to continue moving forward in her life.

Perhaps the fact that I knew it was about to end made our time together even more intense and intoxicating.

Sometimes, she would say, "Perhaps you can come with me to Switzerland."

As much as the idea seemed inviting, I could not conceive of any possible plan to go to Switzerland, which seemed as far away as any other place on Earth. I had never been on a commercial plane, and the amount of money I would have needed to go there was just not obtainable for me at that point.

Soon, the weeks we had left turned into days, and every day, I felt my solar plexus become more and more tense.

She was going to leave. Would I ever see her again?

"Let's make a date," she said the night before she left. "If we don't see each other again, let's meet in five years in Paris."

Although the idea of a tryst in Paris sounded romantic, I knew we were just making stuff up and that I was going to lose her for good.

She was leaving in the morning.

She said, "Tomorrow, I don't want you to give me a hug or come upstairs to say a last goodbye. Let's say our goodbyes tonight. When you wake up, don't go upstairs. I'll leave a note for you in the kitchen that you can read later. Farewells are too painful."

We fell asleep in each other's arms, and when I woke up, she was gone. I knew a taxi was coming to pick her up in the morning, and although she had asked me not to go upstairs to say my last farewells, I could not resist the temptation.

I ran up the stairs as fast as I could, but when I arrived in the house, she had just left. I had missed her by less than a minute, and I could see her shuttle driving away.

As promised, she had left a note in the kitchen that I tore open eagerly and read immediately.

The Mysterious Raw Sickness

Thinking about it now, I can't even remember what she wrote in that final note, but I was heartbroken and lonely, and wished I could see her again.

After Claudia left, I felt an immense void in my life. I had been in love for the first time, felt constant and romantic infatuation for nearly two months, and overnight, the feeling was stripped away and replaced with grief.

I felt such a lack of hunger that I decided to only eat watermelon for five days as part of a little "raw challenge" with David Wolfe.

I wandered alone, going to the beach and feeling barely hungry. Every day, I would listen to the same songs to which we had listened together, mainly the dreamy *Undertow* by Chroma Key and Utraviolet, *Light My Way* by U2.

The lyrics by Chroma Key didn't make sense. Somehow, though, they felt appropriate, and I couldn't get them out of my head:

> *"I know*
>
> *I'll go to Mexico*
>
> *Someplace nothing changes*
>
> *Maybe I'll call on the phone*
>
> *Maybe I'll write you a letter*
>
> *That's what I meant when I said goodbye..."*

After Claudia left, I was still in touch with her by email. We kept exchanging friendly emails, and reminding each other to stay on track with the raw food diet.

Claudia had trouble sticking with the diet and wasn't 100% raw like I was. She would do it for stretches of time, and then fall for European comfort food, namely bread and cheese.

To try to stick with the diet, she would make up a "challenge" with me. She would promise to eat all raw for one whole month, and if she cheated, she said she would buy me a round-trip ticket to Switzerland (which she failed to do, by the way).

In her emails, she kept telling me that all of her friends thought I was so cute, and wished they could all just pitch in to "fly me to Switzerland."

Somehow, I entertained the fantasy that maybe we could still be together again, although I saw no practical way it could work.

After about a month, Claudia's emails stopped coming. She didn't reply to me anymore, and I started to wonder if something had gone wrong with her.

I wrote a few times to ask what was happening, but I still received no response.

Then, one day, I got a crushing email from a man I did not know.

"Hi. I'm Claudia's new boyfriend. We are deeply in love and are about to move in together. We certainly don't want old lovers to come knocking on our door, so please don't contact her anymore."

I was so upset by that email, because there was really nothing I could do about it. It seemed so surreal that she would immediately find someone else just after she had left.

After that event, I became quite sad for a while and did not know what to do to have joy back in my life.

In all of those adventures in California, I had felt less vitality on the raw food diet than what I had initially expected, because of all the excesses I was engaging in, from eating several avocados a day to trying out many high-fat raw recipes.

During that summer with Claudia, I felt I could just live on "fruit and love" and not need anything else. I felt invigorated. After she left, just eating fruit was not enough and left my emotions raw and painful.

I found myself back eating the high-fat, raw gourmet comfort foods.

One particular dish I started consuming with Durian was a "raw cashew cheese" he was buying at People's Market. It was made with cashews, slightly fermented, and seasoned with spices and salt to make it delicious.

Durian would also make a raw version of hummus, where he would simply soak chickpeas, and in the morning get rid of the soaking water, leave them out to sprout for less than six hours, and then blend them up with tahini, lemon juice and seasonings.

My salads were delicious and fatty, made with a lot of lettuce and fresh tomatoes, but also one or two avocados, a few olives, and a generous drizzling of olive oil.

Among the several "sin foods" that Durian was bringing back from the health food store where he worked was Kimchi, a fermented Korean type of sauerkraut, which contained cabbage and plenty of salt and spices.

I had gone from eating a pure, hygienic diet to eating a combination of fruit and gourmet, high-fat raw foods — all for the sake of staying 100% raw. By eating more and more nuts than ever before, I was paving the way for the mysterious illness I was about to experience.

Why You Should Never Eat Raw Beans

Beans in their raw state — even when sprouted — should be avoided. Some kinds of raw beans contain a harmful toxin (the lectin phytohaemagglutinin) that can cause food poisoning-like symptoms. [33,34]

They also contain indigestible raw starch. Even Steve Meyerowitz, an author who wrote many books on sprouting, says:

"Although sprouting makes the large beans easier to digest, increases their protein, and lowers their starch, they are still primarily raw beans. Quantity and regularity of consumption is the caveat here. One should not regularly consume large quantities of raw beans or raw sprouted beans..."

Other Raw Foods to Avoid:

* Buckwheat greens contain a substance called fagopyrin that causes the human skin to become hypersensitive to sunlight. Juicing buckwheat greens should especially be avoided, as it is easy to "overdose." [35]

* Many types of wild greens contain toxic compounds, and therefore, they should be avoided or eaten in very small quantities. This also includes many tropical wild green plants that are popular in Asia as "detox" or "weight loss" remedies. One such plant grows wild in Costa Rica and is commonly called "Katuk," but the name changes in every country. A few years ago, there was a story in the newspapers of a woman following a raw food diet who died after eating some kind of wild green. Although rare, these cases happen once in a while.

* Raw Bok Choy contains compounds called "glucosinolates" that have been found to inhibit thyroid function. One 88-year old woman in the USA was eating two or three pounds of raw bok choy per day and almost died from

33   Venter, F., & Thiel, P. (1995). Red kidney beans--to eat or not to eat?.*South African Medical Journal = Suid-AfrikaanseTydskrifVirGeneeskunde, 85*(4), 250-252.
34   Filho, J., Vizeu, D., &Lajolo, F. (1979). Lectins from red kidney beans: Radiation effect on agglutinating and mitogenic activity. *Journal of food science, 44*(4), 1194.
35   (2010). Poisonous plant.Columbia Electronic Encyclopedia, 6th Edition, 1.

hypothyroidism because of that. This is not to say that raw bok choy should be avoided, but it should be used in moderation.[36]

* Wild Mushrooms are so toxic that simply tasting a bite can lead to death. In 2008, 894 cases of wild mushroom poisoning were reported in the US, including one death. Raw foodists may think they are immune to these effects, but they are not.[37,38]

* Raw potatoes won't harm you, but the raw starch they contain is largely indigestible.[39]

The Mysterious Illness

One day, a cute blonde girl showed up at *Nature's First Law*. She had just started going raw and had befriended Stephen Arlin. She changed her name to Luna and dressed in a gothic style, with mostly black colors, which didn't quite fit with the whole raw food lifestyle, which was supposed to be all about life and liveliness. She picked the name almost a decade before the character Luna Lovegood from the Harry Potter book series became popular!

She was very attractive, and even though she seemed quite depressed and nihilistic, I could not tell how much of it was an act and how much was her true personality.

After her visit, Stephen told me, "You should call her, Fred. I think she likes you."

---

36 Chu, M., & Seltzer, T. (2010). Myxedema coma induced by ingestion of raw bokchoy. *The New England Journal Of Medicine, 362*(20), 1945-1946.

37 Barbee, G., Berry-Cabán, C., Barry, J., Borys, D., Ward, J., &Salyer, S. (2009). Analysis of Mushroom Exposures in Texas Requiring Hospitalization, 2005-2006. *Journal of Medical Toxicology, 5*(2), 59-62.

38 West, P., Lindgren, J., & Horowitz, B. (2009). Amanita Smithiana Mushroom Ingestion: A Case of Delayed Renal Failure and Literature Review. *Journal of Medical Toxicology, 5*(1), 32-38.

39 Mishra, S., Hedderley, D., &Monro, J. (2008).Effect of Processing on Slowly Digestible Starch and Resistant Starch in Potato [electronic resource].*Stärke Starch, 60*(9), 500-507.

I took Stephen's advice, and gave Luna a call.

She worked at *Jamba Juice* (a Californian chain of juice bars), and had just gone raw a few months earlier, after finding out about it through *Nature's First Law's* book. According to her, the hardest part was giving up coffee, which gave her splitting headaches for over a week.

Even though she was about my age, she had gotten married at the age of 18 and was now getting divorced. She lived with her parents, but worked full-time just to pay off her debts for a brand-new car she was leasing and a new computer she had just bought.

"I drive to work with my brand-new car so that I can make enough money to pay for my car," she told me. I kept telling her she should not get into so much debt; otherwise working full-time didn't even make sense.

Shortly after meeting her, I started dating Luna, but I still felt the heartbreak from Claudia.

Luna was a nice girl, but I felt she needed to strip away her whole "goth" persona to replace it with a more "raw-friendly" look. So I would write her some emails to show her some aspects of the raw food lifestyle she probably didn't know.

I tried to be enthusiastic about her, but the truth is that I did not feel the same way with her as I had felt with Claudia.

We dated for a few weeks, until one day, it hit me, and I got seriously sick. I didn't tell anyone what was going on, not even Luna, because raw foodists were not "supposed" to get sick.

The circumstances of this mysterious illness are so strange that even today, I still wonder exactly what happened.

I was walking uphill in the area near Stephen's place, walking towards the bus stop, and suddenly I felt like something hit me. I felt an extreme soreness in my lower back for no apparent reason.

All day at *Nature's First Law*, I had been feeling more tired than usual. It was really a struggle to get through the day. I pretended everything was fine, but something was wrong and I knew it. This was not just tiredness caused by lack of sleep.

When the back soreness hit me as I was walking down the street, I felt like all the energy had been drained from my body. I felt like I had aged 60 years in about 60 seconds, as all of my vitality was drained and my back was aching so badly.

When I got home, I did not have the energy to do anything. So I went straight to bed and rested, even though it was only 4 p.m. I stayed in bed all night.

When I woke up the next day, I noticed something was terribly wrong. One of my testicles had swollen up to around 250% of its normal size, and it felt abnormally firm. It didn't hurt, but it was really, really big. I was confused and terrified.

What was going on? I didn't know who to talk to, and I was literally too afraid to go to the hospital, thinking that they would probably kill me with their drugs.

If I talked to a raw foodist, what would they tell me? The theory of detox would probably not apply here (I didn't see how my testicles could detox anything). And listening to more death metal would probably not help me through this particular crisis as David Wolfe had suggested before.

The only person I confided in was Durian, whom I considered one of my only true friends, and I knew he wouldn't be squeamish if I asked him to take a look.

When Durian saw my enlarged testicle, he said, "Dude, it's huge!" which did nothing to reassure me.

Durian told me I should probably go see a doctor.

"But I don't have any health insurance, and my Canadian insurance won't cover me here!" I said.

"There are some government-subsidized charity clinics that charge very little for a basic consultation."

I looked at Durian and thought about the situation. Everyone else I knew that was a raw foodist had told me it was extremely dangerous to go to the doctor for any reason.

Even Mosséri's books had made me scared of hospitals, where hygienists would often end up after well-meaning family members had called the ambulance on them as they were attempting to do a water fast on their own. Some of these people even died when doctors gave them treatments, unaware that their bodies would react so strongly against certain drugs.

I didn't think that doctors could tell me what was happening, because in my mind, I thought that almost every disease could be explained as a sort of health crisis. I thought that just eating raw would help me avoid getting sick, but I also strongly believed that if I did get sick for any reason, I would know what to do to get better on my own, without doctors.

Of course, if I had broken a leg, I would have gone to the hospital. In this case, the mysterious and sudden illness with the particular symptoms I experienced led me to believe that this was something I could heal myself.

I didn't want to tell any of my raw friends, because it was too embarrassing, and I was supposed to be this super-healthy raw foodist. I preferred to hide and pretend that everything was fine instead of exposing my weaknesses and showing that I had a problem.

I admired these raw foodists and aspired to be like them. At the time, David Wolfe appeared to be a very healthy person, and I could not understand why I was not thriving on his recommendations.

I did not tell Luna, because I was too embarrassed by what was happening. (I stopped calling her, which unsurprisingly drove her away from my life as fast as she had entered it).

My faith in Natural Hygiene was enough to give me the confidence that if anything was going to cure me, it was going to be my own body. No doctor could give me a remedy that would do anything other than camouflage the symptoms, and possibly make me even worse in other ways.

Apart from the enlarged testicle, which caused me no pain, the only other symptom that I suffered was the lack of energy. I had so little energy left that even walking from my room to Morten's house, which was just a matter of climbing about 40 steps, required a great deal of effort on my part.

I had gone away from Mosséri's teachings, but I had not forgotten them completely. So I did the only thing that I thought could heal me, and I fasted.

I did not know enough to do a complete water fast on my own, so I did something close to it. I ate only a small meal of fruit once a day, consisting of a few apples with raisins, or a handful of grapes. Other than that, I just drank water.

Because it was around Christmas time, *Nature's First Law* was taking time off so I didn't even have to make up an excuse to not come to the office anymore.

During my healing crisis, some of my brother's friends came to visit me, and I even managed to pretend that everything was going fine, although I was still struggling to muster enough energy to even walk a few steps.

After about three weeks of eating only a small amount of fruit and resting, I started to feel a lot better. My energy was coming back, and my testicle had even returned to about 90% its normal size. However, it took almost two months for my body to go back to feeling normal.

It took me even longer than that to return to my regular self in health and energy.

Most likely, my mysterious illness was caused by malnutrition. I consulted a family friend, who's finishing a Ph.D. in medicine, who told me that when we are malnourished, our bodies become unbalanced at the cellular level. This can affect the amount and direction of concentration gradients within organs, blood vessels, or body areas. Likely, I was experiencing an imbalance, which caused a blockage or buildup of fluid in this sensitive area. It could also have been hormonal, meaning that the malnutrition caused a hormonal change, which caused the organ to change.

Although I am not certain of what happened to me, I now blame the excess of fat I consumed over a period of several months, including the large amounts of nuts I ate.

Nuts are extremely acidifying when consumed in large quantities, and eating fermented raw cashew cheese, along with raw hummus made with soaked chickpeas, was a recipe for disaster.

Uncooked or undercooked beans contain lectins, which are toxic to the body. Those toxins are destroyed when cooked properly, but when eaten raw, they can provoke a reaction and cause nausea, diarrhea, and vomiting. (Although, if eating raw beans had poisoned me, I wouldn't have experienced an enlarged testicle.)

In all of his books, Mosséri told horrible stories of people who suffered terrible diseases after consuming generous servings of nuts on a regular basis. It has been my experience over the years that the high fat content is only one of the negative aspects of nuts. Consuming an equal portion of fat in the form of nuts will do more harm than getting the same amount of fat in avocados or even olive oil.

Nuts are an excellent food, when consumed in minimal quantities (one or two ounces at a time is enough). By adhering to the concept of "as long as it's raw, it's okay," I overate nuts and fats over an extended period of time, enough to become seriously ill. It is possible that eating too many nuts caused a nutritional imbalance, which precipitated my illness.

There is no doubt that the emotional state I was in at the time was also a triggering factor for this illness, but without the bad diet I was on, it would not have happened.

The Danger of Dogma

At this point in my life, I had been 100% raw for over a year and a half. I had started out by eating mostly fruits and vegetables and practicing Natural Hygiene, and then spiraled down into eating a lot of combo-abombo raw recipes that were heavy with nuts, oil and salt.

Everyone in those days ate whatever and as much as they cared for without any worry about nutrition or calories. Raw recipes were all the rage, and became more like science experiments, to see how gourmet the taste could be made by mixing large quantities of salt, fat and sweeteners together to create the ultimate indulgence.

All of the people I hung out with were raw foodists. We believed that everything raw was good and everything cooked was bad. There was no in between. As long as it was raw, it was good.

We were above everyone else; we were raw foodists. We knew what true health was and how to get there. Anyone eating cooked foods was brainwashed by the media and the government to eat bad foods, and we knew better.

I believed so wholeheartedly in a 100% raw food approach that I did not even question what I was eating anymore. I was eating the best diet in the world.

When I got sick, I didn't know what to do. Everyone says raw foodists don't get sick, and I didn't want to tell anyone I was sick for fear of humiliation.

I now realize how dangerous this behavior was. I was not taking responsibility for my own health. I was letting my peers influence me to the point where I was doing everything they did without question.

I literally gave myself almost no options to get better. I was afraid to go to the hospital, or even talk about my illness to anyone else. No one I knew would have the answer for me anyway, because it wasn't supposed to happen to me in the first place, I was a raw foodist.

I'm very lucky that what I had did not turn out to be life-threatening and that I was able to heal very slowly on my own. I did not even tell anyone what I was doing, and if I had blacked out or even died, no one would have known why! Not even my family.

Now that is really scary.

Sometimes, our dogma or belief systems get in the way of really looking at ourselves and seeing the problems we are causing on our own. I have no idea what would have happened to me if I had continued to eat so many nut recipes, simply because I believed it was healthy raw food, and not gone back to Natural Hygiene and fasted.

In raw foods, we often get brainwashed in the opposite direction to SAD eaters. We think everything we eat is health food. We are superhuman now, and we'll never get sick. Without common sense and a regard for proper nutrition, this is simply not true.

Nowadays, I'm very skeptical about everything regarding raw foods, and I think this is a good thing. If I simply accept everything that people say or what a product promises to offer, then I could put myself in harm's way and not even realize it.

Don't put your health in other people's hands. Often, people give too much credit to raw food gurus, thinking they have all the answers and have experience with every type of situation or illness. It's simply not the case! You need to be in tune with your body, do your own research, and not just blindly believe what someone says because it sounds good at the moment.

If and when you get sick, following your dogma, you'll be the one to blame. Those people you get health advice from will likely never know, and don't have the answers you are looking for. So take responsibility for your health and make sure you are informed.

Know how many calories you need to eat, know your average percentage of fat intake, track your vitamin and mineral intake, get blood tests, etc. Don't just wait until your health has steadily gotten worse so that now you are at a loss for what to do because a haphazard raw diet alone did not help you.

I think it's important to have a doctor or alternative health practitioner that you can trust. This needs to be someone who knows your history and your diet, so that in case anything happens, you will not be afraid to ask questions or seek help.

You don't want to wait around until one day you're so sick and vulnerable that someone around you takes it upon himself or herself to send you to the hospital, where you are unable to inform the nurses or defend yourself from medications that could be potentially dangerous.

It is especially important for raw foodists to let their doctor know that they have high Vitamin K levels (from greens) as this can react with blood thinning medications and increase blood clotting. Kale, collards, mustard leaves, and turnip greens are rich in Vitamin K. [40]

---

40 (2004). Fondaparinux or Enoxaparin for Deep Venous Thrombosis. *Annals of Internal Medicine, 140*(11), 44.

The reason I am more open to different points of view on health and nutrition is because of my experiences, and I can be honest with myself about what is and is not working. I am always open to researching new and even old ideas and using my common sense when it comes to fads in the raw and natural health movement.

I believe that I will always make small changes to my diet and lifestyle as time goes by and not be afraid to admit I don't have all the answers. From my experiences and being around so many other raw foodists, I can sure tell you what doesn't work in the long run and how to avoid making the same mistakes I made.

CHAPTER 12

Cravings and the Raw Food Diet

"Just as the craving of a drug addict for heroin does not arise from the normal physiological needs of his body, so the desire of a cooked-food eater for cooked food, his feeling of hunger, is not the normal demand of his organism; rather it is the demand of his addiction."

A.T. Hovanessian,
"Raw Eating"

In 1999, I was still under the illusion that I was "transitioning" to the raw food diet and detoxing, even though my health was much worse than it had been when I had first started. I thought that if I just kept going, I was going to eventually experience all the wonderful benefits of the raw food diet that had been promised by the gurus and the books I had read.

These benefits included:

- Needing less sleep

- Boundless energy

- Amazing mental clarity

- Clear skin

- Great digestion

Not only did I not experience any of these benefits, I also felt worse than I ever did before. Instead of needing 8 or 9 hours of sleep a night, I needed 10 or 11. The thought of being able to sleep only 5 hours a night seemed like an impossible goal.

Even though I had recovered a lot after my mysterious illness, my energy levels were mediocre at best. I still went through several ups and downs during the day and did not feel high levels of energy.

As long as I did not eat any food, I could focus and work, but as soon as I ate food, my mind became blurry and I could barely concentrate for hours.

My skin was still breaking out, and I would frequently feel as though my stomach was killing me.

Was it that there was something fundamentally wrong with me? What were these other successful 100% raw foodists doing or not doing that gave them such different results?

I thirsted to find answers to these questions, and I knew that I was not the only person in the same boat.

All around me, other raw foodists were complaining of various other issues. There was something else that was often talked about, which was by far the biggest bane of the raw food existence:

Cravings.

My ex-roommate at Morten's place, Scott, had confessed to me that he was still battling with cravings. Late at night, he would often binge on nuts, dried fruits or avocados to try to pacify his unrelenting hunger.

RC Dini believed in the fruit diet, but his cravings were so strong that to calm them, he ate weird fatty mixtures of avocados, honey, hot pepper and almond butter. He also coined the term "Combo-Abombo" to describe these horrible concoctions. There was seemingly no other option but to occasionally eat them, short of going back to cooked foods or summoning the inhuman willpower needed to prevail over these cravings.

The other raw foodists I had met at the potlucks also complained about the cravings. Many of them fell off the wagon and occasionally binged on cooked foods, such as my friend Don the Raw Guy, who confessed to occasionally eating corn chips with guacamole when he was too hungry.

David Wolfe was telling us to simply eat more avocados, but even his recommendation of eating three to five avocados per day was not working. On some level, I knew that eating that many avocados was not healthy, and I could feel the results in my body. But what was the other option? Eat more fruit? I was already eating all the whole fruit I could (or so I thought at the time).

The worst part about it was that the general subtext to the discussion about cravings was that they were a normal part of going raw.

The theory went like this:

Cooked foods were addictive. We ate cooked food all our lives, so we were addicted to it. Breaking the habit required willpower and efforts, and so cravings were a normal part of going raw. Even Joe Alexander, the author of *Blatant Raw-Foodist Propaganda*, one of the first raw food books I had read, had said that breaking the cooked food habit was harder than even quitting cocaine or other hard drugs.

Your body was eliminating all of these bad cooked food cells and toxins, and as part of the process, you had cravings. Weak people just went back to cooked foods, while the stoic long-term raw foodists had learned to go through this initial period of suffering and eventually reached raw food nirvana, where even the smell of cooked food was not enough to make them salivate.

The religious overtones of this philosophy are quite obvious. Cooked food is like the devil or "sin." Raw foodists were like these religious zealots who think that sex is immoral and sinful. The weak people failed and reverted to cooked food (sin), while the pious and courageous ones stayed on the path of raw (virtue).

The Truth About Cravings

Fast forward 12 years later, and the raw food movement has boomed to a worldwide phenomenon, with hundreds of raw restaurants, countless websites and raw food businesses, and an endless number of raw food YouTube channels.

Yet, the vast majority of people who are interested in the raw food lifestyle never manage to fully incorporate it into their lives, because of cravings.

Still today, cravings for cooked food are the number one complaint raw foodists have.

What is going on?

It turns out that the answer is ridiculously simple and obvious.

What I have discovered over the years is that if you give your body what it needs, you will not experience cravings, period. First, let's distinguish two types of cravings:

1- Psychological cravings

2- Physical cravings

Psychological cravings can be more aptly described as *habits.* Since our earliest childhoods, we've been fed certain foods, have developed a liking for these foods, and now have a habit of eating them on a regular basis.

Most people decide to go raw after they've had at least 30,000 regular, cooked food meals since they were little children. Besides this staggering reinforcement of a particular habit, we've also grown up in an environment where certain foods are associated with certain emotions or activities. For example, going to the movies may be associated with eating popcorn, or feeling lonely could be associated with eating ice cream.

Current research has shown that everything we learned and every habit we form in our lives is stored in our brain as a sort of *pathway* of knowledge — a blueprint that tells us exactly what to do at exactly the right time, in order to accomplish all the things we do on a daily basis.

Newer research has discovered a substance called *myelin* that some neurologists now consider to be the holy grail of skill acquisition. It turns out that everything we do –every skill or habit we learn — is created by a pathway or chain of nerve fibers in our brain, a sort of circuit. Myelin is a substance that wraps around those nerve fibers to insulate them and make the signal go faster.[41]

Whenever we practice a skill or a habit, we reinforce the circuit and more myelin gets built around it to make it faster and faster.

That's why if you've been practicing piano for 10 years for 4 hours a day, picking up a Bach prelude and playing it is *automatic.* You don't have to think about every single movement you are making with your fingers while reading the music, because everything is already integrated into a fast circuit in your brain.

---

41 See "The Talent Code" - Greatness isn't Born. It's Grown. Here's How - by Daniel Coyle

The same must be true for habits, whether they are good habits (such as exercising daily) or bad habits (such as smoking or drinking). Once you've done something over and over again, your brain will react appropriately when placed in the same situation that triggers the response.

Once established, such a circuit can never be deactivated, but it can be made much less powerful by simply stopping it from firing. Then, the layers of myelin around the circuit start to break down and the circuit is not as fast to respond.

Going back to our example of the piano player... Imagine that you've played piano for 10 years for four hours a day, but then quit and stop playing for 10 years. When you go back to the piano, chances are that you will have lost most of what you've learned and won't be able to play much. However, like many people who have learned a skill, then forgotten it, then relearned it later in life, you will notice that your reacquisition of the skill (piano) will be much faster than someone who starts from scratch. Therefore, you might be able to get to the same level you were 10 years ago in just one year of practice, instead of another ten.

When we've eaten heavily salted, sweet and fatty foods such as what is commonly eaten on a regular basis in North America or Europe, we have developed certain habits that are difficult to break.

We could call these *psychological cravings*, because they relate to how your brain responds to certain stimuli and generate certain desires.

For example, even if you've been a raw foodist for many years, if something very dramatic happens to you (such as something that causes intense grief or sadness), you might be quickly drawn to reach for the tub of ice cream or the bag of potato chips that gave you comfort in the past. This is a strongly ingrained habit or *circuit* in your brain that you naturally revert to when the stimulus is strong enough.

Another example: you walk down the street and smell a certain type of food, such as a baked good your grandma used to make. The smell suddenly reminds you of your childhood and the countless times you ate the delicious food that your granny made and all the joy those moments brought you. Suddenly, you feel like you want to eat it one more time.

The key to overcoming these psychological cravings is not to fight them with hard willpower. Re-firing the circuit of habits only makes it stronger. The proper way to overcome these habits is to create new positive habits to take their place, and reinforce these instead, in order to create strong, highly insulated circuits in your brain.

So, instead of reaching for the tub of ice cream, replace it with a healthy alternative that would be harmless, such as frozen banana ice cream. Instead of eating granny's cookies again, go buy some raspberries or another fruit your granny fed you, and make a healthy recipe with them. If you just focus on creating new positive habits and reinforcing them, instead of trying to fight and destroy your negative habits, you will succeed.

Physical Cravings

Physical cravings, on the other hand, are a much tougher opponent. A physical craving is essentially a demand from the body for something it needs. If you fail to meet that demand, the need will only grow stronger and stronger, and unless you are a superhuman, you will be forced to respond.

Physical cravings for food are even more difficult to overcome than sexual desire, because food is a biological need that cannot be ignored.

If a man abstains from sex for a period of time, eventually his sexual desires will grow stronger and stronger. After a certain number of days or weeks (depending on his age and other factors), his needs will seek some sort of outlet. During his sleep, he will eventually have sexual dreams that will lead to ejaculation. Although he may have been strong enough to pacify his sexual desires during the day, his body eventually found a way to do what it needed against his will and sneakily during his dreams.

If we abstain from food or undereat for a period of time, our brain cannot make ourselves "eat a giant meal" during the night in our dreams and be satisfied.

In 2005, I fasted on water for 23 days at a fasting retreat in Costa Rica. For the first few days, I was overcome with cravings. After about three or four days of fasting, my body reverted to a state of ketosis, where it started to feed on my own body-fat and to convert it to ketones, as an alternative energy source to glucose from food.

This is a safety mechanism that the body has, which enables us to survive for long periods of time without food. Fortunately, because the body knows it is being starved, the sense of "hunger" eventually turns off during a fast, so we can focus our attention on finding a way to survive.

During my fast, even though my hunger diminished to manageable levels after three days, and completely disappeared after 7 days, I was plagued with thoughts and dreams of food, in which I was eating giant chocolate cakes and giant dates.

Hunger during a complete water-fast mostly disappears after a while, which is not the case during a starvation diet, where you're still providing yourself with some of the nutrients and energy you need, but not all of it.

During World War II, a clinical study was performed at the University of Minnesota on the effects of starvation on the human body. The study is now referred to as the Minnesota Starvation Experiment. The researchers were motivated by the events of the war to help the Allied Forces to provide assistance to victims of famine in Europe and Asia. The purpose of the experiment was to determine the physical and psychological effects of prolonged dietary restriction.[42]

Before the experiment, not a lot was known about the effects of fasting on the body. We now know that a faster undergoes a series of physiological changes, starting with ketosis, and although the process evolved out of the needs of species to survive, it can also cause important health benefits when done properly.

The type of semi-starvation studied in the Minnesota experiment was entirely different. They didn't want to know what happened to humans when they fasted, but what happened to healthy young men when you cut their caloric intake in half over a long period of time.

Thirty-six healthy young men were selected for the experiment. All of them were volunteers and knew what the experiment was going to do.

The experiment was extremely rigorous. First, they followed the subjects for 12 weeks to establish a "baseline" of physiological and psychological observation of these young men.

---

42 Keys, A., Brozek, J., Henschel, A., Mickelsen, O., & Taylor, H. L., *The Biology of Human Starvation* (2 volumes), University of Minnesota Press, 1950.

Then, there was a second phase of 24 weeks, called the "starvation phase," during which the calories in the diet of each participant was dramatically reduced to the point of making each man lose approximately 25% of his body weight.

Finally, the last phase was a recovery phase to analyze what the best diet was to bring these men back to health.

Why did these men decide to be subjected to such a treatment? The incentive was great. If they were selected for the experiment, they could use it as an alternative to military service. That meant not going to war.

Out of a total of 400 volunteers, only these 36 healthy young men were selected.

If you see a picture of these men during the control period, you will notice how fit they looked. Compared to modern men, we could say that the 36 participants selected were quite fine specimens of human beings with great muscle definition and a healthy look.

During the control period of 12 weeks, they consumed approximately 3200 calories per day, which is about the average number of calories that fit, healthy and active young men still need today.

During the 6-month starvation period, their caloric intake was cut to about 1560 calories per day. They were also fed foods that were supposed to represent the types of food commonly eaten in Europe during the war, such as potatoes and other root vegetables, bread and macaroni.

The results of the study were published in 1950 in a large document called *The Biology of Human Starvation*. Here is what was discovered during the experiment:

- "Most of the subjects experienced periods of severe emotional distress and depression."

- They exhibited a constant "preoccupation with food."

- Sexual desire was drastically lowered.

- The subjects reported a decline in concentration.

- They experienced signs of social withdrawal and isolation.

- The participants experienced a drop in body temperature, a lower heart rate, and lower rate of respiration.

They found overall that prolonged semi-starvation created conditions that were similar to those experienced by people with eating disorders, such as anorexia and bulimia. It was suggested that the psychological effects of such disorders were caused by under-nutrition and not any pre-existing psychological conditions.

If you see pictures of the men by the end of phase two, you will be shocked by how they looked. They have the appearance of skeletons, which, unfortunately, is not an uncommon sight in some raw food circles.

Raw foodists commonly brag about how few calories they need to eat, and there are many legends of long-term raw foodists being so clean, they can apparently survive on a few peaches a day while enjoying amazing health.

In my experience over the last 12 years and in dealing with thousands of raw foodists all over the world, I have come to the conclusion that raw foodists experience strong cravings for the simple reason that they are following a semi-starvation diet.

Even though raw foodists feel guilty about the amount of food they eat, the reality is that they simply don't eat enough to stay healthy.

The only reason raw foodists experience physical cravings is because they are not providing their body with what it really needs.

So what is missing?

Two things: carbohydrates and calories.

We know that there are three groups of nutrients that can be used as energy by the human body: carbohydrates, fats, and protein.

Carbohydrates represent by far the most important and most reliable source of energy for the human body. This is why almost all successful cultures on the planet eat a high-carb diet.

Experiments have been done that have shown that foods rich in carbohydrates, such as potatoes, are the best at curbing hunger and create a lasting sensation of satiety, and that is why many people refer to these foods as "comfort foods."[43]

The other group of nutrients that may help people feel full and satisfied is protein. In many experiments, a higher protein intake increases the feeling of satiety.[44] It is no surprise that most weight-loss meal plans focus on protein foods (such as salmon or chicken) with vegetables.

However, we also know from *The China Study* and more modern research that the regular consumption of high-protein, animal-based foods leads to a wide range of health problems, from heart disease to cancer.[45,46] We also know that although eating protein foods may feel satisfying, our needs for protein are very low and can easily be met by eating a variety of plant foods, as long as we eat enough of them to meet our needs.[47]

The last class of nutrient — fat — is universally recognized by nutrition experts to be the worst at helping people feel satisfied.[48] In fact, the more fat we eat, the hungrier we feel, because we are not giving our bodies the nutrients it really needs.

43 Anderson, G., &Woodend, D. (2003). Effect of Glycemic Carbohydrates on Short-term Satiety and Food Intake.Nutrition Reviews, 61(5), 1. Both high- and low-glycemic carbohydrates have an impact on satiety, but their effects have different time courses. High-glycemic carbohydrates are associated with a reduction in appetite and food intake in the short term (e.g., one hour), whereas the satiating effects of lower-glycemic carbohydrates appear to be delayed (e.g., 2 to 3 hours).

44 Solah, V., Zhu, K., Devine, A., Prince, R., Binns, C., Kerr, D., et al. (2010). Differences in satiety effects of alginate- and whey protein-based foods [electronic resource].*Appetite*, *54*(3), 485-491.

45 Bernstein, A., Sun, Q., Hu, F., Stampfer, M., Manson, J., & Willett, W. (2010).Major dietary protein sources and risk of coronary heart disease in women.*Circulation*, *122*(9), 876-883.

46 Micha, R., Wallace, S., &Mozaffarian, D. (2010). Red and processed meat consumption and risk of incident coronary heart disease, stroke, and diabetes mellitus: a systematic review and meta-analysis. *Circulation*, *121*(21), 2271-2283.

47 "Where do you get your protein?" The McDougall Newsletter, April 2007, **http://www.drmcdougall.com/misc/2007nl/apr/dairy.htm**

48 Potier, M., Fromentin, G., Lesdema, A., Benamouzig, R., Tomé, D., &Marsset-Baglieri, A. (2010). The satiety effect of disguised liquid preloads administered acutely and differing only in their nutrient content tended to be weaker for lipids but did not differ between proteins and carbohydrates in human subjects. *The British Journal Of Nutrition*, *104*(9), 1406-1414.

Raw foodists, in their zeal to achieve the most perfect diet in the world, have eliminated the most important sources of carbohydrates, with the possible exception of fruit. There are also very few high-protein foods in the raw vegan diet, so all that is left as a source of calories is FAT.

Most raw foodists are rather vague as to what one should eat in a typical day. David Wolfe did a good job of describing a typical menu in the first edition of the *Sunfood Diet Success System*. Let's take a look at one of the daily menus that is recommended in the book:

Morning: 3 pounds (1.4 kg) of watermelon (not seedless)

Afternoon: 2 mangos, 1 avocado, 3 sticks of celery

Snack: 2 mangos

Evening: One large lettuce, cucumber, tomato, and green onion salad with one handful of raw sunflower seeds, two avocados, and a fresh-squeezed lemon

What is the complete nutritional analysis of this menu? One very positive thing about the menu is that, unlike in most raw food books, it doesn't promote undereating, as it contains enough calories for many people.

If we eat everything that is recommended, we are getting about 2300 calories, which would be plenty for most women, but would fall short for most active, athletic young men.

In the book, David also warns us that the menus represent a lot of food and that many people will probably want to eat less than that. Although it's true that some people would probably need less, especially if they need to lose some weight, many active men and women would need more.

Nutritional analysis of this menu shows that 40% of calories come from fat, 7% from protein, and 53% from carbs, which is not as high fat as many raw foodists eventually reach once they start removing all the fruit from their diet.

In my experience, very few people manage this kind of diet over the long-term.

Eventually, the high percentage of fat in the diet (40%), which is just as high as a standard American diet, creates insulin resistance and makes the body too sensitive to fruit sugar. The natural instinct is to reduce the fruit sugar, instead of getting rid of the fat, which is the cause of the problem. Eventually, as raw foodists reduce the fruit content of their diet, they end up eating a diet that is much higher in fat (60% and up) and too low in calories, which accounts for ALL of their cravings and causes them to eat even more rich foods.

If you eat enough carbohydrates and enough food in general, you will NOT experience physical cravings. I repeat, you will NOT experience cravings.

But how much food is that? Following the same example, let's say we reformed the Sunfood menu to make it lower in fat, what would it look like?

Morning: 6 pounds of watermelon

Afternoon: 6 mangos, 3 sticks of celery

Snack: 2 mangos

Evening: One large lettuce, cucumber, tomato, and green onion salad ½ an avocado, OR one handful of sunflower seeds, and a fresh-squeezed lemon.

If we follow the menu above instead, we get between 2200 and 2400 calories (depending on whether you choose the sunflower seeds or the avocado), from 9 to 13% fat, and 5 to 7% protein (the higher numbers are for when eating 2 ounces of sunflower seeds).

The above menu would be perfect for a lot of active women, but it could be deficient for many active, athletic men.

If you are completely blown away by the quantities of food consumed, keep in mind that different fruits can be more or less concentrated in calories. Watermelon is not very dense, so to get enough calories one must eat a lot of it.

Eating large quantities of fruit, lots of vegetables and not too much fat (if you eat a fruit-based diet, I don't recommend going beyond 15%) is what is required to succeed on a 100% raw food diet and eliminate cravings completely. It's as simple as that.

In the DVD accompanying this book (for more information, go to www.rawcontroversies.com/dvds), I go into more detail about the specific nutritional aspects of the diet. Also, later in the book, I will give you more options, for those who prefer not to eat 100% raw.

CHAPTER 13

How I Became a Gourmet Raw Food Chef

"If I told you you'd never have to count calories, fat grams, or whatever, that you could eat whatever or whenever you want, eat banana cream pie for breakfast, enchiladas for dinner, and a chocolate dessert... and you'd feel better than you ever felt in your whole life - nobody has ever said "No" to that challenge!"

Alissa Cohen,
Raw Food Chef

In early 1999, I went to a raw food potluck somewhere in Southern California and met an Idaho-born wanderer named Andrew, a few years my elder, with whom I would form a very deep friendship that would last for years.

Andrew was a modern-day nomad, a self-proclaimed truth-seeker, who was inordinately well-spoken and erudite. His brother Paul was a rock star (a music with which I would eventually develop a deep connection and love), and his dad, an inventor, but Andrew hadn't yet settled to any one path. He had studied music, had experimented with fasting, had spent many years studying Objectivism (the philosophy of Ayn Rand), and displayed a wide range of skills in a variety of fields, yet did not seem committed to any one of them, except for this personal search for truth and knowledge.

He had recently relocated to San Diego, where he was extremely keen on the idea of starting or being involved in some sort of raw food community.

At the potluck where I met him, Andrew told me he was looking for a place in San Diego. I told him about the weird place where I was staying in City Heights, and said, "Well, if you find anything, let me know, because I'm looking for someplace better too."

A few weeks later, Andrew called me and said he might have found a place where I could stay. He had befriended an older woman by the name of Tera, who lived in a decent neighborhood and had a room for rent. For $400, I could have the room.

I gathered from the conversation that Andrew wasn't renting that room himself because he was sharing a space in Tera's bed. However, this fling wasn't going to last, and he could not afford the room anyway.

For me, it turned out to be perfect. Finally, I could live in a house, with a real room and a real bed, not some kind of shack down a canyon in a shady neighborhood. Instead of having to walk up a canyon to get to the kitchen and the toilet, I could just step out of my room. I was also looking forward to a good night's sleep without the disturbance of dogs barking or police helicopters flying over my head. Tera seemed like a decent lady, although a bit excessively paranoid about everything. She quickly accepted me as her new renter, and so I moved in with my modest possessions.

At the same time, Stephen at *Nature's First Law* had bought me a used iMac on eBay, one of those Bondi blue models that were so popular in the late 90s. Although I was to pay him back from what the magazine would earn, I was extremely grateful for his generosity and desire to help me succeed. The iMac was also my first computer ever, one that I could use to unleash my creative powers, start my own websites, and take *Just Eat an Apple* to the next level.

In exchange for helping me find a place to stay, I helped Andrew find some work in San Diego by convincing *Nature's First Law* that he would make a great part-time employee. David's business had grown to the point where he needed more help, so Andrew was there at the right time.

He still hadn't found a place to stay, though, and although he would visit Tera's house, and even camped in the backyard sometimes, he eventually stopped seeing her altogether. For a week, his best option was to sleep in a canyon near *Nature's First Law's* offices.

I could not believe my eyes when I saw him in the morning, his hair a mess and his face covered by ant bites. "You slept in a canyon?" I asked.

For almost a week, Andrew slept in the canyon, until he could not take it anymore, and found refuge at a Buddhist temple in San Diego. During that time, we were joking that he was probably the only homeless person in the world *with an actual job!*

At Tera's house, I started making dinner every night for everybody — Tera, Andrew when he was there, and other friends that would stop by. At that point, I had gathered a lot of ideas by watching what all those people were doing in various raw food restaurants in California, and I felt confident enough to start making my own creations.

The nickname of *Raw Demolition* was serving me well once again. Andrew claimed that whenever I entered the kitchen, I left it a complete mess and disaster half an hour later, but I redeemed myself by serving him the most delicious salad he ever had.

Compliments like this convinced me that I should probably start putting these recipes together in some kind of book. Then, I got an idea.

I asked David Wolfe, who was coming out with his book *The Sunfood Diet Success System* what he thought of the idea of me writing a companion recipe book called *Sunfood Cuisine*. David thought the idea was terrific, and told me something that sounded familiar again. "Write the book, Fred, and we'll publish it!"

Suddenly, I became a mad scientist in the kitchen every day. Although I had never figured out how to cook in my life, the raw food diet unleashed my creative power, and I suddenly understood how to make foods taste good.

Even though I had been extremely sick a few months before and had to heal myself by fasting and avoiding fat completely, I did not know for certain what had caused my sickness. So I went right back to eating raw recipes. I decided to limit the quantity of nuts, though, or avoid them for a while. However, I still wanted to be a raw foodist. In California, all the raw foodists were still eating raw recipes, so I didn't know what else to do.

I discovered that by combining certain basic flavors, I could make anything taste amazing. My formula for making a tasty salad was to combine the following categories of ingredients together:

Crunchy/Bitter — Green vegetables

Tangy/Sour — Lemon juice, lime juice, or apple cider vinegar

Fatty/Creamy — Avocado, oil, or nut butters

Salty — Sea salt, sea vegetables, Nama Shoyu, or tamari sauce

Sweet — Fruits, dried fruit, or honey

Spicy — garlic, onion, or hot peppers

Unsurprisingly, my "amazing discovery" was one that most chefs in the world have made at some point or another. Even Thai cuisine explicitly advises this sort of flavor combination in most dishes (in particular sweet, sour, salty, and spicy altogether).

Although I was trying to reduce my consumption of nuts and seeds after my mysterious illness, in order to make those raw food recipes taste great, I felt I needed to use good amounts of oils and plentiful avocado. Eventually, my "no-nuts" policy went out the window, and I also started to make use of nuts and seeds in my recipes.

What recipes could be made raw, besides salad?

I became famous for my raw pizza with sprouted wheat, Nori Rolls, Thai coconut soup, and a few other dishes. I had tasted each of these recipes somewhere and tried to reproduce it in my kitchen without a recipe or ingredient list, giving it my own personal twist.

In June 1999, David Wolfe and Stephen were generous and kind enough to invite me to attend a raw food retreat on the island of Maui, organized by raw food author and chef Jeremy Safron. In exchange for attending the retreat, I just needed to help in the kitchen.

To me, that was a perfect exchange, because working in the kitchen with experienced raw food chefs in Maui was not work, it was mentoring!

All the raw food chefs I met were concerned about one thing only: making the food taste good. They felt that the "health" aspect of the food was already taken care of by eating everything raw, so now it was just a matter of trying out different combinations of foods to make them more appealing and tasty.

In Maui, I learned many new recipes, such as Jeremy's famous sprouted wild rice salad. It consisted of raw wild rice, soaked almost a day to make it soft (until the rice "opened"), and then seasoned with a good amount of olive oil and avocado, vegetables, some salty seasoning, such as Bragg's Liquid Aminos, and the sweetness of maple syrup (which is not really raw, but is widely used as a vegan alternative to honey.)

Jeremy also had another signature dish: a raw pizza that actually tasted good! The crust was not dry like the one I used to make, but rather moist and filling. He made a peculiar mixture of some kind of raw grain, sprouted and ground, with nuts, vegetables and seasonings, and then partially dehydrated it before adding the other pizza toppings.

Almost every dish we made contained oil, avocado or nuts and seeds. I did not realize it, but I was fully back on track with the high-fat raw food diet, which was the only trendy way to eat raw.

Fortunately, I also discovered some amazing tropical fruits that I had never tasted before, such as the famous *canistel* or eggfruit, which has the consistency of cooked egg yolk, but is sweet. I ate so much of it that eventually just the thought of eating another eggfruit made me feel sick.

I continued to bathe in the raw food lifestyle day after day, and my inspiration to continue being raw was not at all changed by my mysterious illness. I did not really know what to think of it. Why did I get sick? Maybe it was a healing crisis. Maybe I had done something wrong (I suspected the raw chickpeas, which I quit eating from that point forward). Maybe it was the emotional distress, or maybe a combination of all of the above. One thing I never suspected was the raw food diet itself. How could going back to natural foods make you sick? I refused to even entertain the notion.

After the Maui retreat, I felt much more confident in my skills as a raw food chef. One person I had learned a tremendous amount from was Suzie Bohannon, who worked as a chef under the tutelage of Jeremy and who also lived in Maui at the time. At the end of the retreat, we all stood in a circle and publicly thanked everyone and said one thing we appreciated about someone else. Suzie stood up and said, "Well, there's someone I'd like to acknowledge... and that's Frederic!" She then looked at me and said, "...for your taste buds!" I felt incredibly flattered by what she said, because I had worked hard to improve my skills as a raw food chef and because I now felt that I knew what kinds of raw foods tasted good together and which ones didn't.

I continued working on the book *Sunfood Cuisine* until I finished it in January 2000. It was then published in 2002 by David Wolfe's company, where it remained in print and distribution until 2008, when it was discontinued. When the publishing rights reverted to me at that time, I decided I would no longer publish and distribute it, but instead I made it available as a free bonus on my website.

Why? Although there is great information in *Sunfood Cuisine,* and the recipes sure taste good, I then went through many painful years of trial and error to realize that gourmet raw food cuisine is fundamentally unhealthy. Gourmet raw food cuisine is based on the false premise that raw foods are always better than cooked foods, and just switching to eating all-raw is enough to make you healthy regardless of how much fat you eat.

What's Wrong with Raw Food Recipes?

Until experience proved me wrong, I used to explain the idea of the raw food diet as follows:

We should be eating a raw food diet because raw foods are foods in their natural state, while cooked foods are damaged foods. No other animal in nature cooks its food, and also no other animal is as sick as we are. Raw foods contain vital energy, such as enzymes, that are completely destroyed in the cooking process. When we eat raw, we keep all of the vitality that these foods would have lost being cooked. Also, cooked foods are all toxic to some degree because of the damaged molecules and carcinogens that are created during the cooking process.

As human beings, we've eaten raw foods for most of our history on this planet, so going back to raw is just going back to the natural order of things.

When I look at the description above, I now find that almost every single concept is just plain false and misleading. Yet, I still recommend a raw food diet for optimal health. So what has changed? Here's how I explain the concept of the raw food diet today:

Eating a raw food diet is optimal because fruits and vegetables are the most biologically appropriate and clean foods for the human body. Raw foods are also superior to cooked foods because they tend to contain more nutrients, and by eating raw, we avoid the common and potentially carcinogenic toxins that are sometimes created in the cooking process. But the main advantage of the raw food diet is that it forces us to eliminate sub-optimal foods that are making us sick. These foods include: animal products (including meat, dairy products, fish and eggs), refined sugar, grains (especially bread and gluten-containing foods), and industrialized foods and condiments (including salt). With these foods out of the way, and by providing the body with what it needs (an abundance of fruits and vegetables), the healing process can take place. The raw foods themselves have no healing power, and the absence of disease-producing foods is what does the real magic.

However, to get the full benefits from a raw food diet, it is absolutely imperative to eat enough calories to maintain your energy levels and to get those calories in the form of fruit, instead of large quantities of fat (found in avocados, nuts, seeds, and oils), which should be limited to no more than 15% of total calories.

Because raw food chefs are only concerned with the *rawness* of foods, they don't tend to calculate the amount of fat or the nutritional profile of a meal.

They tend to want to reproduce the tastes and qualities of cooked foods by using raw ingredients, and to do that, they end up using large quantities of fat.

When a raw food chef creates a raw version of a common dish, such as mashed potatoes, by replacing the potatoes with pureed cauliflower, we tend to automatically think, "Oh, how healthy! Eating cauliflower instead of those evil cooked potatoes!"

However, no one would eat a dish of mashed "potatoes" if it was made with some chopped up cauliflower and a few vegetables. It wouldn't have any of the creaminess that we associate with mashed potatoes. So, the raw food chef will add copious amounts of something fatty like cashews and oil, as well as seasonings and salt, to transform the plain vegetable into a mighty powerful dish.

But what happened in the process? We replaced the relatively healthy carbohydrates in the cooked potatoes with *fat*, and added nothing else to replace the missing carbs. And as we already know, vegetables like cauliflower are very low in calories and thus are low in carbs.

We're ending up with a dish that, nutritionally speaking, is almost 100% fat (by percentage of calories).

Yes, the food is raw, but is it healthy? Long-term health simply cannot be achieved on such a high-fat, low-carb diet. It would be better indeed to eat a dish of cooked potatoes, processed in a food processor without any fat, to make mashed potatoes, rather than the raw version of "mashed potatoes," which is essentially nuts and fat disguised as something else.

If you look at any other raw recipe, you will find the same process in action. For example, you could make raw spaghetti by replacing the pasta with zucchini noodles, but the result would be only a few calories' worth of vegetables. Even if you covered it in a special, tasty tomato sauce, you would at best get a salad that might delight your taste buds, but it would do nothing for relieving your hunger and satisfying your need for food.

So, raw food chefs will solve the problem by making the dish more "consistent" and "satisfying," which usually involves a different sauce made with... guess what? More nuts, seeds, nut butters, avocados, or oil (like in a rich pesto sauce or a creamy cashew Alfredo). Again, we've replaced the carbohydrates of pasta with a calorie source that is almost 100% fat.

So what can be done? I will discuss the details of the diet later in this book, but for now, suffice it to say that raw food chefs would benefit from a lesson or two in nutrition.

First, it is just not possible to replace familiar cooked food dishes, such as pizza and macaroni, with raw dishes without making those raw dishes full of fat. The taste buds simply have to get used to new tastes and try new foods instead.

Otherwise, it would be like the vegetarian that insists on eating meat substitutes all the time, but not changing his diet otherwise, continuing to eat hot dogs, hamburgers, and turkey... except all vegetarian! The real vegetarian doesn't need all of these meat substitutes, although he may eat them occasionally. Instead, he prefers to focus on vegetarian foods, such as lentils, vegetables, beans and potatoes for calories.

Likewise, the real raw foodist does not need to eat foods that resemble or taste like cooked foods. Instead, she focuses on healthy raw foods, such as fruits and vegetables, with limited quantities of nuts, seeds, and avocados.

What about the taste? How can you eliminate the fat and still make a delicious raw meal?

The answer is simple: by using more fruit. Raw food chefs know how to use vegetables, but they don't know how to use fruit.

In my new version of raw food cuisine, I have limited my use of nuts and seeds and other fats, and instead, I use more fruits and vegetables than ever, with an emphasis on fruit to add flavor. I now easily combine fruits with vegetable fruits *together* in one dish for interesting and delicious results.

For example, I may make a raw soup by using vegetables, such as tomato, cucumber, dill, etc. In the past, I would have added some fat to cream it up, and salt to make it savory. Now, I rely on the natural taste of the vegetables and herbs, and instead, I add a sweetener (usually a whole fruit like peach or mango) to totally transform the taste of the soup and make it more satisfying at the same time. No fat is used, yet the result is surprisingly good.

Where was the boundless energy? When was I going to experience those amazing benefits of the raw food diet? What was wrong with me?

I was asking myself these questions on a regular basis. By the summer of 1999, I had been eating 100% raw for over two years, without any exceptions. The theory that "over time, the cooked food cells will be purged from your system, and you will feel amazing" did not hold much water anymore.

I was left with one possible answer: I needed to fast.

I became convinced that the one thing I had never tried that could possibly turn my health around was a long fast.

I had read about water fasting, about juice fasting, and other detox programs, but I had not done any of them, except a short three-day fast, back when I had first gotten started in Natural Hygiene.

By reading more about fasting, I became convinced that a 14-day fast was what I needed to finally get my health back in order.

Unfortunately, I looked online at all the different retreats that offered hygienic fasting, and all of them charged rates I simply could not afford. I was left with one option: to fast on my own.

My little room in San Diego wasn't appropriate for a 14-day fast. Tera would probably freak out and wonder what I was doing, maybe worry about my health and send me to the hospital.

So I called Barbara in Escondido and asked her if she would mind if I came to visit for two weeks and fasted. Barbara was well-versed in some of Shelton's work, so I was sure she would be sympathetic to my quest for health and desire to fast. I told her I could repay her by doing work on her property--before or after the fast, of course; not during (as I intended to spend the whole time resting in bed and drinking water, as Shelton had advised).

Barbara had access to some good distilled water in huge glass jugs, and her ranch was peaceful and relaxing. I felt I had found the perfect location to fast.

I was very excited to see how this fast would transform my health. I honestly thought that at the end of the 14 days, I would be a transformed version of myself — purer, healthier, and finally where I had always wanted to be.

The first two days of the fast went well. However, I felt quite hungry all the time, and I couldn't stop thinking about food.

On day three, I started feeling very weak, and my cravings for food grew stronger and stronger. I kept walking in front of Barbara's kitchen, and seeing her stash of Reed avocados, grapes and oranges made me salivate.

At the same time, Barbara became extremely preoccupied with my condition. "Are you sure you're okay?" "Do you think you're doing the right thing?" Her tension was palpable, and as my fast went on, I realized she was just not comfortable with the idea.

On day four, I started feeling unwell. I was hungry, drained of energy, and something was happening in my body that I did not understand and did not like. (I had gone into the stage of ketosis, where my body started to feed on my meager fat reserves).

On day five, I could not take it anymore and broke the fast. I had fasted for a total of 4 days. Barbara was relieved to hear my decision, and confessed to me that her main worry was that I was drinking all the water, and she only had limited supplies of distilled water!

I spent a few more days eating fruit (and some avocado, I admit) at Barbara's place, and then headed back to San Diego.

When I saw David again, he was not surprised to hear that I had broken the fast after four days. He told me that he had made a bet with other people that I would give up after this exact number of days.

I did not ask him why he was so sure I couldn't stick with my initial intentions, but the truth is that I had no idea what I had gotten into. Maybe this was why all the professional Natural Hygienists who supervised fasting always advised people never to attempt a long fast on their own.

If water-fasting was too extreme for me, then maybe some other form of cleansing was what I needed.

In the summer of 1999, I got invited to participate in a raw food retreat organized by David Jubb and his wife Annie in the heart of Oklahoma, on a site previously occupied by Native Americans and now used by spiritual and other kinds of self-improvement retreats.

David Jubb was an interesting character from New York City who was the archetypal raw food guru. Originally from Australia, he had relocated to New York City, where he practiced alternative medicine and advised people on his special type of raw food diet. He would often come to San Diego to give talks, so I had already seen him several times.

Jubb looked quite healthy, and he looked more like the type of metrosexual guy who dresses trendy and works out at the gym than your typical hippie raw foodist. Yet at the same time, he often dressed in ponchos and other Native American attire, wearing feathers and random trinkets.

His health philosophy was unlike anything I had ever heard before. He claimed to be a liquidarian himself, living on nothing but limited amounts of liquid foods, even borderlining toward becoming a breatharian.

Among his various heresies was the belief that certain commonly-eaten, heavily hybridized raw foods, such as carrots and bananas, were evil because they contained a type of sugar that "hurt the liver."

He was also was a big proponent of the liver flush, a type of cleanse where one would drink an entire cup of olive oil with a lot of lemon juice, as well as making a few other preparatory changes, in order to get rid of a surprising number of "gallstones" that most of us mere mortals, having previously lived on the Standard American Diet, were harboring unknowingly. Users of this liver flush reported a great feeling of enhanced health when they finally got rid of these gallstones (which required several flushes).

He also consumed and advocated a large number of special powders and supplements that no raw foodist I knew would ever touch with a ten-foot pole. Things like MSM, supplemental enzymes, seaweeds, Celtic sea salt, green powders, various medicinal herbs, and other strange items were all part of his arsenal of tools for optimal health.

His health philosophy was a lot more complicated and complex than the typical advice of "Just eat raw foods, and you will be healthy." He made advanced concoctions, such as raw soups and smoothies, where every single ingredient had some kind of specific purpose.

His recipes were no longer indulgences where the idea was to simply turn a cooked dish into a raw one, but instead, they became a prescription for health. "That energy soup that you're drinking? It's no longer just food — it's a remedy, an elixir for health." The same went for his famous raw pizza, which contained a perfect balance of raw ingredients and superfoods, such as spirulina and seaweed.

Before David Jubb, I had never even heard the word "superfoods" or seriously considered things like spirulina and seaweed. But the more he visited San Diego to give his lectures, the more his influence began to be felt in the raw food movement.

David Wolfe himself, a simple eater of mostly whole raw fruits and vegetables and avocados at the time I met him, was now becoming influenced by Jubb's philosophy. He started experimenting with all those superfoods, started using Celtic sea salt (even though he had always been against salt before that), eating seaweed, and even tried some of the supplements that Jubb recommended. Whenever I would go to David's home, I would see him carefully reading and analyzing one of Jubb's books, taking copious notes, obviously mesmerized by his information.

Through Jubb, I got introduced to the New York City raw food scene, which was quite a sophisticated bunch compared to the raw foodists of the California scene, whose diet seemed somewhat primitive by comparison.

Jubb's influence started to be felt. Every other raw foodist I met had given up carrot juice and bananas, because they were trying to avoid "hybrids" like Jubb had recommended (even though they could not exactly explain the reason why.)

There was certainly something attractive in Jubb's philosophy — even though it was something that contradicted all the reasoning of Natural Hygiene that originally attracted me to the raw food diet.

I was very surprised when David's wife, Annie, invited me to come for free to their $2000 two-week long event in Oklahoma. "Why don't you just come?" she said. "We'll figure out some way for you to help."

Two weeks with David Jubb and his crew? I could not refuse the invitation, so I booked my flight to Oklahoma, a place I knew nothing about.

The retreat was set on a gorgeous piece of land that featured a lake, a complete playground with ropes and harnesses and obstacle courses (I suspected that we would make use of these items during the retreat, but why?), as well as a large building with an industrial kitchen and enough space for many people to hang out, complete with couches everywhere and a fireplace.

Again, I was put to use in the kitchen, where I concocted my favorite raw food recipes, but this time, I added the special David Jubb twist, by including his favorite ingredients, like Celtic sea salt and pumpkin seeds, and avoiding the evil ones, like carrots and bananas.

The retreat started full of romance and intrigues worthy of a soap opera — this time, a raw one. Jeremy Safron was present at the retreat, but this time as Annie Jubb's boyfriend. Apparently, Annie and David had broken up, but they were not officially divorced and were still working together. Jeremy was the new boyfriend, and apparently, David didn't mind having him around.

The retreat itself featured a combination of various "self-improvement" exercises, where we had to go through our fears by accomplishing feats that seemed dangerous but were completely safe. For example, we were asked to climb a tall telephone-pole looking thing and stand on top, where there was a tiny square, just big enough for one person to stand. We were then asked to jump to the other side to grab a trapeze. Of course, we were fully harnessed, so it was safe. But it was still really scary!

In between those days of exercises, David Jubb would give cryptic lectures at night, where he would talk for long periods about strange topics, ranging from cellular nutrition to his philosophy on life and spirituality. Everybody seemed mesmerized, even though not much of what he was saying made sense. Sometimes, I would be asked to play my guitar during the evening, while David was conducting a type of meditation.

Everyone who followed David Jubb had a special tribe name. For example, the man who hosted David when he came to give his lectures was also known as Fred Silverbear. There was also a pretty woman who went by the name of "Raven."

During the retreat, I even received my own animal name from Jubb himself: *Goodvoice Elk*. Jubb told me that I had the elegant and unassuming qualities of the Elk, and that my path in life was to continue to spread my message.

Another activity of the retreat was a sweat lodge, an ancient spiritual ritual learned from Native Americans. Over the course of the two weeks I spent there, we did about five sweat lodges, which was a tremendous amount. Fortunately, each sweat lodge was done on a small scale and organized properly and safely.[49]

The retreat culminated in a fire walk — another native ritual. The ground would be filled with hot coals, and we would have to walk on them. Proper preparation and the power of the mind would enable us not to get burned. (In reality, if you walk at a steady pace, you will generally not get burned. It has nothing to do with the power of the mind.)

During the retreat, everybody seemed to be having a good time, but I knew something else was going on behind the scenes. I heard Jeremy Safron express a lot of criticism towards David Jubb, saying that everybody was just being "brainwashed" and didn't realize what was really going on.

I could now see another side of Jubb that I had not known before. Was he really who he claimed to be? Jubb considered himself to be so advanced that he almost claimed he was a breatharian.

---

[49]   In October 2009, the self-improvement guru James Ray led a $10,000 sweat lodge retreat in Arizona that led to the death of three participants and the hospitalization of 18 others.

Yet, in reality, his friends told me that he couldn't live without Starbucks coffee, as he loved to drink strong espresso. He also smoked tobacco (for "spiritual reasons"), and regularly ate all kinds of junk food, as he said that "nobody could be 100% congruent."

I had no problem with Jubb not being perfect, but it was disturbing to hear that when in most circumstances he claimed to be some kind of superbeing that could live on a few ounces of juice a day. This made the rest of us feel inadequate and aspire to be at his level, destroying our health in the process.

Although I did not fully accept Jubb's philosophy as truth, I had gathered some interesting ideas from the Oklahoma retreat, and I was eager to put them into action.

Who knows, maybe I needed to do a liver flush. I also wanted to try a long juice fast to see what would happen. During the retreat, I spent a good part of my free time hanging out with Raven, who was a beautiful brunette in her thirties who lived in New York City and was at the heart of the raw food scene there. I had so much fun in her presence, laughing and eating fruit, that I started to feel something for her. Again, it was another one of those impossible love stories that I was building, and somehow, unconsciously, I was following the same process I had gone through with Claudia. I kissed Raven the very last day of the retreat, just when we were about to leave for the airport. "I hope to see you again, Fred," she said with a smile. I just loved how she said my name with her East Coast accent.

After the Oklahoma retreat, I knew I was ready for something new, but what?

In my travels in California, I had met a British guy named Michael, who had become a good friend. I first met Michael at the *Raw* restaurant in San Francisco.

Michael claimed to have once been part of the British Special Services, having been raised in a military family. He had fought in wars on several occasions and had killed people. After his military career, his desire for adrenaline manifested in his pursuit of *base jumping*, an unusual use of "parachuting," where you jump off buildings with a chute and hope to make it alive at the bottom. According to his story, he had jumped from the Empire State Building once, a feat that put him on a major US evening talk show. After a series of similar life experiences, he was now a follower of eco-living and raw foods, and quite militant about it too. I suspected him to be an eco-terrorist as well.

Although I seriously doubted that everything Michael said was true, he seemed real enough, and who knows, maybe his story was too. One thing was for sure: Michael had a charismatic personality and could convince anyone of anything. He told me that he was moving to Arizona to work at Gabriel Cousens' raw food retreat there, called the *Tree of Life*.

He had managed to end up as the managing Chef at Gabriel's retreat in Arizona, even with his limited experience, and he was in charge of all the menus for the chefs. He told me I could move there, help in the kitchen, and get free room and board. It would be a perfect situation for me to continue working on my magazine *Just Eat an Apple.*

I already knew of Dr. Gabriel Cousens, because his giant book, *Spiritual Nutrition,* was one of the first raw food books I had come across.

So I showed up there in the fall of 1999, and then immediately started making raw food recipes in the kitchen with Michael and his long-haired assistant.

Tree of Life was a fairly new retreat center set on a large piece of land in Patagonia, at the very south of Arizona, close to the border with Mexico. There was a main building where the kitchen was, where the guests came to eat their meals, another building where they slept, as well as buildings just down the road in town, where Gabriel's offices were located.

On the actual land of *Tree of Life*, there were also several Native American tipis, where Gabriel would conduct his meditations, as well as mini-sweat lodges, as he was a believer in Native American spirituality.

When I first showed up, they didn't know where to put me, so they decided to place me in an entire unfinished building down the road near town. It looked more like a big room in a warehouse, but it had been cleared out, and had a bed. I also had a desk, where I placed my Bondi Blue iMac to work on the magazine.

In the kitchen of *Tree of Life*, they had an extremely well-organized set of raw food menus for the month. Each day of the week had a different theme, for example "Indian Recipes" or "Asian-Inspired Recipes." They followed a pattern, and the same recipes would be repeated over the course of the month in cycles as the weeks went by.

Breakfast at *Tree of Life* consisted of a limited amount of fresh fruit, along with soaked dried fruits with some spices and nuts added, and nut milk. Lunch was the main meal of the day, and it consisted of various kinds of salads, according to the menu, and usually one kind of heavy main course such as a nut pâté. Dinner was supposed to be light and sometimes non-existent, as Gabriel himself only ate two meals a day and skipped dinner altogether (although he sometimes ate some fruit or soup at around 3p.m.).

The staff that worked in the kitchen often complained of this heavy fare of nuts and fats, and Michael's assistant often fasted on grapes (eating only grapes for a few days) and avoided eating most of the heavy recipes they were making. This behavior was consistent with other raw food chefs I had met, who prepared all of these heavy gourmet raw foods for people, but did not eat them themselves. This was something that I had only witnessed in the raw food movement, and it was frequent.

Gabriel was excited to have me as part of his team, as he had heard of my reputation via Michael and knew I was already involved in the raw food movement. He also wanted me to be part of his community and come to the regular meditation sessions and sweat lodges they organized, which was not of great interest to me.

Not so long after my arrival at *Tree of Life*, my friend Andrew joined our little team and easily secured a job in the accounting department.

Almost all of us ate the nut-rich foods served at *Tree of Life*, and we felt worse and worse as the weeks went by. It did not seem logical to me that this was the food we served to guests as the healthiest diet in the world, and yet all of us working in the kitchen were trying to avoid it, because it made us feel sick and tired.

I started to think that perhaps the reason Gabriel and the rest of the *Tree of Life* staff felt compelled to stop eating after 3 p.m. was the fact that the lunches served were so heavy in fat. Many guests and staff would often eat a very large serving of nut pâté with vegetables for lunch, and follow it with a generous amount of raw pie (complete with cashew frosting). The amount of fat contained in those two dishes combined must have been at least 100 grams (or the equivalent of three avocados). How could they feel hungry for dinner after eating that kind of lunch?

To see how I would feel, I started skipping dinner like Gabriel. I discovered that in spite of doing that, I would still feel the effects of eating all this fat-heavy food the next day.

The more time I spent at *Tree of Life*, the more I started to question this approach to raw foods and health. Many guests who came to *Tree of Life* for a few weeks also left with a giant box of supplements to take home. Yet, in Gabriel's first book, no mention was ever made of all these supplements that were recommended at the retreat center that he ran.

I felt that Gabriel was genuine, but at the time, I thought his prescribing of supplements and other pills did not seem any different from the regular medical profession, except that it was combined with raw foods and a form of spirituality.

Speaking of spirituality, the more time I spent at *Tree of Life*, the more pressure I got from Gabriel for not attending the spiritual meetings with the rest of the community. I would sometimes show up for a meditation session, but I preferred to spend most of my free time working on my magazine *Just Eat an Apple*.

Although I had nothing against meditation, my goal in coming to *Tree of Life* was to learn to become a better raw food chef, and I had no intention of adopting their special brand of spirituality, which combined Native American rituals and Eastern teachings.

There were a few activities led by *Tree of Life* that interested me. One was the monthly juice fast, where guests came for a week to drink nothing but juice, and spend an inordinate amount of time meditating inside tipis. After this "juice fast," many reported feeling amazingly well.

I felt more than a little "blah" from eating all of these gourmet raw foods, so I decided I would give the juice fast a chance.

My experience trying to do a water fast on my own had been a failure, but perhaps juice fasting would be easier, because I would still be providing my body some nutrients, albeit in a liquid form.

For the juice fast, I decided to follow Gabriel's program, at the same time that he was leading the juice fast for his guests. However, I could not attend all the meditation sessions, since I had to work in the kitchen preparing the juices.

Two types of juices were prepared for the juice fast:

Green juices — which combined celery, kale, parsley, and other greens, with a touch of lemon, and perhaps a little carrot.

Fruit juices — like apple or grapes, which were to be diluted with an equal amount of water. According to Gabriel, this made the sugars easier to assimilate.

In the green juices, it was also possible to add some spices, such as curry or cayenne.

My first few days on the juice fast went well, but on the third day, I felt like my blood sugar was all over the place. As soon as I drank a juice, I would feel a rush of sugar to my brain, and I felt hyperactive and was unable to concentrate. Then, an hour or two later, I would "crash" and feel depressed.

Gabriel suggested that I switch to green juices only instead, but when I did, I felt I had absolutely no energy to do anything at all.

Finally, I was forced to end the juice fast on the morning of the 6th day, because I was simply not able to muster enough energy to keep working in the kitchen. After eating a few whole grapes, my energy came back, and I completed the last two days of work for the guests who were juice fasting.

Although this juice fasting experience was not a complete failure, it made me realize the direness of my situation. For over three years, I had been following the path of raw foods, initially with Mosséri's diet, and then with the 100% raw diet in California.

Yet, I felt worse than I ever had in my life, and every attempt I made to improve things by cleansing and following the advice raw food experts gave me had failed.

Was there one thing I hadn't tried?

CHAPTER 14

My Meeting with a Breatharian

"Anyone who wishes to live entirely on prana can do it."

Jasmuheen

When I first met my friend Andrew, he told me he was a vegetarian. I asked him how long it had been since he had eaten meat.

"Over 10 years, but last year, I did eat some burgers."

"Why?" I asked.

"I was learning about breatharianism, and I met Wiley Brooks."

"Who's Wiley Brooks"? I wondered.

"He's a breatharian... well, he claims he is."

"So... he lives on air, but he eats burgers?"

"Well... he says he doesn't need to eat but *chooses* to. He wanted me to get over my obsession with healthy eating, as a first step towards becoming a breatharian. So I followed his recommendations and ate some junk food."

"Burgers?"

"Yes."

This Wiley Brooks character puzzled me, so I did some research on him. Apparently, the guy had been promoting breatharianism since the early 80s, when he appeared on the TV show *That's Incredible*, apparently lifting an insane amount of weight, something like 10 times his body weight (Wiley is a tall skinny guy who only weighs 135 pounds).

After claiming to be a breatharian, he was caught on one occasion leaving a convenience store with a big Slurpee, a hot dog, and Twinkies in his hands. On another occasion, he was caught with a *quarter-pounder burger with cheese* from McDonald's. Shots from his junk food binging habits were apparently published in a local newspaper, with a headline like "Breatharian Caught!"

Wiley believes that he has the capacity to live on nothing but air, but that electro-magnetic and other types of pollution are preventing him from doing so for an indefinite period of time. Therefore, he lives on air most of the time, except when he's having a quarter-pounder cheeseburger and a diet soda from McDonald's.

Wiley believes that our world is a three-dimensional universe in which people must eat. But in other dimensions, specifically the fifth dimension, everybody is breatharian and no one needs to eat anything. (Apparently, the sex is also awesome there too.)

Therefore, he offers private workshops to teach people how to reach the fifth dimension and learn to be a breatharian. This private workshop is available for the low price of only one billion dollars!

On his website, **www.breatharian.com**, Wiley claims to have lived past lives as a number of famous people, including Jesus and Zeus. Apparently he does not remember ever having a past life as a person who was not famous.

Brooks explains why he consumes McDonalds' food. According to him, the *double quarter-pounder with cheese* from McDonalds is a fifth-dimension food (5d) and "possesses a special base frequency." That's why he recommends it for breatharians over fruits and vegetables. Brooks also thinks that diet coke is "liquid light" and says:

"The 5d qualities in the diet coke acts as a type of binding agent which binds all other sugars and toxins (after-effects) in the meal being digested at that time to the beef in the burger. The beef acts as a catalyst that draws these toxins to the digestive tract and escorts them out of the body as waste."[50, 51]

That's how my friend Andrew ended up eating a cheeseburger after almost a decade as a vegetarian.

---

50 Reference: http://www.breatharian.com/breatharians.html
51 For your information, a Quarter-Pounder Burger with Cheese yields 420 calories and contains 28 grams of fat, and 730 mg of sodium. Surprisingly, that's less than most raw food recipes.

211

When I was in San Diego, one day, the phone rang at Morten's house. I picked it up, and it was Wiley Brooks on the other end. He wanted to talk to one of my friends.

"Hi, this is Wiley Brooks, the breatharian."

"You're a breatharian?" I asked.

"Yes. There's a few of us out there…"

After hearing about Wiley Brooks, I did not think much about breatharianism until David Wolfe invited Jasmuheen, a famous Australian breatharian, to come give a lecture in San Diego.

Jasmuheen had just written a book called *Living on Light* that *Nature's First Law* carried. David seemed to have developed a fascination with breatharianism.

"Do you think it's possible?" I asked him.

"Oh, I think it's possible…once you've reached a certain level." he said.

I attended the seminar that Jasmuheen gave in San Diego, along with a few dozen motivated truth-seekers. David was even hosting her in his home. I was curious to find out if she really did live on air as she claimed.

"She drinks tea," David said, "with honey. Sometimes, she'll eat something else, but the whole time she stayed with me I didn't see her eat anything."

David was even embarrassed to have to go to the health food store to buy Jasmuheen her favorite brand of tea, as this was not a *Nature's First Law* "approved" item (i.e. raw).

When Jasmuheen arrived in San Diego, she had a cold that lasted throughout the seminar weekend. Her immune system was probably so weak from eating so little that she got sick very easily, but at the time, she rationalized her cold in some other way.

She looked frail to me, but not dying. She did have good concentration, but was not vibrant. She also left the seminar with over $4000 in cash as her fee.

Over the years, I've met many people who have tried to become breatharians, or claimed they could live on air. In all instances, these people occasionally ate food, usually claiming they only did it for "pleasure" and not nourishment.

It's not surprising that the human body can live on very little nourishment. Wiley Brooks is now 74 and looks healthier than most people of his age. He walks a lot and lives on a diet of occasional McDonald's cheeseburgers and diet coke. Without knowing it, he is practicing caloric restriction, which is the only proven method to extend the life of any animal.

When Jasmuheen visited San Diego, she claimed to have gone for a few years without food. She admitted that sometimes she ate food for "pleasure," and like most breatharians, it was not always the healthiest fare (chocolate chip cookies were her favorite). She always claimed that she could indeed live without food or water indefinitely, and had done so many times in the past.

Her claim was put to the test in the Australian TV show *60 Minutes* in 1999. In this episode, she came across as a complete lunatic while explaining her methods, but remained adamant that she could prove herself. When the *60 Minutes* team challenged her to go without food or water for 7 days under supervision, she didn't hesitate for a second. "So you're happy if we lock you up for 7 days and watch you die?" asked the show host. "Oh, you wouldn't watch me die. I'd come out smiling and laughing; it'd be a holiday", she replied.

They secured a hotel room overlooking a beautiful part of Brisbane, with a team of security guards watching her 24/7, to ensure she didn't eat or drink anything. Her progress was also checked onsite by a doctor.

By day two, there were already problems: she was dehydrated. By day three, Jasmuheen was complaining that city pollution was limiting the nutrients she could obtain from the air. After she complained of the bad air quality, they moved her to another location (Clear Mountain, 20 kilometers outside of Brisbane), surrounded by trees and nature.

However, even in this pristine environment, Jasmuheen started to look gaunt. By day four, she had lost 6 kilos (13 lbs.) Her blood pressure was down, and her pulse rate was over twice as fast as when she started. Her eyes were sunken, and her dehydration had passed the 10% level. She also started to talk crazy, like a little insecure child instead of a grown adult. The doctor monitoring her warned her she could suffer from severe kidney failure and that it would be too dangerous to continue, so the experiment was stopped.

At the end, Jasmuheen continued to defend her case that the "pollution" from the first hotel room in Brisbane had prevented her from getting enough nutrients from the air.[52] However, in another interview, she claims that breathing polluted air in big cities has no effect on "her being nourished by prana," and that she spends 50% of her time in cities.[53]

From meeting Jasmuheen in person, I believe she is a deluded person, rather than just a liar looking to make a quick buck. Her willingness to appear on television and put her claims to the test showed that she did believe she could live on air. Like all breatharians, she does not take into account that her sparse diet of tea with honey and chocolate cookies is actually what is keeping her alive, and not prana.

---

52 A recording of this TV show episode has been posted on the Internet at: **http://video. google.com/videoplay?docid=-8060648983626971848#**
53 http://www.lifepositive.com/Mind/Holistic_Living/Living_on_love_and_fresh_ air12010.asp

According to the press, at least three people have died from following Jasmuheen's advice.[54] I believe that the total death count attributable to breatharianism in general is much higher. I personally know at least one person who died after following this type of advice (a case that was never reported in the media).

Jasmuheen has also claimed that her DNA has changed shape from 2 strands to 12 "in order to absorb more hydrogen." A group of skeptics offered her $30,000 to prove it via a simple blood test, but she declined the offer, saying "I don't know the relevance for it." Later, another skeptical group, The James Randi Foundation, offered her one million dollars to prove her claim.[55] Wouldn't it be easy money for Jasmuheen, if she were so convinced that she could live on prana?

She refused this offer as well.

Some might wonder what the folly of breatharianism has to do with the raw food diet. Unfortunately, there remains a common thread in the raw food movement that eating is "bad", and that as we get healthier, we should be able to live on less and less food. Many raw foodists actually believe that one day, they will be able to live as breatharians, the ultimate enlightened beings.

It's fair enough to say that "overeating" is bad, but what bugs me is that those who condemn this practice never bother to define exactly what overeating is. They simply state that overeating is eating more than the body needs, without defining exactly what the body needs and how much. This leads their followers to imagine that they are overeating when they are eating a large meal of fruit, even though that meal might only be 400 calories (barely enough as a meal for a grown adult)!

---

54   Sect Madness: Disciples starve themselves to death **http://www.rickross.com/ reference/breat/breat11.html**
55   **http://www.randi.org/jr/070105quality.html#14**

Some raw foodists have claimed to be able to live on less than 1000 calories a day, thereby encouraging inadequate calorie and nutrient intake, which can lead to disastrous results.

For example, here's an excerpt from an interview with Loren Lockman, director of a fasting center in Panama:

Question: What might you eat in a typical day?

Loren: Today was typical for this time of year. I had a large cantaloupe for lunch, and 4 or 5 peaches for dinner. Of course, with so many delicious fruits available right now, there are many possibilities. 2 or 3 meals a week are usually green salads.

Question: And for breakfast?

Loren: I almost never eat breakfast.

Question: That doesn't sound like very much food. Can you get enough calories that way?

Loren: I can, and have, for 5 or 6 years. When I went all-raw in 1991, I ate three times as many calories as I do now. Typically, as the body cleans out, and adjusts to the much higher quality of a raw vegan diet, it gets more efficient, and is able to operate on much less food. The metabolism drops, and the body is able to accomplish the same amount of work as before, with far less energy expended.[56]

Let's analyze what Loren supposedly eats in a typical day. A large cantaloupe might be 300 calories (if it's sweet enough), while the average large peach might be 75 calories (if you're lucky). This means that in a "typical day," Loren eats around 675 calories, or let's say 700, to give him the benefit of the doubt (maybe he found a super-cantaloupe). A man like Loren probably has a basal metabolic rate of 1600 calories per day[57]. This means that if Loren does nothing all day except sit in front of the computer in his pajamas, he will need at least 1600 calories to

---

56 http://www.tanglewoodwellnesscenter.com/loren-lockman-interview.php
57 Calculated with the basic *Harris-Benedict formula*, one of the many methods to determine BMR from known data.

maintain his weight. In the interview, we hear that in a typical day, Loren eats barely half that amount.

What I have found over the years is that anytime someone pretends to live on almost no food at all, they only tell you about the days they ate a few pieces of fruit. They conveniently forget to mention the 3000-calorie meal they had binging on nuts and seeds or cooked foods, and tend to inaccurately keep track of their caloric intake over the long term.

If someone wanted to prove that a grown man could live on 700 calories a day and thrive, perhaps they should submit to a voluntary experiment and be monitored for a month, to see how their theory holds water. Remember that caloric restriction is measured over a period of time and is accomplished by consistently eating less food. It does not mean eating less some days and more on other days.

Because this kind of magical thinking is so common in the raw food movement, most people who try to follow this diet are unable to make it work in the real world and usually quit, while blaming their lack of discipline and willpower for their failure. Those who persist in trying to live on almost no food often see their health deteriorate, sometimes beyond the point of no return.

Although calorie restriction is a proven method to increase longevity and improve health, most calorie-restricted diets cut down only 10 to 25% of total calories. This reduction in calories is not from base metabolic rates, but rather from what people normally eat in a typical day.

Tonya Zavasta, a Russian-born engineer, wrote a book called *Quantum Eating*, where she advocates a plan of not eating after 3 or 4 p.m. as well as caloric restriction. From looking at her in her videos, she is clearly thriving on her diet, with a youthful appearance that is remarkable for her age. When my wife contacted her to ask how much she eats in a typical day, she estimated between 1400 and 1600 calories.

For a short woman like Tonya, now 52, a diet of 1500 calories a day can qualify as a calorie-restricted diet, but not a starvation diet. Although Tonya openly talks about her calorie-restricted diet, she also emphasizes that young people under 40 should not attempt to live on such a diet. As we get older, it may be beneficial to eat less food and fewer total calories, as long as this plan is not too drastic and takes into account our individual needs.

The problem with calorie restriction is that when young people or even older people with eating disorders or anorexia hear about these raw foodists who supposedly thrive eating almost nothing, they get the idea that they should do the same.

Although raw foodism does not necessarily lead to eating disorders, anyone with an eating disorder or with a history or anorexia should only follow a raw food diet with proper supervision, to ensure they are eating enough calories. Until someone can learn to eat enough on a healthy whole food diet (containing cooked carbohydrates, such as potatoes), they should not venture to a raw food diet with a pre-existing eating disorder.

CHAPTER 15

Don't Be in a Rush to Flush

"Most people in the developed world have accumulated hundreds, if not thousands of stones in their liver. You will see them come out after doing your flushes and will be amazed!"

Andreas Moritz,
The Amazing Liver and Gallbladder Flush

By November, the staff at *Tree of Life* had fallen apart. Michael had left, apparently upset at Gabriel's staff for reasons that were unclear to me. Andrew also disappeared, disillusioned and ready for something different. A few other staff members working in the accounting department with him also quit.

During my stay at *Tree of Life*, Raven had visited me for a few days, and had also invited me to come visit her in New York City for a few weeks.

After everybody left *Tree of Life*, I stayed for a little while and decided the time had come to set my sights on a new horizon, and I left for New York City to go meet Raven.

I was quite excited to go spend some time with Raven. She lived in a little apartment that she loved in the East Village of Manhattan, close to all kinds of cool health food shops, yoga studios and fruit vendors.

Being in New York was so different than being in California. I could see the East Coast/West Coast rivalry, as every New Yorker thought that New York City was the best place ever and considered himself or herself more sophisticated and cultured than the bums living on the West Coast.

Raven was quite involved in the Jubb/Raw scene of New York. She had started a company with her previous boyfriend to sell all kinds of raw food products and supplements. Besides raw foods, she was also interested in yoga and other Eastern forms of philosophy and spirituality.

At Raven's place, I started drinking copious amounts of green juices made with her Green Power juicer. Green juices represented another ray of hope that perhaps I could turn my health around and experience the fabled benefits of pure raw foodism.

I was not new to green juices, though. Even in San Diego, I had drunk lots of green juices, and eaten lots of kale in all of its forms, to make sure I was getting enough minerals. I thought of green juices as a form of "antidote." Because they were so alkaline-forming, I thought they were the perfect way to counterbalance the acidity created during the digestion of nuts and seeds. But I was wrong.

Besides green juices, I tried E3-Live, a form of liquid blue-green algae, sold in a bottle and frozen. It tasted nasty, gave you a little boost in energy initially, but otherwise, it did nothing else positive that I could notice. I now think of E3-Live as basically a supplemental stimulant and don't recommend it.

There was one thing left that I hadn't tried: the liver flush.

David Jubb was a proponent of this naturopathic method and, according to him, several liver flushes were necessary to rid the body of these nasty gallstones.

The liver flush involved a special procedure. First, you had to drink a lot of apple juice for a few days, which according to Jubb, would help "soften" the gallstones and make them easier to pass.

In addition, or in preparation for the flush, you could also do a coffee enema, which I did. The coffee enema is quite simple: it's like a regular enema, but instead of water you stick coffee up your butt! The results are brutal — an enema with a caffeine buzz!

Then came the moment of truth: the drinking of the olive oil and lemon. According to Jubb, you had to drink no less than one cup of olive oil and one cup of lemon juice. You used the lemon juice to chase down the oil. Other types of oil, such as flax oil, could also be used.

The drinking of the olive oil was really disgusting — an experience I don't recommend to anybody. But surprisingly, I managed to drink it all down with the help of the lemon juice. Once I was done, I felt some nausea and was afraid it would all come out the same way it came in, but I was able to hold it down.

After a few hours of drinking all this oil, your body is shocked into "flushing" the liver, thus getting rid of all those nasty "stones" that had been cluttering it.

The stones came out in your feces, and some religious devotees of the flush would even spend some time fishing them out of the toilet bowl, as a sort of gross trophy to show other people.

The next day, when I saw my "stones" come out of my body, I was shocked. There were at least 12 of them, and some were as almost as big as a golf ball, but most were less than half that size.

My first thought was "No way!"

I did not have a strong background in physiology, but I knew that these "stones" were not what they were claimed to be. They looked bright green, just like the olive oil I had drunk. Wouldn't it make sense that they were merely the olive oil I had just drunk, in a sort of weird solidified state?

I asked David Jubb that question. He looked at me angrily and said, "Are you a microbiologist, Fred? No! Well, I am, so I can tell you that these stones are not just oil. It's your liver flushing them out."

I wasn't sure why being a microbiologist would be a requirement for common sense, but I knew something wasn't right with the liver flush theory.

I talked to some people who told me they had done the flush and kept their stones, and found to their amazement that the stones had melted overnight. Wasn't that a proof that they were nothing but oil?

Others had done the flush with different types of oil, and found that the type of oil one drank affected the color of the stones.

Could this be true?

What I knew is that after this flush, I did not feel any better. Actually, I did feel a lot better, but only in the same way that one feels better after having food poisoning and then recovering from it. It was a relief to know that it was all over with.

For a long time after the flush, I could not smell, be near or even think about olive oil. Just the thought of oil made my body quiver and my stomach turn upside down.

The Truth About Liver Flushes

Why do people think that drinking down a cup of oil will flush out their livers? This type of cure is not new. It's been around for decades and possibly longer.

Proponents of the liver flush claim that the procedure can improve digestion, eliminate allergies, and even get rid of all kinds of body aches and pains, in addition to being energizing.

The theory of the liver flush is that by eating a Standard American Diet, we eat too much processed fat. Because of that, our gallbladder ends up being cluttered with small calcified "stones." This causes a great variety of health problems. When you flush out the liver a few times to get rid of the stones, all of your health problems will magically go away.

In reality, if these giant gallbladder or liver stones were so common, they would be detectable by a simple ultrasound, which is a common procedure. (Do not confuse these with gallstones, which can develop in the bladder.) Yet we never hear about these stones outside of the Naturopathic world, as if it's some kind of conspiracy.

So what are those mysterious stones that are found in your poop after a flush? Sometimes, there are so many of them that to hold them all you would need a gallbladder the size of a purse! I even heard people say they passed hundreds of stones at a time. I've heard of others who kept a collection of giant stones they passed in their freezers (so they do not melt, obviously).

The bile duct itself could never accommodate a stone the size of a golf ball and pass it.

A medical study published in the Lancet in 1999 concluded: [58]

A 40-year-old woman was referred to the outpatient clinic with a 3-month history of recurrent severe right hypochondrial pain after fatty food. [Note: Here "hypochondrial" means "below the ribcage," not as in "hypochondriac."] Abdominal ultrasound showed multiple 1-2 mm gallstones in the gallbladder.

She had recently followed a "liver cleansing" regime on the advice of an herbalist. This regime consisted of free intake of apple and vegetable juice until 1800 h, but no food, followed by the consumption of 600 mL of olive oil and 300 mL of lemon juice over several hours. This activity resulted in the painless passage of multiple semisolid green "stones" per rectum in the early hours of the next morning. She collected them, stored them in the freezer, and presented them in the clinic.

Microscopic examination of our patient's stones revealed that they lacked any crystalline structure, melted to an oily green liquid after 10 min at 40°C, and contained no cholesterol, bilirubin, or calcium by established wet chemical methods. Traditional fecal fat extraction techniques indicated that the stones contained fatty acids that required acid hydrolysis to give free fatty acids before extraction into ether. These fatty acids accounted for 75% of the original material.

Experimentation revealed that mixing equal volumes of oleic acid (the major component of olive oil) and lemon juice produced several semi solid white balls after the addition of a small volume of a potassium hydroxide solution. On air drying at room temperature, these balls became quite solid and hard.

We conclude, therefore, that these green "stones" resulted from the action of gastric lipases on the simple and mixed triacylglycerols that make up olive oil, yielding long chain carboxylic acids (mainly oleic acid). This process was followed by saponification into large insoluble micelles of potassium carboxylates (lemon juice contains a high concentration of potassium) or "soap stones".

58   Sies, C., &Brooker, J. (2005). Could these be gallstones? *Lancet, 365*(9468), 1388.

In other words, the stones are nothing more than the product of the olive oil drunk for the flush! They are just saponified oil.

CHAPTER 16

Back to the Land of Snow, and Cooked Food

"Steamed vegetables are inorganic sulfur deposits, devoid of any life-giving properties. Steamed vegetables do not feed the living cells that make up your body. They are not nourishment; they are poison."

The Raw Courage Vegetable Man,
aka RC Dini

After my month-long stay with Raven in New York, we broke up, and I went back to San Diego to finish my book, *Sunfood Cuisine*.

I felt my options were running out, and that I had pretty much accomplished what I wanted to accomplish in my travels south of the border.

I had learned to become a raw food chef. I had amassed an impressive amount of knowledge on health and the raw food diet, tried everything, failed and tried again, and learned with the leaders of this movement all over the United States.

I had now finished writing my first book (a recipe book and food encyclopedia) and had published my magazine *Just Eat an Apple* for almost two years. I was ready for something new.

I decided that I needed to go back to live permanently in Canada, start my own business, and finally achieve some kind of balance in my health.

In spite of the difficulties, I was still extremely passionate about the raw food diet. I didn't yet have clarity about what had happened to me, and hadn't quite realized that the raw food diet had been mostly a personal failure and not the great success story I was hoping for.

My final stop before getting back to Quebec was New York City. From there, I took a Greyhound bus back to Montreal, and I chose a really bad day to do it.

It was February 14th, Valentine's Day, and the North East was facing the worst snowstorm of the year.

On the bus with me was a man from Sri Lanka who was on his first night of a visit to Canada. He looked at the gloomy sight of snow and dark sky outside and asked me with a terrified voice and a thick Indian accent, "Is it like this all the time?"

I laughed and reassured him that no, Canada was not a land of snowstorms all the time (only some of the time...). He could not believe his eyes. For someone who had never seen snow before in his life, this was probably a disturbing and shocking experience.

It was a big shock for me too, since I'd managed to escape three Canadian winters. Although the snow was nice to see and the temperature was decent *while* it was snowing, I knew that within a day or two it would get extremely cold, and I didn't like that idea at all.

When I got back to Canada, my brother and my dad were waiting for me at the Greyhound station. My brother was still 100% raw and had maintained the diet all those years, so as soon as we got back home, he made a giant salad full of veggies with some tomatoes, dulse, tahini and avocado.

One person that was no longer raw, however, was my friend Dominic. I had inspired Dominic to go 100% raw in summer 1997. He was the one who, a year prior, had told me about food combining. I had followed this lead and found out about Natural Hygiene, and then raw foods.

Dominic went 100% raw at that time, and he never looked back. After I left for California, we stayed in touch, and he would tell me how he still considered eating raw to be the *foundation* of his path of personal development, because it was what was going to bring him health and energy.

Two years later, he told me he was having doubts about it. He didn't really like being raw anymore, but he was afraid to eat any cooked foods because of how his body would react.

David Wolfe and other raw foodists had written that if you were raw for a long period of time and then ate cooked foods, your body would *violently* reject them, and you would get very sick.

Dominic didn't want that to happen to him, so he stayed raw, even though he didn't like the diet anymore and felt he wasn't getting the results he was after.

Finally, one day, when I was living at Tera's place, I talked to Dominic on the phone, and he told me he had broken his raw food streak.

I asked him what happened. He said, "I wanted to see how my body would react the next day. So I ate half a donut."

I was kind of shocked that Dominic would go for half a donut after such a long period of eating raw. I would have thought that some steamed broccoli and potatoes would have been better. So I asked him, "And... what happened?"

"Absolutely nothing happened," he said.

After that, Dominic stopped eating raw, little by little. He was smart enough not to gorge himself with cooked foods, and he slowly reintroduced them into his diet.

Although I had discovered gourmet raw food in California and indulged in it, Dominic did not have that "opportunity," and continued eating the way we ate when we first went raw together. That meant whole fruits and vegetables, eaten throughout the day, with big salads with avocado and green onion, but absolutely no salt, oil, or condiments. He also ate lots of nuts, but he did not know anything about nut butters and other such items.

His diet wasn't perfect, but it was a lot better than the one I had followed in California. Yet, his raw food experiment was also a failure. Although he didn't destroy his health like I did, he experienced none of the famed health benefits that were attributed to raw foods, such as amazing energy, needing less sleep, and feeling great. Dominic was only 21 at the time.

My brother, on the other hand, seemed to be faring quite well on the diet. To me, Sebastien was a strange case. He had always had a stronger constitution than I did, perhaps because he was much more active and athletic (running sometimes), and foods did not seem to affect him the way they affected me. Therefore, he said he felt "great" eating raw, even though he consumed lots of avocados (three a day!) and tahini.

When I got back to Montreal, I continued eating raw. However, there was a thought in my mind that kept growing. *How would I feel if I ate cooked foods?* Going back to eating some cooked food was the *only* thing I hadn't tried, it seemed.

I was so used to eating raw that I wasn't even craving cooked foods. My cravings were for heavy gourmet raw food recipes, which I ate to try to pacify my hunger.

Until I could find an apartment in Montreal, I went back to live at my mom's place, exactly where I had first discovered Mosséri, then spent my first winter on a mostly raw, hygienic diet, and later the summer on a 100% raw diet.

Getting back there brought back many memories, and suddenly, I felt like these two worlds, Quebec and California — the first being a place I wanted to escape, and the second representing my dream life — were finally brought back together.

I decided right then that I was going to eat something cooked.

As a first experiment, I bought a sweet potato and baked it in the oven.

While the sweet potato was cooking, I could not help feeling like a naughty boy who was doing something very bad, hiding away in a secret place to do it.

As I took the sweet potato out of the oven when it was done, I could feel my heart beating faster and faster.

"It's just a stupid sweet potato!" I wanted to think, but all that came to my mind was this thought: "You're about to eat some *cooked* food."

It made me laugh how American raw foodists used the word *cooked*. Unlike the French word "cuit", the sound of the word *cooked*, with three consonants in only one syllable, is very staccato. When you add a little wind to it and some anger, it can almost sound like an insult. In fact, that's how the Californian raw foodists used the word.

"Dude, that guy is soooo *cooked*," I could hear them say.

Now, I was about to become seriously *cooked* by eating some evil *cooked* food, for the first time in who knows how long.

I almost felt like an alcoholic, who after a long streak of abstinence, decides to have a drink again. Hopefully, I wouldn't turn out like that Clint Eastwood character in the movie *Unforgiven* and go berserk…

I decided to eat my sweet potato plain. I didn't even know what you could put on a sweet potato, and I figured it would be just as good the way it was.

I waited for it to cool down, because I knew that I could burn my mouth, being used to eating cold foods for so long.

When it was ready to eat, I cut a large slice and put it in my mouth.

It tasted like… wow! It was absolute amazing, creamy and sweet, warm and delicious: it melted in my mouth. It didn't even need any salt or fat. It was just perfect the way it was.

I could feel a little drop in energy after I was done, but surprisingly, I didn't grasp my chest in convulsions and fall down on the floor, writhing in pain, like I had been led to believe.

In fact, I felt a lot better than after eating a nut pâté or even a big avocado salad, which would usually leave me *out of service* for about two hours while digesting it.

I could not help thinking that I had done something *bad*. I was supposed to be this pure raw foodist, and now I had just eaten cooked food. What kind of person was I?

After this episode, I went back to eating raw for another month, without trying anything else cooked again.

Eventually though, the specter of cooked food would come back to haunt me.

Rediscovering Cooked Foods

In 2000, I was invited by the Fresh Network to give "uncooking classes" in London. There was a huge demand for more education about raw cuisine in England, and because I was one of the first people to publish a raw food recipe book and publicize it on the Internet, I was invited by Karen Knowler, one of the founders of the Network, for a series of events.

Although I was still mostly raw and passionate about raw foods, deep in my heart I knew that I was no longer "pure," having broken my several-year streak of eating 100% raw.

As much as I loved the raw food world, I also felt pulled towards the "the dark side of the force:" cooked food.

Ever since I had eaten that baked sweet potato, I had trouble considering cooked food as bad and evil as I once did. I realized that I had closed my mind to the possibility that cooked food might have some positive aspects. That disturbed me, because I had always prided myself on having an open mind.

My first cooked food experience in years opened all kinds of new possibilities. I realized that from the moment I became independent and left my parents' home at the age of 20, I had been a raw foodist. Never once in my life had I tasted Japanese, Indian or Thai food. I felt that there was an entire world out there that I had not even known! I knew the raw food world very well, but what about the rest of the *modern world*?

A few months prior to my trip to London, I had met a woman in Arizona at David Wolfe's Y2K party (for New Year's 2000). Her name was Marianne. She was quite a few years older than me, but looked super youthful. She had been a raw foodist for over a year, but the one thing she never gave up was her morning Starbucks Soy Latte! She was quite happy eating all-raw, but she was not about to give up her beloved coffee, no matter how many arguments she heard about the dangers of caffeine.

In London, I spent a lot of time with Marianne, and for the first time in my life, I discovered that coffee could be delicious, invigorating, and surprisingly... pleasantly addicting!

Although I had never really drunk coffee in my life, I discovered why everybody raved about these gourmet coffees: they really tasted amazing, and they gave me a jolt of instant joy that lasted for hours.

One of Marianne's health gurus had told her: "It's okay to have one cup of *poison* per day." She certainly wasn't fooling herself into thinking that coffee was healthy, but she felt that this small indulgence gave her more pleasure than negative side effects. I started to feel the same too, and I enjoyed some Starbucks soy lattes.

When I got back to Montreal, I quit the coffee, but now I was interested in trying something else. Besides baked sweet potatoes, what was there to eat?

Little by little, I introduced other cooked foods into my diet.

At first, I would go for steamed vegetables, as I did not really know what else to try. I could only think like a raw foodist. Most of my meals were raw, but sometimes, I would add something cooked to them, such as creamy chickpea hummus.

At first, I did not really notice negative effects from eating those things. I even felt a lot better eating potatoes and cooked vegetables than I did eating gourmet raw food recipes!

I continued a mixed path of raw and cooked, where I would still eat fatty raw food recipes, but also try out different cooked foods. Things like steamed vegetables, bean soups, lentils and potatoes. I would go raw for a week or two, then go for a week eating some cooked things, and then go back to raw again.

I didn't really know what I was trying to accomplish. Initially, I felt drunk with the excitement of being "liberated" from the strict philosophy of the *100% raw at all costs*. Now that I was no longer living in California and most people around me were *normal*, I no longer had the judging eyes of other raw gurus over my shoulders. I felt free to do whatever I wanted.

I only knew Natural Hygiene and vegetarianism, so I would revert back to that for anything I ate cooked. Whenever the cooked foods I was eating weren't simple baked potatoes or steamed vegetables, I would make cooked soups with lentils and other recipes that I still remembered from my cooked vegetarian past.

Most of my culinary skills were still with raw food recipes, so my diet became a curious combination of fruit, salads, gourmet raw foods, and cooked vegan foods.

The more time went by, the more I didn't feel trapped by any rule or restriction.

I returned to Europe to travel. I started learning Spanish, German and Portuguese, and I was making progress in these languages at an incredible pace. I suddenly thought that there was an entire realm of possibilities outside of *raw foods* for my life in the future. After all, I was only 24. There was still time for me to maybe go back to University and pursue a real career, instead of forever dabbling in the crazy raw food world and getting nowhere.

Over the two years that followed, I continued my language studies and went back to Europe over eight times.

As time went by, I felt increasingly disconnected from the raw food movement, and instead, I became interested in other things. At the same time, I started eating more and more cooked foods.

Suddenly, I noticed something strange happening: I did not feel amazing at all.

I felt cheated that I had spent all that time going raw, never achieved the positive results that I'd expected, and when I went off the diet, I started feeling worse, but in a different way.

On the raw food diet, the main problems were the cravings and the lack of energy.

On cooked foods, I had no cravings, and my energy levels were much better. However, I started feeling frequent depression and irritation.

From eating mostly raw with some steamed vegetables and a few baked potatoes a week, my experimentations with diet went out of control, and eventually my diet devolved to the point that I was eating everything, short of beef and chicken.

I felt like a Buddhist monk who had spent years in a Monastery, only to give it up and live a life of excess with gambling, women and alcohol. Except this was food — vegetarian food.

One year after getting back to Canada, I was eating fruit and gourmet raw food along with things like bread, cheese, yogurt, soy ice cream, organic chocolate, pasta, or sandwiches for dinner. I would even drink wine sometimes, as well as coffee, a new habit I had first developed with Marianne in London.

At some point, I realized that because of these changes, my health was really suffering.

I was fooling myself into thinking that it was just a question of quantity or ingredient quality, or that I could balance the negative effects of these things by eating more raw food.

My health would go through ups and downs, just like my diet, and it got worse and worse with time.

At some point, I would be so depressed some days that I could barely get up in the morning. I felt like my brain was forever falling into one dream after another, and upon waking up, I experienced this horrible sleep inertia that lasted all day, which made me irritable, depressed and unable to concentrate.

I noticed, however, that on some days, I would skip breakfast altogether and eat fruit all day. At night, I would eat something simple, like a potato without fat, and then the next day, I would wake up and feel great.

I was almost ready to make the radical changes in my diet I had needed to make for years, but a new obstacle was about to come my way.

CHAPTER 17

The Reward of Raw: A Mouthful of Cavities

"Dude, you have to brush your teeth."

Stephen Arlin

When I first read Herbert Shelton, I was captivated by his coherent philosophy of Natural Hygiene. Even though I eventually felt more enticed to follow the raw food path instead, a lot of what I originally read in those Natural Hygiene books impressed me.

On the topic of dental health, Shelton had very unusual advice. He claimed that toothbrushes harmed the gums and were not helping our teeth. In his reasoning, cavities were caused by over-acidification of the system, and they were a symptom of something that was going on in the entire body. In other words, if you get holes in your teeth, you probably have them in your bones too. Your body is trying to get the calcium it needs to neutralize all the acidity created by the Standard American Diet. Brushing teeth tended to do more harm than good. Instead, he claimed that when we ate raw foods, we didn't need to brush our teeth anymore because all the high-fiber foods we were eating had a natural cleansing effect on the teeth. I knew there was probably some truth in this, because even some dentists had told me that eating an apple was good for our teeth because the fiber and water in the apple naturally "brushed" our teeth. On the other hand, soft foods like bread and porridge just get stuck to the teeth and are not tough enough to exercise our weak jaws.

So I took his advice and got rid of my toothbrush, and started to eat a lot of apples and carrots instead.

In California, raw foodists had mixed feelings about this. Stephen Arlin told me, "Dude, you have to brush your teeth." David said he brushed without any toothpaste, but he agreed that maybe it wasn't necessary; after all, "Gorillas don't brush their teeth!"

For over three years, I rarely brushed my teeth with a toothbrush. I did not share that decision with anyone, because everybody was convinced that if you didn't brush your teeth, you would automatically have terrible breath. Instead, I found that on the raw food diet my breath was naturally sweet and not bad-smelling at all, even though I didn't brush.

I also had all of my teeth, so I could easily crush apples and exercise my jaw that way.

But my diet wasn't just apples and carrots. I also ate lots of nuts, gourmet raw foods, and, at times, dried fruit. On top of that, I ate large amounts of soft sweet fruit, such as mangoes, cherimoyas and bananas.

By the summer of 1999, I could already feel that my teeth were not doing so great anymore. When I looked at my mouth, I could see a few brown spots in places where my teeth had previously been white. I knew I needed to get them checked, but procrastinated doing it. Then I started brushing my teeth again, just in case.

The occasional pains and discomforts in my teeth continued, and it was Fall 2000 when I finally decided to go to the dentist.

When the dentist looked at my mouth, spending a few minutes poking my teeth with his tools, he kept saying a few names and numbers aloud to his assistant. "17, left M third molar...19 left M first molar."

I could not understand what these codes meant, but I knew it was not good news.

After a few X-rays were taken, the dentist came back to me and said, "Well, my friend, you have 19 cavities."

I was utterly shocked and stupefied. "19 cavities! How much is this going to cost?"

This mouthful of cavities required four subsequent visits to the dentist, and the constant drilling in my mouth left me in pain for several months after. I refused to even swallow an aspirin, so I stoically endured the stabs of pain that would often keep me up at night.

I knew that I had done something very, very bad to deserve that many cavities. I could not attribute it to detox or any other raw food theory, and I was forced to admit that not brushing my teeth for so long, while eating so much fruit and nuts at the same time, were the most likely causes of the decay.

Fortunately, it didn't get to the point that I needed any root canals or anything serious, but my teeth had officially been destroyed by the raw food diet and my own ignorance in following advice from books written in the 1940s.

Was it just the lack of brushing that caused the decay?

My brother, who had been a raw foodist throughout the time I had been one, and was still raw when I came back to live in Canada, also visited the family dentist around the same time. Unsurprisingly, he also came back devastated, having learned that he had 13 cavities. Yet, my brother had kept up his dental hygiene routine during the whole time he was raw, and he did not quit brushing his teeth like I did. So what caused the decay? Only the diet could explain it.

My other friend Dominic also had the nasty surprise of a mouthful of cavities after a few years on the diet (although not nearly as many as we did). What was more shocking to him was the fact that never in his life had he had a cavity before!

After this dental catastrophe, I continued brushing my teeth religiously. I also did my best to avoid dried fruit. I thought that this would be enough to prevent any further decay, but just two years later, I would be in for a nasty surprise.

Going Back to Natural Hygiene

Although I was still shocked by the dental disaster I had experienced, I attributed most of it to my own mistakes and my throwing away my toothbrush to replace it with an apple.

As far as my health was concerned, I was starting to make some observations. I started to realize that these first years of 100% raw had been almost a complete failure.

I also noticed that going back to regular "cooked comfort foods," like most of the things I was indulging in, was having some serious negative consequences. Another thing I noticed was that coffee was making me depressed (after an initial period of euphoria).

I also noticed that whenever I ate simple fruits and vegetables, whether raw or cooked, I felt better.

Could it be that Mosséri, my first teacher, had been right? I had forgotten about his teachings all these years, and during that time my health had degraded, not improved. When I remembered my first months on Mosséri's diet, I had had cravings at the time, but was doing so much better overall.

In early 2002, I went on a trip to Costa Rica and brought with me an entire suitcase of books by Mosséri, Shelton, and other Natural Hygienists. I was not going to blindly apply every single piece of advice they gave, like I had done in the past, but would try to understand the main principles behind this philosophy.

When I got back home from this trip, I had made many reflections and assimilated a lot of information. I came to some realizations:

By blindly accepting the raw food ideals, I had put aside the principles of health that really make a difference. The main principle I had forgotten was to give my body the optimal fuel it needed!

1. I came to the conclusion that just because a food is raw, it doesn't make it healthy. All those gourmet raw foods I had eaten in my raw food days are what made me sick. In comparison, eating steamed potatoes would have been infinitely better. Therefore, raw was NOT law.

2. Abusing nuts and fatty foods in general is what had done the most damage to my health. To gain it back, I had to focus my diet on fruits and vegetables and minimize all concentrated foods, raw or cooked.

3. Since junk cooked foods were not working either, I had to go back to the principles of Natural Hygiene as laid out by Mosséri and Shelton.

4. Just by following my own advice and applying these principles in my life, I finally got rid of the health problems that had been nagging me for years, such as lack of energy, waking up in the morning tired and groggy, blood sugar imbalances and irritability.

I started writing my thoughts down in an article that I called "When 100% Raw is Not 100% Healthy."

My article grew and grew, and I decided to add more parts to it, as I kept doing research and realized everything I had done wrong over the past years.

Eventually, my friend Andrew had moved to Montreal with me, and together, we had decided to revive my magazine *Just Eat an Apple*, but this time outside of the tutelage of *Nature's First Law* and as our own masters, promoting the principles of Natural Hygiene that I had been studying over the past months.

When Andrew saw what I was writing, he said: "Dude, you have a book right there."

"What do you mean?" I asked.

"Keep writing more chapters. It'll become a book."

Encouraged by that idea, I kept writing and writing until, as Andrew had predicted, I had written a book.

My old friend Dominic suggested calling it *The Raw Food Secrets*, and then finally it became *The Raw Secrets*.

The book was a success from the moment it was released in the fall of 2002. In just two weeks, we had sold out of our first printing, and I had to increase the size of our original order to make it available to more people.

The book was the first one to have been written for raw foodists, by a raw foodist (or at least someone who had been there and done it), that was casting a critical eye at the raw food diet.

I went against the trend of "As long as it's raw, it's healthy" to say, "No, raw food is a double-edged sword. It can really benefit your health, but it can also destroy it if you do it incorrectly."

I also said clearly that some raw foods are NOT as healthy as some cooked foods. The book was one of the first to criticize the modern raw food diet, advocate a low-fat raw food diet, and present important principles of Natural Hygiene, all under one hood.

I did not expect a lot of the positive responses I got from that book. Suddenly, all of these raw foodists from all over the world were coming out of the closet and admitting that they had gone through the same problems as I had, and declaring that my book had been the turning point in their lives.

It seemed like the mistakes I had exposed in *The Raw Secrets* were very common. But my little book did not please everybody.

I had hoped that *Nature's First Law* would want to distribute my book, as their philosophy was to carry every raw food book ever written; yet their response was:

"We've decided not to carry your book, because we don't feel it contains any original or new information."

"No original information?" I exclaimed! That was quite a bold thing to say, especially coming from them and their commitment to "carry every single raw food book ever printed." Their catalog was filled with many repetitive titles, including lots of nonsense, such as books on how to live on air and become a breatharian…

It was clear, however, why they refused to carry the book: it was too much an overt criticism of the diet they promoted, especially since their main business now was selling supplements and miracle superfoods, rather than just books.

I did not write the book *The Raw Secrets* as a reaction against what I had learned with *Nature's First Law*, but as a reflection of my personal experience with the raw food diet. I thought my information was valuable, and I felt totally cut off from people I considered to be my friends. At the same time, maybe I was just "spitting in the soup that fed me," as we say in French.

I really appreciated David and Stephen's generosity in providing me with so many opportunities to get involved in the raw food world, which had been my dream. However, I had to recognize that some of the ideas they had led me to believe in were not working, and that many other people would benefit from learning from my experience.

Fortunately, I did not need anyone's help to sell the book. The orders kept coming in, as the popularity of the book grew by word of mouth.

Over the next year, I continued my promotion of Natural Hygiene and raw foods through my magazine and my book.

By the summer of 2003, my book *The Raw Secrets* had been around for almost a year, and I had completely transformed my health from the disaster of my first few years of raw and its low levels of energy to having overcome these problems and feeling much better than ever before.

Even though I was struggling to apply the principles I promoted in my life, and would often mix some of the old (gourmet raw food) with the new (Natural Hygiene), I still managed to get rid of most of the problems that had afflicted me for all these years.

However, starting from the summer of 2003, I embarked on a year-long period of new doubt and skepticism towards raw vegan concepts, and during that time I even started eating animal products, such as eggs, fish and even meat.

What caused this change of attitude?

More Dental Troubles, and Going Back to Meat

Why, almost two years after writing a book (*The Raw Secrets*) did I start doubting some of the very concepts I had just espoused, namely the *vegan* part of the diet, as well as the high-fruit approach?

The answer is simple: another dental health crisis made me rethink the *entire* philosophy of raw.

I explained my first 19 cavities as being due to my own ignorance in blindly following the advice of Shelton and not brushing my teeth for so long, coupled with a diet high in sweet fruit, nuts and dried fruits.

After these cavities were repaired, I knew I had done something wrong. I was very careful with dried fruit, and no longer ate the large quantities of nuts I used to eat. I also brushed my teeth three times a day.

For the next two years, my teeth would continue to bother me on an occasional basis. I attributed it to all the drilling I had gone through, and I did not think my teeth could continue to decay as long as I brushed them and was careful with what I ate.

During this period of time, as I explained in the previous chapter, I had also stopped being 100% raw and eaten cooked foods for over a year, but eventually, I reverted back to what I felt was a better version of the raw food program, the one I described in my book, *The Raw Secrets.*

This new version of the raw diet I was following no longer included the massive amounts of avocados, nuts, seeds and oils I used to eat. Instead, I ate two relatively large fruit meals a day, with a salad at night,

247

but sometimes I also ate steamed vegetables or potatoes, and avoided condiments and spices.

I also ate Iranian dates, which I felt were not as bad as other dried fruits, because they had not been artificially dried. I organized raw food potlucks at my house. People would bring all kinds of raw dishes that included nuts, and occasionally I ate some of that, too. The combination of what I felt was the ideal diet (Natural Hygiene) with the gourmet raw food I was still preparing and eating might seem like a contradiction. Yet, it is still part of the raw food philosophy today that although gourmet food is not as ideal as fruits and vegetables, it's a great form of transition to raw eating, a good way to overcome cravings, and certainly acceptable to eat occasionally.

Unbeknownst to me, my diet was still much higher in fat than it should have been (probably around 20 or 25% fat), but this was still a major positive change from how I was eating before (up to 60% fat) and was the main reason why I was able to finally overcome the health problems that had plagued me during the first years I was eating raw in California.

By the summer of 2003, I was spending time with my girlfriend Julie, a famous French-Canadian nutritionist who had recently converted to the raw food diet. She believed in the blood type diet, which contains the idea that different people should eat different diets, and the same diet does not work for everybody. She was an extremely bright girl and would always challenge my belief systems and often shake some of my firmly held convictions.

Although our relationship did not last, a result of it was the idea that she planted in my mind that *perhaps the raw food diet I was trying to follow was not the best for me.* This idea would continue to grow and expand and lead me to doubt everything all over again.

The triggering event was my next dental exam.

I had avoided seeing a dentist again since my last round of drilling. The pain and the humiliation I associated with visits to the dentist made me procrastinate making another appointment. But one day when I was with Julie, I crunched a grape seed and instantly broke a filling that was located at the bottom of one of my canine teeth.

I knew I had to go back to the dentist and get everything checked. Julie gave me the address of an alternative dentist in Montreal, who did not use any toxic compounds like mercury. So I summoned all of my courage and decided to go.

As I was sitting in the dentist's chair, I experienced the familiar scene of the dentist checking all of my teeth with a pick and giving a series of names and numbers to the assistant. It did not sound good at all.

The dentist told me I had many cavities, but she needed to do a complete X-ray to be certain. After the X-ray was done, I got shocking news again.

I had 21 new cavities!

I could not believe what I was hearing. In a period of almost three years since I got over 19 cavities repaired, I now had even more. I didn't understand what had happened. How could I get so many cavities, if I had been brushing my teeth since then? I thought that was enough to save me.

I told the dentist my story of the book I had read and how I had gone for so long without brushing my teeth. Surprisingly, she said that they had had another client who had done the same thing, and ended up with a mouthful of cavities. "I wonder if you guys read the same book!" she exclaimed.

The dentist then explained to me that it was possible that I had a very high bacteria count in my mouth, which led to my first round of cavities. Since then, although I had started brushing again, I had still not taken care of the bacteria problem, as they were probably very entrenched, having been undisturbed for so long.

"Are you eating a lot of sugar?" she asked. I admitted eating a lot of fruit and dates.

Again, I was in for quite a while to repair all of those cavities. I had to go back to the dentist four times, each time getting 5 or 6 fillings done. By the time this was all over, I was trying to analyze my emotions. I definitely felt ashamed. My mouth was now a war zone, where almost every single tooth had one or two fillings. This was a visible testimonial that reminded me of the consequences of following the wrong advice and not having enough critical thinking.

I also felt angry. I felt angry at the raw food movement, at myself, at those Natural Hygiene books, and at the fact that this diet was simply not working. But going back to cooked foods hadn't worked either. I was doomed to this sad life of raw eating, where it was impossible to get the best of all worlds. I could feel healthy eating fruit, but if the inevitable result was that my teeth were going to fail, this was not sustainable. After all, if I kept getting this many cavities year after year, my teeth *were going to fall out.*

After this experience, all of my beliefs in the raw diet were completely shaken. Even my own book, *The Raw Secrets,* which seemed to have helped so many people worldwide, was possibly mistaken. What was going to happen next? What needed to happen next?

In November 2003, I decided to go to Brazil for one month. For the past two and half years, I had been studying foreign languages as a hobby, and in that time, I had been able to master Spanish, German, and Portuguese, as well as studying other languages like Russian. I was eager to go to Brazil and practice my Portuguese, as well as meet some of the raw food people there. Maybe along the way I would be able to find an answer.

When I first arrived in Rio de Janeiro, I met with Maria Luiza, a raw foodist I had met at the Portland Raw Food Festival the year before. She lived with her Swiss husband on a beautiful farm with lots of fruit trees, in the mountains near Rio.

They were very welcoming and happy to have me around for a few days, but it seemed that our diets clashed. The raw food diet they were following was more inspired by Ann Wigmore, with an abundance of sprouts, featuring meals that combined vegetables, a little fruit and sprouts, nuts or some avocado. The diet seemed to be working for Maria, who was a small woman with lots of energy, but her husband was lacking energy and strength and was overly sensitive to sugar, to the point where even consuming a little honey would send his blood sugar flying high.

I could not live on the types of lunches they were eating (I tried one day, and I was hungry half an hour later). I was looking forward to eating some jackfruit instead — an all-time favorite of mine, which was in season in Brazil when I was there. In Maria Luiza's household, fruit was used more like a condiment rather than as the main element of the meal.

I had told her that, after all those years of eating all-raw, I was no longer doing it 100%. Maria Luiza believed firmly in the 100% raw diet, having been influenced by Victoria Boutenko's philosophy of green smoothies in the USA. She thought that to get the real results of the raw diet, you had to commit to it 100%.

I had done it, and it had not worked. I could not just eat sprouts either. Secretly, I was still so shocked by what had happened to my teeth that I was looking for real answers. Maria Luiza suggested that I look into Dr. Doug Graham's philosophy, because I had talked about him in my book *The Raw Secrets,* and his work had certainly influenced my return to Natural Hygiene. Over the summer, I had attended a lecture by Doug in which he discussed the main reason why raw foodists fail, which was the high fat content of their diet. That certainly corresponded with my own experience. I was tempted to give the 80-10-10 Diet a try, but I was too scared that I would end up with a mouthful of cavities once again.

Even though she didn't follow Doug's program, Maria Luiza advised me (in Portuguese) that I should commit to a 100% raw path such as Doug's program. I was not going to achieve health if I continued to mess around between raw and cooked, she said.

I seriously thought about what she said, but I was not ready to commit to 100% raw again after what had happened to me before.

All over Brazil, the raw food scene was dominated by the sprouting and *living foods* philosophy. One woman advocated a drink that was some sort of concoction of sprouted sunflower seeds, blended with apples and greens, and then strained manually in a cheesecloth. She claimed this drink had completely transformed her health. I tried it, but gagged after drinking a few sips — it was simply unpalatable to me.

Eventually, I found my way to Brasilia, where I stayed with some friends who owned a vegetarian restaurant. There, I found comfort in cooked vegan foods, and ate in their restaurant every day.

The main change in my diet that occurred in Brazil is that I started eating cooked food for lunch. For years and years, I had always eaten fruit for breakfast and lunch. When I stopped being 100% raw in 2000, I still continued this pattern, and only ate cooked foods for dinner on the days I ate them.

For the first time ever, I cut down my fruit intake for the day by eating a regular cooked lunch, but kept eating fruit for breakfast. I wanted to see what would happen to my teeth with this kind of pattern, which was much lower in sugar.

During my trip, I spent time on the internet researching the raw food diet. I read endless blogs, medical studies, e-books and discussion forums, trying to gather some useful common threads.

I discovered that there was very little medical research to guide me, since very few researchers had taken an interest in the raw food diet. In one German study that I found, on a group of raw foodists in Germany, it was found that the high acid fruit intake among these people had caused abnormal enamel erosion.[59]

Some ex-raw foodists and Natural Hygienists were coming out on the Internet and telling their stories. Many reported experiences similar to mine. Some of these people had started eating animal products and experienced improvements in their health and their teeth.

Little by little, the thought planted in my mind that *"Maybe the raw food diet was not the right diet for me"* started to grow bigger and bigger. I was starting to think about eating animal products, which brought me right back to 1997 when I had met Bodhi and heard about the raw meat-eaters. This time, I realized it did not need to be raw. Maybe I could try eating some cooked animal products to see what would happen.

When I returned to Canada in December 2003, I continued eating cooked vegan foods, and did not immediately experiment with animal foods. I was torn between wanting to give up the raw food diet entirely and eat meat, and still feeling it was a great diet that I just hadn't learned properly. I kept reading about Dr. Doug Graham and his high-fruit, extremely low-fat diet. However, I was still afraid to try it 100%, because of the dental issues with eating so much fruit.

Shortly after I got back from Brazil, Gillian, a girl I had met in Portland at the raw food festival, invited me to come to her hometown of Vancouver to give a conference to her raw food group.

Gillian, a tall brunette of about my age, had gone raw a year or two earlier, and she was involved with the BC Raw Food Society. Now she wanted me to come over to give a conference. She would pay for the flight and give me part of the profits, and I could stay with her for a week.

---

59   Ganss, C; Schlechtriemen, M; Klimek, J (1999). "Dental erosions in subjects living on a raw food diet." Caries research 33 (1): 74–80. doi:10.1159/000016498. PMID 9831783.

It sounded good, but I wasn't sure what I could talk about during the conference. I was no longer the perfect raw foodist I once could claim to be. However, everything I had written in the *The Raw Secrets* was still true, except that I couldn't figure out why I got so many cavities on the diet and hadn't been able to stop the decay.

I decided I would give a general introduction to the raw food diet, explain the mistakes I had made along the way, and give people a good list of tips that I wished I had known when I first got started.

The raw food diet would always be the light in my life, and would always be with me. Even though I had gone through periods of extreme doubt about it, I would always rebound with enthusiasm at the idea of trying it again, but this time differently.

In preparation for the Vancouver conference, I went raw all over again, following my own advice and thinking to myself I would continue my research on dental health and my experimentations with diet after it was over. I just didn't want to show up in Vancouver with a belly full of rice and give a conference on the benefits of eating raw.

When I arrived in Vancouver, Gillian asked me if I was okay with doing some TV and Radio Shows to promote the conference. "Uh... Sure!" I said, even though I had never done that before.

The next day, I was all over the news in Vancouver in some local morning TV shows. A few days later, she managed to get me on the Vicky Gabereau show, one of the biggest afternoon talk shows in Canada. On the show, I showed Vicky and her audience a display of delicious-looking gourmet raw foods, such as raw vegan sushi, raw chocolate cake, and a few other all-time favorites.

The producers of the show had warned us in advance that they wanted to see a raw chocolate cake. They insisted on it. It was not going to be about discussing the philosophy of raw foods, but rather, the aim was to make it look like an appealing diet, with gourmet recipes that are, surprisingly, all raw.

Vicky was the most gracious TV personality I had met. She made me feel so comfortable to be seen in front of 250,000 people, and surprisingly, I was not nervous at all. She seemed keenly interested in the raw food concept and kept repeating, "This is wonderful!" and that I should come over to stay a week at her place to make her food.

She asked me in front of the camera: "So do you eat only raw foods?"

I answered no, I did not eat 100% raw.

I had taken the vow never to lie about my diet. I had been misled by so many people who claimed to be something different from who they were that I was certainly not going to be ashamed to talk about things the way they were.

After the TV show, I prepared for my conference. One of the guys who was helping Gillian put together the conference had looked at my slides the day before.

I had included all kinds of slides on the mistakes of raw foods, how raw foods can destroy your health and your teeth, possible deficiencies, and more along those lines.

He told me, "You can't have that in there! It's too negative. People won't have the proper context to judge the information and will end up not wanting to try it at all."

So I revised my slides to avoid being too negative about the results of eating raw improperly, and instead focused on the positive.

But I was still constantly preoccupied with the potential problems of the raw food diet.

The conference turned out to be a success. Over 400 people came from all over British Columbia, and some even drove all the way from Washington State to attend.

After the conference, I spent a lot of time with Gillian talking about the raw food diet. She confessed to me that she felt amazing during the first year of eating raw, but now she just felt indifferent. "I don't feel bad, just not amazing anymore. I also gained back all the weight I initially lost going raw."

I felt Gillian was on the verge of quitting the raw food diet altogether. She said, "I feel the outcome of our conversation will decide whether I continue being raw or not!"

I told her about Doug Graham and the 80-10-10 diet, and she said that she had some raw friends that went that way and "lost a million pounds," but she could not imagine giving up avocados and just eating fruit.

I noticed that Gillian ate a lot of fat. Once, we stopped at *Whole Foods* to get a meal, and she ate a big salad with dressing and an entire, very large avocado to accompany it.

"This diet is already strict enough. I gave up the other foods that I liked, so if I have to give up fat on top of that, I'm really not interested in continuing."

When I got back to Montreal after this Vancouver adventure, I was determined to get some more clarity about this entire raw food diet confusion. A few weeks after my return, I got a call from Gillian, who told me that one of her raw food friends had died.

This was a lovely woman who was involved with the BC Raw Food Society. I had just met her and spent some time with her while I was in Vancouver. She lived in an affluent neighborhood with her son and her husband, and she had been raw for a while.

Apparently, she got into the idea of eating less and less, which is very popular in the raw food movement even now. She was already so thin. "Why?" I thought to myself. Eventually, she started to feel weak. She ended up in the hospital, where doctors could not figure out what her problem was. At that point, she entered the medical system, where doctors were not aware of how sensitive she was. Her body was so weak and "pure" from all those years of eating raw and calorie restriction that possibly some of the drugs they gave her killed her.

I was in shock. This was someone I had just met weeks ago, and now she was dead!

I decided I needed to madly research what was wrong with the raw food diet and why so many people were not succeeding. One thing that I did was to contact some of the people I had read about when I browsed the web in Brazil, while I was doubting the raw food diet and looking for answers.

One guy I had come across called himself "Nazariah." I had first read some of his comments on a discussion forum where he talked about all the health problems he had endured while going raw vegan, including a severe B12 deficiency that left him almost paralyzed. He also claimed that most influential raw food leaders he knew were secretly binging on cooked foods and suffering from all kinds of mental health problems caused by deficiencies in their diet.

I thought that what Nazariah had written was very interesting, and I wanted to know more. So I located his email and arranged a telephone interview with him.

I then transcribed the interview and posted it on my website. In the interview, Nazariah described his failure with the raw vegan diet, claimed that most raw food leaders were not actually raw, and also claimed that the raw vegan diet was deficient and animal products were necessary for most people, for optimal health.

At that moment, the interview sent out shock waves in the raw food community. All over the web, people were posting about it, either criticizing it or using it as proof against raw veganism.

I started getting strange emails from all over the world.

One couple I had met in Germany at a conference emailed me. The woman had experienced serious dental problems on the raw diet, while her husband was too skinny and did not have the energy to exercise. After reading my interview with Nazariah, they decided to stop being raw vegans, and instead ate what they called a healthy vegetarian diet that included tofu, rice, steamed vegetables, and some yogurt. After changing their diet, she said that her husband finally had the energy to work out again, and they both felt much better.

Other raw food leaders were emailing me in disgust, as they said that my interview had caused them to lose many of their followers and customers, who decided to quit the diet and follow Nazariah's advice instead.

Whenever I would go to a raw food potluck, I would meet someone who had read the interview, and they thanked me for it. Many times, it was a scrawny, unhealthy-looking raw foodist I had met previously, who finally saw the light and stopped trying to survive on a semi-starvation diet and stopped being raw vegan.

My friend Gillian in Vancouver told me that just after I left, she also stopped being raw. She then read my interview with Nazariah and told me I should become the "world's foremost anti-promoter of the raw food diet."

Gillian told me she had realized that her problem was that on raw food, she had an eating disorder. She had read a book by a psychologist who helped women recover from such disorders after going on too strict a diet. The book claimed you could eat whatever you wanted, as long as you ate it mindfully.

"At first," Gillian told me, "I got super sick from eating cooked foods. I felt absolutely terrible. But I realized that after these two years of being raw, my body needed time to adjust."

Gillian told me that after a few weeks, she already felt much better. She could now digest cooked foods, and she noticed many improvements in her health.

"First of all, I don't feel bloated anymore. On raw, I always felt bloated like I was pregnant. I also don't have to eat so much anymore. I can eat a plate of noodles, and I'm fine for hours."

She also told me that there were some negatives to going back to cooked.

"Now, I need to put on deodorant. On raw foods, you don't need deodorant, because you don't have much body odor anymore."

It seemed like my article had triggered some serious questions from raw foodists worldwide. Victoria Boutenko, a well-known raw foodist, told me that when I published the interview with Nazariah, she constantly received phone calls from raw foodists who were afraid they were going to get sick on the diet.

For one thing, it proved that raw foodists worldwide were not healthy. The healthy ones did not care that some long-bearded dude in a toga was telling them you should not be raw vegan. If the diet really worked for them, it would have as much effect as telling a convinced and healthy vegetarian that they were going to die if they did not get enough meat protein.

But raw foodists, though a motivated bunch, were not convinced by their own real-world results. Therefore, my interview with Nazariah was enough to make some of them doubt their convictions and quit the diet, if they could find something better. It was like shaking a building with no foundations. A modest little kick had made the entire structure crumble.

The interview with Nazariah also had an important impact on me. For one thing, I decided to continue with the plan of eating only one fruit meal a day, instead of two.

For lunch, I generally had a big vegetable stir-fry (cooked in water), often with rice or rice noodles, and some tofu. Alternatively, I might make a big salad that contained some cooked ingredients like beans. For dinner, I might have a combination of cooked potatoes, salad and other combinations of cooked or raw vegetables.

I started eating some eggs, often hard-boiled, with my salads. I also ate yogurt with my fruit in the morning, and occasionally I had some grilled fish with my dinner. I did not feel ready to have any red meat yet, though.

I also started working out with weights, and I found it much easier to get the necessary energy to complete the workouts than I ever had in the past.

Over the course of the next months, I continued my experimentations with animal products. At some point, I mustered all of my courage and decided to eat some red meat. Surprisingly, it didn't "destroy" me and make me feel bad like all of those gourmet raw food recipes did in the past. Instead, I felt slightly more invigorated, calmer, and more grounded on the days I ate meat.

Along with these experimentations, I continued to madly search for information and question the raw food diet. I continued interviewing raw foodists from all over the world who were questioning the raw vegan diet. Many of them were mostly raw, but consumed some animal products on a regular or occasional basis.

I wasn't sure what the future would hold for me. If I came to positive conclusions that the raw vegan diet was not ideal, I would need to come out and expose the truth to my list. Then, I would have to think of something else to do for a living as well.

Since my last visit at the dentist, I had radically changed my diet. Although I still ate more fruit than most people, I had stopped eating two large fruit meals a day, and my lunches and dinners were now cooked or partly cooked. Initially I was still a vegetarian, but since my return from Vancouver I had started to eat eggs and yogurt, then some fish, and now, meat.

Yet, I was still worrying about my teeth. When I looked at them in the mirror, I noticed some brown discoloration spots that I suspected were cavities.

In panic, I scheduled another appointment with the dentist.

I told him about the brown discoloration spots and my fear of getting new cavities. He examined my teeth and told me,

"Well, it doesn't look like you have any cavities."

"What about the brown spots?" I asked.

He said, "It looks like your enamel has solidified and in the process left some of these brown spots. It looks to me like you had some more benign cavities developing and suddenly, you did something that made your teeth build back some enamel and prevented those benign cavities from turning into full-blown cavities."

"What do you mean by these benign cavities?" I asked.

He said, "Once a cavity has started, it's impossible to stop it, and we have to drill out the decay and put in a filling. But sometimes, if a cavity is stopped in the very early stages, the tooth can build back some enamel and repair it naturally. But that can only happen in when the decay is just starting."

I was flabbergasted.

Getting off the raw food diet had actually *worked,* and I now had the proof that my raw food diet was the cause of all this decay.

Could I attribute this remarkable recovery to the cooked foods I'd been eating or to the animal products?

I had also made some changes in my dental hygiene. I started using *toothsoap* twice a day, a product that claimed to help teeth re-enamelize themselves by keeping them clean and free of glycerin, an ingredient found in all toothpastes, that stays on the teeth and, according to the inventor of toothsoap, prevents them from building more enamel.

In my desperation, I had also started occasionally using a fluoride-based toothpaste once a day. Most natural-food people were radically anti-fluoride and made sure they purchased only fluoride-free toothpaste, claiming that fluoride is toxic.

After doing my own research and comparing the two camps, I came to the conclusion that the use of fluoride *topically* was one of the only things that was proven to reduce the incidence of decay. Taking fluoride *internally*, such as in fluoridated water, could have some negative consequences and isn't necessary, since all the teeth need is to be exposed to fluoride on their surface.

I was done with the idealistic theories of raw foodists. I had finally done something radically opposed to all their ideas, and I had gotten positive results by taking action.

After that checkup, my convictions were even more shaken. How could I continue being a raw foodist, or even *try* to be raw, when the inevitable result was a mouthful of cavities, low energy, and constant difficulty maintaining the diet?

I was forgetting the health improvements I had experienced since lowering the fat content of my diet and getting rid of the nuts and oils I was eating. The dental problems that seemed to be inevitable on the raw diet scared me so much that that I questioned whether to even try to make it work again.

I also knew I was not the only one.

I had met so many raw foodists who had experienced similar dental issues. Many had even worse problems, needing root canals and sometimes losing some teeth.

I did not buy the reasoning that *everyone has dental problems, not just raw foodists.*

So many people I had met had never had a cavity in their life, until they went raw. Even one of the only scientific studies ever done on the raw food diet showed that enamel erosion was one of the negative consequences of this diet.

Why Raw Foodists Have Problems with Their Teeth and What to Do About It

Raw foodists have, on average, more problems with their teeth than the national average in Western countries. This has been shown in one study done in Germany on a group of raw foodists, but can also be inferred from the number of discussions and concerns about dental health in various raw food groups.[60]

When I was in Costa Rica, I saw the following sign at a National Park. This is a word-for-word transcript of part of the sign.

Contrary to the stereotype, bananas are not the preferred food of monkeys in the wild. Bananas, especially those containing pesticides, can be upsetting to the monkeys' delicate digestive system and cause serious dental problems that can lead to eventual death.

60 Ganss, C., Schlechtriemen, M., &Klimek, J. (1999).Dental erosions in subjects living on a raw food diet. Caries Research, 33(1), 74-80.Excerpt from the study: The aim of the study was to investigate the frequency and severity of dental erosions and its association with nutritional and oral hygiene factors in subjects living on a raw food diet. As part of a larger dietary study 130 subjects whose ingestion of raw food was more than 95% of the total food intake were examined. The median duration of the diet was 39 (minimum 17, maximum 418) months. Before the clinical examination, the participants answered questionnaires and recorded their food intake during a 7-day period. Dental erosions were registered using study models. As a control 76 sex- and age-matched patients from our clinic were randomly selected. The raw food diet records showed the median daily frequency of ingesting citrus fruit to be 4.8 (minimum 0.5, maximum 16.1). The median intake of fruit was 62% (minimum 25%, maximum 96%) of the total, corresponding to an average consumption of 9.5 kg of fruit (minimum 1.5, maximum 23.7) per week. Compared to the control group subjects living on a raw food diet had significantly ($p</=0.001$) more dental erosions. Only 2.3% of the raw food group (13.2% of the controls) had no erosive defects, whereas 37.2% had at least one tooth with moderate erosion (55.2% of the controls) and 60.5% had at least one tooth with severe erosion (31.6% of the controls). Within the raw food group, no significant correlation was found between nutrition or oral health data and the prevalence of erosions. Nevertheless, the results showed that a raw food diet bears an increased risk of dental erosion compared to conventional nutrition.

The reality that all raw foodists refuse to admit is the simple fact that *a fruit-based, raw food diet is more cariogenic than many other types of diet.* (Cariogenic means "causing cavities or caries".)

The culprits are the high sugar content of the diet (in the form of fruits and juices), the number of dried, sticky items consumed (from dried fruits, nuts and raw crackers), and the tendency for raw foodists to snack constantly during the day, rather than settle for an average of two or three meals a day with no snacks. The latter is partly caused by the low caloric density of the diet, which makes it difficult to eat only two or three meals a day without some planning.

Let's not put the blame on fruit-based diets alone, but also include in that category most other types of raw diet, with their high nut and dried fruit content.

Even the typical cooked food diet eaten by most people is more cariogenic than the diet our ancestors ate, prior to the cultivation of grains and the widespread use of cooked foods.

In the Paleolithic and Mesolithic ages, caries (dental decay) were not prevalent, and only started around the Neolithic age.[61] Dietary culture changed throughout history — mainly because humans started to eat more foods containing carbohydrates and cooked them, which made them softer and more likely to stick to teeth.

Native Americans also saw an increase in dental decay when their hunter-gatherer diet was changed for one that included a greater amount of maize. It is also possible that dental decay appeared in Native Americans through contact with the Europeans, who brought the disease with them.[62]

The biggest increase in dental caries occurred in the period starting in 1850, when there was a greater availability and use of refined sugar, refined flour, bread, and sweetened tea.

---

61 Whittle, A., & Whittle, A. (1996). *Europe in the Neolithic : the creation of new worlds.* Cambridge University Press.
62 Mullin, M. (n.d). Iroquoia: The Development of a Native World (Book). *American Indian Culture & Research Journal, 27*(3), 112-114.

It's important to note that the fact that certain diets are more cariogenic is not a judgment on the healthfulness of these diets. Also, dental decay in itself is not an indication that the overall health of the person is failing. Although this is contrary to what you'll hear in some natural health circles, dental decay is generally not related to any other health problem, except in some rare cases when someone is not producing enough saliva, for example.

There are many positive aspects to the raw food diet, and the issue of dental health is the real weak link. This is not to say that these problems are inevitable, but more that *it is easier to create the conditions that will lead to an increase in dental decay on the raw diet than on most other diets.*

The Two Culprits

It's important to understand that decay is a transmittable disease. It is caused by the proliferation of the bacterium *Streptococcus mutans* in the oral environment, and it can be transferred from mother to child in the early stages of life (through kissing, sharing food, etc.)[63]

The bacteria metabolize sugars and produce acids, which start to break down the enamel surface of teeth. As the destruction of the enamel goes deeper, a cavity is the result.

The process is reversible if it is caught early enough, before the enamel has been affected too deeply. This is how I was able to stop my rampant dental decay by taking aggressive action (by eating fruit less frequently and using toothpaste until the cavities healed).

The bacteria will tend to accumulate in a sort of "colony," an intro-oral biofilm called *plaque*. It's a sticky substance that is a breeding ground for those bad bacteria, and that's why we must disrupt it daily through proper dental hygiene and regular cleanings.

Sugar and carbs are the food of these bacteria. In this regard, the sugar in fruit is no different than the sugar found in any other food.

---

63 McAuliffe, K. (1993). Contagious cavities. *Omni, 15*(9), 29. DNA testing found that the leading bacteria responsible for tooth decay originates primarily in our mothers' mouths. The culprit, Streptococcus mutans, is passed in saliva from mother to child following the eruption of molar teeth at about two years of age.

It wouldn't be fair to say that fruit is just as bad for the teeth as candy. A piece of fruit, full of water and fiber, will not be as cariogenic as a sticky substance like candy. The action of the fiber against the teeth certainly contributes to some natural cleansing, especially when we're eating a harder type of fruit like an apple.

On the other hand, dried fruit is just as bad for our teeth as candy, because it tends to stick to the teeth and feed bacteria for longer periods of time. Nuts, however, have been found to have no positive association with dental decay.[64]

A big cause of dental decay is the *frequency* with which teeth are exposed to cariogenic or acidic foods.

Every time we eat something, the bacteria in the mouth will start to feed on the sugar and produce acidity, which will lower the mouth pH. Given a little time, the pH will return to normal with the action of saliva.

Every time we put acidic foods in our mouths (including oranges and limes), or eat sweet foods, the bacteria will consume the sugar to produce more acidity. Some portions of the mineral content on the surface of teeth will start to dissolve, and this state persists for up to two hours.

Therefore, the more often we eat (especially fruit), the more we will encourage the development of dental decay or enamel erosion.

That is why experts today say that the frequency of sugar intake is more important than the amount of sugar consumed.[65]

But on the raw food diet, we automatically have the tendency to eat more often because the foods are lower in calories. People are afraid to eat a lot of fruit at once and tend to spread out their intake over the course of the day, which can have disastrous consequences for their teeth.

So the high sugar content of fruit is not the problem. The problem is that we eat fruit or sweet foods constantly!

---

64 Llena, C., &Forner, L. (2008). Dietary habits in a child population in relation to caries experience.*Caries Research*, *42*(5), 387-393. In this study on Spanish children, sweet snacks, industrial bread and soft drink consumption showed a positive association with caries while cheese and nuts showed a negative association.

65 Cann, R. (2006). Health Food Mystery Reveals the Tooth Decay Culprit. New Life Journal: Carolina Edition, 7(7), 8.

For example:

- Drinking coconut water throughout the day

- Drinking other types of freshly pressed fruit juices

- Snacking on fruit every few hours

- Sipping smoothies throughout the day

- Snacking on dried fruits

All of the above can have disastrous consequences for your teeth, even if you are very diligent about dental hygiene. Ideally, we should be eating a maximum of three meals a day with no snacks.

The Only Solution

The only way to prevent dental decay for life and reverse a bad situation is to take active control of your oral environment.

First, you have to reduce your exposure to sugar by eating fewer times a day and avoiding snacking. On the raw food diet, this requires some training to be able to consume the necessary amount in fewer servings.

But just controlling your diet does not address the root of the problem, which is bacterial proliferation and plaque, which are organized into "colonies" or hotbeds, rather than being in a free-flowing state.

The problem is that most dentists don't teach you that you can actually reverse this process and keep your teeth mostly free of plaque and the bacteria at an acceptable level. They just say, "Floss once a day, brush twice a day and use a fluoride toothpaste!"

This kind of advice is not very effective.

What you need to do is to move from a regular hygiene program to a *super* hygiene program.

This means:

Increasing the Time You Brush

I recommend brushing before going to bed with an advanced electric toothbrush, such as the Oral-B Triumph, and letting it run for 4 minutes — one minute for each corner of the mouth. Then also brush right after you wake up in the morning and after your lunch. That's a total brushing time of around 8 minutes per day. Make sure you brush softly; otherwise, you could be hurting your gums and causing them to recede. If you don't know the new conservative brushing technique, ask your dentist. If he doesn't know, or repeats what you've already heard, find another dentist!

Using an Oral Irrigator

The Waterpik is the most popular kind. I prefer the Vita-Jet. They work extremely well to remove food particles that may not have been caught through brushing and flossing. You don't need to add any substance to the water.

Using a Tongue Scraper

It's used to clean your tongue, once or twice a day. You can now find them in most pharmacies.

And of course, floss using the right technique (again, ask your dentist).

That's the only effective way to prevent dental decay and gum disease for life.

CHAPTER 18

The Raw Curse

"The longer you are raw, the more sensitive you become. Processed foods you ate before are no longer tolerated. I have been on a raw diet for almost 7 years. I am convinced that half a hamburger would put me in the hospital. If you were to give Dr. Fred Bisci, 40-year raw foodist, the same half hamburger, it could be fatal."

Matt Monarch,
of The Raw Food World

When I completely moved away from the raw diet for a period of a year, I noticed a lot of improvements that I enjoyed.

For one thing, I felt that this new diet was having a much better impact on my teeth.

I also gained weight, going from a weakling at 139 pounds (at 5 foot 10) to a more respectable 150 pounds. Was it all muscle? No, but the weight gain alone was enough to make me feel better about myself.

My digestion was also better. Having to eat less often, my body seemed to be able to better process the foods it was eating.

On the negative side, I felt less vitality or "joy" eating this way. This should not be confused with physical energy. On any raw diet, even the high-fat ones, I have experienced a certain lift in mood and overall vitality. This is not just a personal experience but also a widespread phenomenon. Eating raw food relieves depression in general.

On any cooked diet (unless cooked food did not represent more than 20% of calories consumed), I did not feel the same level of "joy."

When I no longer viewed myself as a raw foodist, I opened the doors to all kinds of new culinary experiences. I avoided overt junk foods and processed foods, but suddenly, all kinds of cooked foods I never thought I would eat again crept back into my diet.

Seeing my weight and my energy levels go up, I started to think that perhaps I had underestimated the importance of protein. For all these years, I'd always thought that the obsession with protein was a "myth" and that I could get all the protein I needed from fruits and vegetables.

The interview with Nazariah made me rethink that position. Although I still had an aversion to eating meat (I only ate it on a few occasions), I started including more eggs and fermented dairy products in my diet.

For breakfast, I would often eat an omelet. Sometimes, I would eat scrambled eggs with beans for dinner. I would often put some tofu in my salads, and I would eat kefir or yogurt with my fruit in the morning.

The more time went by, the more "cooked" and high-protein my diet became.

The surprising thing is that I would often get complimented on how I looked when I went to raw food potlucks. One day I had eaten a lot of bread, and the next day my face looked a bit more puffed up than usual. People said I looked "great," probably because I had gained some water weight.

But in spite of these superficial results, I started to feel worse again.

At the end of summer 2004, I decided to go to the Portland Raw Food Festival just to see what was happening there. Even people like Fred Bisci, a raw food nutritionist I had met a couple of years earlier at the festival in my skinnier days, said that I looked "much better" than when he first met me. However, I did not feel as great as I may have looked to him.

I felt a real physical depression, a sort of dark cloud in my mind and heaviness in my brain, but at the same time, I had energy. I wasn't lethargic, but I felt like doing nothing for days.

At the end of the summer, I came to a very sad realization: the raw food diet did not work, but cooked foods did not work either. What was I going to do?

The Raw Curse

When I met RC Dini back in 1997, he told me that he had gone back to cooked foods a few times during his first year or two of raw eating. Every time, he got so sick that he created a term called *the raw curse*. He said that once you go raw, there is no going back. Even if you want to go back, you can't. Your body has gotten used to a new state of health, and you will get sick.

In my book *The Raw Secrets*, I talk about something I called the *Law of Vital Accommodation.*

From my book:

"Understanding the Law of Vital Accommodation may be one of the most important lessons in this book. It will help clarify many blind spots. This law states that when a poison is introduced into the organism on a regular basis, to a degree beyond the body's capacity to expel it, the body adapts to this invader by insulating itself from it. This is done at the expense of normal body functioning. For example, if you smoke, your body will prevent absorption of the toxic fumes by hardening the lung membranes to avoid intoxicating the body beyond a certain level of toleration.

If you take a less-than-fatal dose of poison every day, after six months you could take a more-than-fatal one and survive. The body will resist the poison by avoiding absorption at all cost. But this also means that general nutrient absorption will be diminished.

In Orthobionomics, Shelton wrote, "Toleration to poisons is merely a slow method of dying. Instead of seeing in the phenomena of toleration something to be sought after, it is something to seek to avoid the necessity for."

A Purer Body

When you begin a clean diet based on fruits and vegetables, you are no longer taking in a lot of popular poisons: coffee, chocolate, cigarettes, spices, food preservatives, etc. Your body rejects accumulated poisons and goes back to a more original, pure state — like that of a child. In other words, you will be like a beginner, before he starts to take his daily dose of poison, which means that you will be much more affected, and penalized, by small doses of poisons than most people. A cup of coffee could have the same effect on you as five cups on your neighbor. You will be more affected by what you eat, especially if you go off your new diet.

Here are some examples of this law in action:

If you go on a pure diet without garlic and onion or hot peppers, next time you try to eat these things your body might react negatively, and you might strongly dislike the experience. However, if you go back to eating them a little bit at a time, eventually you will be able to eat them without problems. This is the reason why children often do not like strong or spicy foods.

If you don't use any salt at all for a while, having just one salty thing, like a bowl of soup, will make you feel extremely dehydrated from it. However, if you drink a little bit of soup every day, in just a week or two, your body will adapt to the higher salt intake, and you'll be able to have entire bowls of soup without feeling affected.

If you don't eat any meat at all for years, and then go back to meat by eating a 6-ounce piece of meat, you won't be able to digest it. It will literally come out undigested. However, if you start slowly and have a little piece of meat at a time, every day, then in a matter of weeks, your body will adapt to the higher protein intake, and you will be able to digest a 6-ounce piece of meat.

This strange law of adaptation explains why raw foodists feel so sick when they go back to cooked food. Because of their raw diet, their bodies have literally lost most of the ability to digest complex carbohydrates, handle higher protein intake, and possibly handle salt intake, too. When they go back to cooked foods, they get a much stronger reaction than what would be considered "normal."

I'm not saying that there are not certain substances in cooked foods that are toxic, such as all the preservatives and MSG in prepared food. The Law of Vital Accommodation also works for them. That is why a heavy drinker can handle much more alcohol than someone who drinks only once a year.

The Law of Vital Accommodation works in reverse too, from cooked foods to raw foods. It mainly has to do with the fiber content of food. When someone is used to being on a cooked food diet with a very low fiber content, and then switches to a high-fiber, raw food diet, he might experience all kinds of digestive issues, especially with big salads and greens consumed in all forms. Again, if he starts slowly, by having a little bit of green smoothie every day and increasing the amount gradually, he will eventually be able to digest these vegetables without problems.

Fruits require almost no digestion, as the energy they provide comes mainly from simple sugars, with a very low fat or protein content. They do contain some fiber, but not as much as vegetables. Therefore, people who live on fruit alone, with nothing else, experience the most violent symptoms if they go back to cooked foods, and even if they eat heavier raw food recipes.

So the Law of Vital Accommodation works from raw to cooked, from cooked to raw, and within the raw diet itself.

If someone goes for a time eating only fruits and vegetables without fat, and then eats an entire avocado, she might conclude, overhastily, that avocado is bad, because she has a negative reaction to this large amount. This happens quite a lot with people who eat no overt fats or strive for a 90/5/5 type of diet (an extreme form of 80/10/10).

Some people have taken this Law of Vital Accommodation very seriously. The author Fred Bisci, whom I mentioned earlier, often talked about the danger that raw foodists face when going to the hospital.

He claimed that because raw foodists eat such a pure diet, they become ultra-sensitive to every drug. Therefore, if they are given the same amount of anesthetic or other drugs as other people, they could get seriously ill or die.

Some raw foodists are excessively obsessed with purity. Any sign that the human body is "working," such as feeling a little tired after a meal or any gas, is viewed as "bad." They want to feel completely pure, so as time goes by, they tend to keep simplifying their diet.

For example, in 2003, I met a guy in Spain who was a complete fruitarian. He looked extremely skinny and had no energy, yet he continued his restrictive diet. He got to the point where he felt that even certain fruits like bananas and figs were too "heavy" and only consumed the light, juicy fruits like melons.

This kind of approach is not healthy. Here's how to stay healthy, while avoiding the main consequences of being too pure:

Get enough calories

Whether you're eating 100% raw or not, it's important to make sure to eat enough food to get enough calories. As you can probably tell by reading my book this far, my main mistake over the years was undereating. This mistake tends to be easiest for young men to make, as they need more calories. If you consistently undereat, your body will eventually become weak.

Be consistent

Although a low-sodium diet with no added salt is best, going back and forth from a high sodium intake to a no-added-salt diet is worse than eating just a little bit of salt every day. In general, it's better to be consistent and reasonable than to go back and forth between two extremes. This is not to say that you should just live the philosophy of "everything in moderation," but that avoiding the extremes of a "yo-yo" diet is important.

Don't be too pure

The tendency towards extremism is strong in the raw food movement. If we find that a low-fat diet is great, then a no-fat diet must be even better, right? Just feeling more pure should not be the only goal. We must give our body everything it needs. I do not recommend a diet that includes no added fat. Having a small amount of nuts and seeds on a regular basis is beneficial (one ounce at a time is usually plenty).

Exercise

Exercise is a form of stress on the body. Muscle tissue is broken down and lactic acid is released. However, this stress does not weaken the body. With adequate recovery, it makes it stronger. That is why being athletic improves every other area of health, including your ability to digest food.

If you can understand the Law of Vital Accommodation, you can use it to your advantage. For example, some raw foodists are worried that if they find themselves in a situation where they cannot maintain their diet, such as a long trip somewhere, they are going to get extremely sick if they eat any cooked foods. Knowing how the Law of Vital Accommodation works, you will no longer experience stress about such situations.

Let me give you an analogy from something I discovered while studying foreign languages. Over the years, I've studied many foreign languages, including Spanish, Portuguese, Italian, German, and Russian. I've gotten to be fairly fluent in many of them, especially the ones I used the most. Right now, I couldn't prove to you that I speak any Russian, because I haven't practiced it for years. However, the previous knowledge I built comes back very fast if I immerse myself in the language again. On my last trip to Germany, I realized how bad my German had gotten in the last few years through lack of use. But after just a few weeks in Germany, I was speaking fairly fluent German again.

If you're a strict raw foodist and you ever find yourself in a situation where you cannot maintain your diet for a period of time, you can always rebuild the ability to digest cooked foods by training your body to digest them.

What really shocks the body is going from a very pure diet to a cooked meal, with no transition in between. As my friend Dominic discovered, you can retrain yourself to digest cooked foods by eating just a little bit at a time, increasing the quantities slowly as necessary.

This is to say that raw foodists are free to choose. The raw food diet can bring great rewards, and this doesn't have to come at the cost of extreme sensitivity.

I find that it's best to follow a diet that brings you as close as possible to the state of health you desire, while not being so strict that you become sensitive to everything and paranoid about your diet. On a diet without any overt fats, your ability to digest fat properly will be temporarily compromised. Remember that you need essential fatty acids, and that no fat is no better than too much fat!!

I recommend the consumption of 1-2 ounces of nuts or seeds a few times a week, consumed in the form of salad dressings. Athletes can increase these quantities, while sedentary people or those seeking to lose weight can eat less. Other raw foods rich in essential fatty acids, such as avocado, durian, and coconut, are also good to eat in moderation and can be used instead of nuts and seeds if you like.

CHAPTER 19

My Fast in Costa Rica

"When the stomach is full, it is easy to talk of fasting"

St. Jerome,
Father in the Early Church. 340-420 AD

In 2004, I spent a great deal of time doubting the raw food diet, questioning it, and then giving up on the ideal of 100% raw completely. By the summer, I came to the realization that once again, I had failed in my attempt to achieve optimal health, and that perhaps I had thrown the baby out with the bathwater.

Eating raw had benefits, but the way I had done it for so many years had not worked. The thing I had done that worked the best was going back to Natural Hygiene, the way I ate for my first years of raw, while following Mosséri's principles. However, even in those days, I was still plagued with cravings and had difficulties maintaining the diet.

Going back to a mostly cooked diet (including animal foods) made me depressed and sick, so that did not work either.

I reckoned that there must be some kind of balance in between. I had met so many people who seemed perfectly healthy and happy on an 80% raw food diet, finding an ideal balance between eating super healthy, and allowing themselves some leeway and eating some healthy cooked foods.

My experience showed that trying to restrict myself in that way did not work for me. Eating steamed squash and broccoli and baked sweet potatoes eventually led to bread, cheese, sandwiches, and pizza.

I had not tried to fully live out the "balanced" path of 80% raw, but there were also some other things I had not tried.

In my book *The Raw Secrets*, I quoted Doug Graham, with his thought-provoking ideas on the failure of the raw food diet and his own brand of the raw food diet that he called *80/10/10*.

At the time, Doug Graham had not fully expressed his ideas in a book, and the only way to get the full scoop was to participate in one of his live events.

So I went to the raw food festival in Oregon in 2004, and attended some of Graham's talks, where he presented his approach to raw food in more detail.

"I have analyzed the diet of hundreds of raw foodists," explained Graham. "Many of them think they follow a low-fat diet, when in reality the fat content of their diet is close to 40%, sometimes more!"

Doug explained that it's quite easy to eat more fat than you should without realizing it. He also explained that to fully succeed on the raw food diet, you have to eat quantities of fruit that would seem excessive to the average human, and even the average raw foodist.

"Whenever I meet someone who tells me they have problems because they are eating too much fruit, upon close examination I often find out that their problems were actually caused by not eating enough fruit!"

All those years, I had eaten plenty of fruit, but perhaps Doug was right, and I was just not eating enough. Maybe this is what caused me to have all of those cravings, which led me to binge on gourmet raw foods, and later led me back to cooked food.

At the event, I met people who were following Doug's 80/10/10 diet, and they looked quite healthy and athletic. One girl of my age ate only fruits and vegetables, and yet, she was training for a marathon. Surprisingly, she did not even look super-skinny like many other raw foodists.

Although extreme weight loss was one of my concerns, I decided that maybe I could give the low-fat 100% raw diet another try. But after all the damage I had done to my body over the years by eating raw incorrectly, maybe I needed to do something else, too.

Doug was a big proponent of fasting, and every year he organized a fasting retreat in Costa Rica. I had read about fasting for all these years, and I was convinced of the health benefits of a properly-supervised water fast. However, I had never fasted myself, except for those few occasions where I tried to fast on my own, only to quit after a few days.

Doug's retreat seemed exceptional, because it was undertaken in a beautiful tropical country during the winter, so getting cold was of no concern. His fasting retreat required an entire six-week commitment, including an average of three weeks of fasting and three weeks of recovery and refeeding. If I went, I would share a room with another faster and be under professional supervision.

To me, it sounded like paradise. I could take six weeks of my life to just *rest*. Do nothing, lie in bed, and give my body a chance to heal.

Right after the fasting retreat and in the same location, Doug organized a two week "walking tour" of Costa Rica, which featured lots of hiking and more health education. This sounded like a perfect thing to do to get in shape after the fast.

I decided to sign up for both events, as he was offering a deal for doing both at the same time. "Why don't you come to my *Health & Fitness Week* as well?" he asked.

The *Health & Fitness Week* was his main yearly event, an exciting week of fitness and health education, "gourmet" 80/10/10 meals three times a day, and *lots* of exercise. I thought this was just for raw vegan athletes, but Doug explained to me that he had people of all ages and abilities that participated.

I didn't need much convincing to give it a try, and after he offered me a very generous discount for taking all three events in the same year, I signed up for the package.

Right after I got back to Montreal, my German friend Rachana, got inspired by my plans and decided to sign up for both the fasting retreat and the walking tour. "Great!" I thought, "I won't be going there alone."

In preparation for the fast, I decided to clean up my diet and go on a hygienic diet similar to the one I had followed years ago, before I went raw. I ate only fruits and vegetables, but I also included potatoes and steamed vegetables. In the process, I lost about 10 pounds, and I got to

Costa Rica in late December 2004, back at my scrawny weight of 139 pounds.

It had been a few years since I had first visited Costa Rica, and just arriving at the international airport in San Jose made me realize how much I had missed the tropics. The warm air greeted me in Alajuela, and with my open ticket, I could stay in Costa Rica as long as I wanted and miss most of the Canadian winter.

The plan was quite simple: we would spend one night at a hotel near the airport, and then the next day a shuttle was to take us to the town of Uvita, about five hours away on the beautiful Pacific coast, where the fast was going to take place.

On the morning we were leaving, we had breakfast at the hotel. Doug had instructed the staff to serve us fresh pineapple and papaya, without the usual rice and beans that Costa Ricans eat for breakfast. I ate a bit of pineapple, but decided I was going to save my appetite for the lunch we would probably have in Uvita.

When our shuttle left, I asked Doug what time our fast would start tomorrow. He replied "Tomorrow? What do you mean tomorrow? The fast has already started!"

"You mean..." I said, "This morning's breakfast was our last meal?"

"Yep," he replied.

I was quite disappointed at that moment... I had expected a nice "last meal," a sort of mental preparation for the fast. Had I known that we were going to start the fast right after breakfast, I would have eaten more than those few slices of pineapple!

"Oh well..." I thought, "That's what you signed up for."

My Fasting Journal

What follows is the exact digital journal I kept during my fast in Costa Rica, never published before. I do all my personal writing in French, so what follows is my own translation into English of what I originally wrote in French when I was fasting.

January 3rd, 2005

It's the second day of the fast. I feel tired. My tongue is not too white. I feel quite similar to when I fasted in the past: fatigue, a little dizzy, but otherwise it's going well. I feel like I have a headache coming on, but it doesn't come.

My weight was 139 pounds this morning. I was at probably 141 before I left, and maybe 144 a few months ago.

It's going pretty well, and I'm not too hungry. Now I'm going to sleep.

January 6th, 2005

It's the fifth day of the fast. Yesterday, it started to become difficult, and today it is even more so. My weight is now down to 130 pounds, without having drunk any water today. I'm really tired, and I just feel like lying down. I do not want to talk too much, or walk, or read. In the afternoon it's better, and I have more energy.

Day 9

I went through some pretty tough days. It started with a sort of sore throat, and then that was followed with more discomfort in my jaw. This morning it's going better, and I feel more relaxed. I just want to stay in bed and rest. I listen to music to kill time. My tongue wasn't too white when I started the fast, but now it's white as snow. I had a sort of light headache (not a migraine), but it went away pretty quickly.

Day 10

Extreme fatigue, especially in the morning. I feel like staying in bed, listening to music, and that's it. My sore throat is 92% healed.

Yesterday I couldn't stop thinking about what I wanted to do in my life after my fast for 2005.

Day 12

Good day yesterday. Today I feel less inner peace. It's okay. My throat and mouth feel really dry. I have a really bad body odor. I stink...

Day 15

I had some weird dreams about food. My dreams have become very lucid and clear, almost like a movie. I dreamed that I was eating some kind of giant chocolate cake and dates the size of mangoes (even though that's not possible). The sore throat is gone. My complexion is getting better. I sleep pretty well with lots of dreams. I've been having really bad breath in the last few days.

Day 18

I've experienced many changes. My breath is better. My weight is down to 120 pounds. My skin is getting much better. I'm counting the days still to go: I can't help it. I sleep less. I have great mental clarity. My tongue is not as white. I brushed my teeth and my gums were bleeding a little. I watch DVDs in the afternoon to pass time.

I've been thinking a lot about my life after the fast, how I'm going to gain back the weight, how I will go back to raw foods after all these years of problems, such as dental decay and doubt. I saw the movie Touching the Void, and I just have to think about this story to find courage to go at it one step at a time. One day at a time, this is what I have to do. Now, I'm fasting.

Day 19

I had weird dreams last night.

Day 20

I'm feeling strange tingling on my tongue. I thought it could be a Vitamin B12 deficiency, but Doug doesn't think so. I'm continuing the fast for now. Apparently my breath is still bad.

Day 21

Lots of dreams.

Day 22

My tongue feels weird... like a little numb? I talked to Doug about it. He reassured me everything was fine, but I'm not so sure myself.

Day 23

Still the same numbness in part of my tongue. I decided to break the fast tomorrow if everything goes well. I had a dream in which I was eating giant dates and then realized I had just broken the fast by doing so, and I was disappointed in myself.

Day 24

I broke the fast at 14:00. I ate watermelon: four slices in four hours. It was amazingly delicious. I still feel like I'm fasting though. My gums bled a little when I was eating. I should have brushed more often during the fast to strengthen the gums, but Doug told us not to. Now they're too weak.

Day 25

I still feel like I'm fasting. I only ate melon today.

Day 26

The weird numbness in part of my tongue is still there, but it's going away. Today, I only ate papaya, and probably more than I should, since Tyler kept bringing me more servings in spite of Doug's orders to give me only a smaller amount.

Day 27

I ate too much papaya, and I got a stomach-ache yesterday. Today, I skipped breakfast and at 11:30 had four mangoes. The first one was delicious, but I can find better mangoes in Montreal. I look like a skeleton. I'm pretty weak, but the strength is coming back little by little.

Day 28

Doug thinks the numbness in the tongue and the other things I was feeling may have been from lack of B vitamins (not just B12), so he recommended that I should start eating more greens.

Day 29

My elimination is slowly getting back to normal. I feel stronger, but I still don't feel like myself.

Day 33

I never thought this would be such a difficult experience psychologically. I slept better yesterday, with lots of dreams. I still have a weird tension in my left arm, but it's getting better. This is the 10th day since breaking the fast.

Day 34

Today I feel very tired. I did not have any energy to walk up the hill. But it's the first day that I've felt normal otherwise, in a good mood. The tension in my arm is gone. I feel waves of dizziness, and I'm not sure I'm tolerating all of this fruit sugar. I think it's going to take me a while to get back to normal. I started working out my upper body and feel better. Today, I was craving guacamole. I think a lot about my return home.

Day 36

Day 12 after the fast...

My digestion got really bad, with liquid and urgent stools. I suspect that all of these wild greens they've been feeding us for dinner have been making me sick. Tonight, we had a black sesame tahini dressing: it also made me feel sick, I think. I think it would be easier to recover from the fast if I had more blended foods, but right now there is none available.

Otherwise, I definitely have more energy. I still feel a little spacey though.

Day 38

I feel better in general. I feel more like myself. I'm looking forward to going back to Montreal, but not the winter.

Day 43

I've been feeling a lot better for the last 4 or 5 days. I'm no longer spacey. I still sleep a lot though; about 10 hours a night, and I don't have a lot of energy when I get up. I also get up to go pee about 4 times a night; with these big fruit and salad meals we have for dinner. The evening meals have included some avocado, but my digestion is still not good.

After the fast, I participated in the *Walking Tour of Costa Rica*, and after that was over, I traveled a little bit with Rachana. After that, I spent another month on my own.

Rachana and I were the only participants in the walking tour that had also done the fast. Everybody else came specifically for the walking tour.

To my surprise, our energy and endurance was better than everybody else's (the only person that was in better shape was a girl who worked at a national park and hiked several hours a day). All these people had been eating three meals or more per day when we were fasting, and yet we were faster and fitter than they were.

This was probably the main health benefit I noticed from the fast.

I had hoped that the fast would heal my myopia, but there were absolutely no changes in my vision. I still needed my glasses.

During the fast itself, the one thing that impressed me the most was the mental clarity I had after 7 days. I had some of the most vivid dreams I'd ever had in my life, and during the day, I would write down elaborate plans and ideas for things I wanted to do after my fast.

The most difficult thing about the fast itself, apart from the lack of energy, was the constant self-observation. I'm the kind of person who already spends too much time overanalyzing, so whenever I'm put in a situation where all I have to do is observe my thoughts and my body, I start to freak out.

A year prior to the fast, I had participated in a 10-Day Meditation Retreat with a Vipassana group, and I absolutely hated the entire experience. Meditating 10 hours a day just put my mind into overdrive and achieved the exact opposite effect of what most people hope to get from these programs.

In many ways, the fast was a lot easier than the 10-Day Meditation Retreat. All I had to do was rest, talk to other guests, and rest some more.

At the end of the fast, I weighed 115 pounds, and my body fat was around 5%. My height is 5 foot 10 inches (178 centimeters). A few days later, I quickly gained back 10 pounds (most of it as water and stored glycogen), and it took me a month or two to get back to 135 pounds. After that, it took me several months to get back to my normal weight (at the time) of 145 pounds. (I now weigh 155 pounds.)

When I started to eat fruit after the fast, I felt like all the sugar was hitting my brain at once. I felt a rush of excitement, but very little energy to do anything. I also felt very spacey and initially felt very little mental clarity, compared to what I experienced during my fast. After a week or two, this "spaciness" went away, and I felt back to normal.

It took about two weeks to regain my energy levels, and after three weeks, I was doing surprisingly well in terms of having the physical endurance to walk all day. Recovery continued. I started doing pushups and other body exercises to build my strength, and found that I wasn't as weak as I expected. After just four weeks, I could do about 40 pushups in a row.

The most difficult thing with the period after the fast was getting adjusted to eating again. I continued to experience digestive disorders, gas, bloating, cramps, and really bad elimination.

The main cause of that was the sudden transition from fasting to eating a lot of fruit, and then to eating large quantities of salad with nut dressings.

At the time, Doug had only one assistant for the fast, a Canadian guy named Tyler who did not completely agree with his philosophy. So instead of feeding me the amount of fruit that Doug had recommended, he would feed me more.

Since then, Doug has fired Tyler and changed his system to include better follow-up after the fast. At the time, this overfeeding after the fast caused me many problems.

It was also very difficult to get enough calories by eating whole fruit. It would have been a lot better to have access to easily digestible smoothies, in addition to whole fruits.

Dinner meals were also a problem, and after eating dinner I felt an urgent need to go to the bathroom.

There's a green that grows in Costa Rica called katuk, a tropical plant that can be planted in any garden and spreads like crazy. Its leaves are edible and tasty. After the fast, katuk was part of our evening salads, and I suspect it made me sick. Two years later, I was living in Costa Rica for the winter, and my girlfriend and I had a pet bunny. We fed the bunny katuk leaves, which he seemed to enjoy, every day. After a few weeks, the bunny died. A local living in the area told us that rabbits can get poisoned by eating too much katuk. I also learned that some years ago in Thailand, a green preparation made with katuk leaves was sold as a natural remedy for weight loss. After a few people died from overdose, the katuk-based product had to be taken off the shelves.

In any case, I found my post-fast recovery was slower *because* of these digestive issues, which could have been caused or made worse by katuk consumption, which they served us at the retreat.

A few days after the fast, the dressings for these salads contained nut butters. Because they were served buffet-style, it was difficult to limit and restrain myself, which contributed to more digestive problems.

At the time, Doug's philosophy was to feed us fruits and vegetables in their natural state. So, for breakfast, we were served big slices of watermelon, and for lunch, it was usually whole bananas.

My problem was that I had difficulty eating enough bananas at once. I was hoping that we would be served some banana smoothies, which was an easier way for me to eat my bananas, but unfortunately, it was not part of the plan. I had to wait until the entire fasting group left the premises, when only Tyler, Rachana and I were left on our own for a few days until the next event started, the *Walking Tour of Costa Rica*.

During that time, Tyler made us giant banana smoothies that we deeply enjoyed for lunch, as well as avocado-based salad dressings for dinner, which were my favorite and the easiest to digest.

A long water fast is not an experience one can have without proper supervision. I knew that when I started the fast. What I did not expect was how vulnerable fasting would make me emotionally and physically.

Vulnerability During the Fast

After about 4 or 5 days of fasting, the body becomes very weak. It seeks to conserve its energies by doing less and less, and resorts to burning its own reserves of body fat to produce ketones that it will use as fuel.[66]

Doug warned us to "not make any major life decision" during the fast, because when the brain runs on ketones, our thinking is not the same.

I did experience great mental clarity during the fast, but I also felt extremely concerned about each little thing that was happening in my body.

---

66 Garruti, G., Triggiani, V., Ciampolillo, A., Giorgino, R., Santoro, G., De Pergola, G., et al. (1995). 34-day total fast in an adult man.*International journal of obesity and related metabolic disorders : Journal of the International Association for the Study of Obesity, 19*(1), 46-49.

The vulnerability that is associated with fasting comes from the fact that the faster is indeed *in great danger* during this critical period. As the body burns through its reserves, it becomes weaker and weaker. When the fast is broken, extreme care must be taken over the refeeding. (There are even historical stories of people who starved by force of circumstances and then gorged so much when food became available that they killed themselves.)

During the fast, you must have 100% trust in the person taking care of you. If, for any reason, anything were to happen, you would not be able to take care of yourself as usual. For example, you can't simply decide to break the fast on a whim, pack your bags, and leave. The further you go into the fast, the more delicate the situation becomes, because the body is weaker and weaker, and increasingly sensitive. Any drastic influence (such as the reintroduction of a food it is not ready to digest) can have dire consequences.

A person who is fasting is extremely vulnerable to drugs: a small quantity could have devastating effects on their hypersensitive body. Therefore, it is absolutely critical not to end up in the hospital for any reason during the fast, as doctors who have no experience with fasting might make drastic decisions that could have fatal consequences.

The mental state of the faster is as important as her physical state. Any amount of fear during the fast will make fasting that much more difficult and dangerous.

Past the 14-day point of my fast, I experienced daily fear and doubt about continuing the fast. This partly came from the fact that Tyler, the assistant in charge, had a different health philosophy than Doug. He would often tell us that he disagreed with Doug on many topics. This induced a certain level of doubt in the safety of what I was doing there.

After about 16 days of fasting, I started noticing strange sensations in my body. I noted some of them in my fasting journal, such as a strange sensation of "heat" and numbness in my tongue and lip, and micro-spasms. After the fast, I also noticed a strange tension in my left arm that popped up for no apparent reason. Most of these symptoms persisted for about two weeks after I broke the fast.

It could have been a Vitamin B12 deficiency (some of the symptoms corresponded to that), or it could have been my imagination. The important thing was that I felt that something was wrong, and I didn't want to continue the fast beyond that point.

Fasting in a tropical third-world country also brings some challenges. I was in the tropical heat of Uvita, sitting in bed all day and barely moving. I sweated a lot, but I did not have the energy to take frequent showers (I managed to take one a day on average). This made my skin worse, and after the fast I had a huge breakout on my back, where I have had a tendency to bad skin for most of my life. I also had a very bad case of dandruff, confirmed by a hairdresser who cut my hair after the fast. She suggested a one-time use of a medicated shampoo to get rid of the dandruff, which worked. The wet heat of Uvita certainly did not help my skin at all.

Although it was great to never experience cold during the fast, I believe a drier type of weather would have been more appropriate (since then, Doug Graham has moved his fasting retreat to this type of location).

What I Ate After the Fast

After the fast, I spent about six weeks traveling Costa Rica, first with Rachana, then on my own. During that time, I was 100% raw. I was very eager to gain back some of the weight I had lost, and this led me to eat more avocado than what was recommended.

Every night, I would eat a big salad with Costa Rican ingredients (such as lettuce, big tomatoes, cucumber, lime juice, etc) and add an avocado or two to it.

Even though avocados and nuts had done me in before, it was hard to think rationally after breaking the fast. I was starving. I ate all the watermelon I could for breakfast, but I was hungry a few hours later. For lunch, I ate 7 or 8 medium Costa Rican bananas (not like the Cavendish variety), and I could not eat any more. Two hours later, I was starving again. So, when it came time for dinner, I couldn't help myself. I ate a bunch more fruit and then a large salad topped with lots and lots of avocados or nut dressings. I had this insane craving for vegetables, which I think I probably needed to remineralize my body. However, the greens we had in Costa Rica were often tough, bitter, and wild, along with some regular green-leaf lettuce. They did not taste good by themselves at all, so to force them down, I had to cover them with dressing.

I did this every day, and it created this vicious cycle of starving all day, overeating at dinner, and then feeling sick and going to the bathroom with very urgent and painful stools.

There's no doubt that the avocados I ate helped me gain some of the weight I had lost. I would eat at least 2000 calories a day, but with my level of activity, I was probably burning more than that, so the weight gain was slow. Because I did not have a blender, all I could do was eat whole fruits, and I found it difficult to eat enough to get sufficient calories after the fast.

During the fast, my life was entrusted to someone else. I had no physical energy, which meant I was very weak and vulnerable.

For the first few days of the fast, I still had enough energy to walk to the pool, which was about 50 meters away from my room and down a few stairs. After 5 or 6 days, I didn't feel like going there anymore, and did not bother. After around 14 days of fasting, I needed to use a chair to take a shower; otherwise, I could black out from the sudden drop in blood pressure if I stood up after picking up a bar of soap.

The conversations about food with my roommate were constant. During the first 7 days of the fast, we were really hungry, and we avoided mentioning anything about food. During the second week of the fast, we started talking about food, what we would eat after the fast, our favorite fruits, our favorite recipes, and so on. These discussions would generate some desire and sometimes made me feel hungry, but after about 18 days of fasting, talking about food was like talking about something very abstract, like computer science. I felt totally disconnected from food and no longer had any sense of hunger, yet I still missed the connection with food and the pleasure I used to get from it.

I spent six weeks in the same room, sometimes walking a little in the surroundings. I spent most of my time in bed. I would sleep at least 10 to 12 hours a day, and I would spend most of the remaining hours laying down, reading, writing, listening to music, or most likely, doing nothing. It was literally a game to see how I would be able to kill time and avoid getting bored. The only thing I could look forward to each day was Doug's evening lecture, which provided some intellectual stimulation.

Some people recommend fasting with your eyes closed and avoiding any stimulation like music or watching movies. I initially went with that mindset, but the boredom of fasting was so intense that eventually I gave up and allowed myself one movie a day and as much music as I wanted. Fortunately, a fellow faster had brought a giant collection of

DVDs with her, and I would borrow a different one every day to watch on my 17-inch MacBook.

I noticed that during the fast, some people did amazingly well and were very energetic. Some were walking around like zombies, like me, and others were somewhere in between.

Just as Mosséri had said, people who started the fast with the most weight to lose had the easiest time during the fast. One person lost over 30 pounds during the fast, from a starting point that could be considered quite overweight. At the end of the fast, she looked at least 10 years younger.

Ken, who worked for Doug as a programmer for his website at the time, was a very athletic and muscular guy who had let himself go a little bit and had gained some weight. During the fast, he was able to shed all of that excess weight, and at the end, he looked like he had just been training for a body-building competition.

Rachana, my German friend, started out with an average weight, and ended the fast looking like a model!

The skinny people (and I was the skinniest of all) didn't have the same experience. Because we were already at a normal weight, it seemed like the fast was much more profound and difficult for us. We had no energy and were zombies in comparison with the heavier ones, who were walking around full of energy and seemingly unaffected by the fast until they started to lose significant weight at the end.

My roommate Dan, who was about my age and started the fast with twenty pounds more, looked amazing after the fast. He weighed 139 pounds at his lowest, which was the weight I started out with!

Now that my normal weight is around 155 pounds, I wonder what would happen if I tried another fast...

What I discovered is that my fast did not help me to deal with "food issues" at all. Doug Graham had already warned us that if you want to learn how to eat raw, you have to practice eating raw. Fasting does the opposite, because you have to be extra careful after the fast.

Because my body was so hungry after the fast, I had a really hard time trying to stick with eating raw. The only thing that made me stick with the diet for long enough was my fear of getting sick if I ate anything else. It was not an unfounded fear, since my body was so sensitive that it would violently reject anything that was less than optimal.

During my fast, I kept thinking about food. After my fast, I thought about food even more. I was obsessed with food.

When I got back to Canada, I wrote a letter to Albert Mosséri, telling him about my difficulties with the "after-fast," and he wrote back a classic response, telling me, "your fast was ended too brutally."

He suggested reducing the amount of fruit I was eating temporarily, avoiding raw salads, all nuts, seeds and avocado, and instead eating a few steamed vegetables and potatoes at night. I was supposed to follow this very bland diet for a week or two. After that time, it would be okay to start eating more fruit and introduce salads.

I followed Mosséri's advice and felt instant relief, as the digestive issues went away. I stayed on his bland diet for a little while, and then added more fruit to my diet. This time, I felt a lot better.

Overall, the fast was an incredible experience, but it was also a very demanding one, both physically and mentally. It took me a few months to get back to normal, but once I did, I had more energy than ever. However, my digestion was still poor.

While in Costa Rica, I wrote down many notes about my life after the fast. Once I got back, I was very inspired and energized to put all of my ideas into action.

This made 2005 one of my most productive years ever. I moved from Montreal to a nice town in the countryside, where I had always wanted to live. I finally got over my fear of driving and bought a car, which enabled me to make this move. (Having lived as a vagabond for so many years, I only got my driver's license when I was 28.) I totally changed my business and turned it around beyond my expectations.

I attribute this extraordinary productivity to the level of clarity that I got from the fast.

Fasting, to me, was like dying and then being reborn again. It felt like I had just spent a year in prison, brewing in my head how I was going to enjoy my freedom once I got back.

Back Home After the Fast

One would imagine that Costa Rica, being a tropical country, has an incredible variety of fruits and vegetables. The availability of fruits in tropical countries is very seasonal, so there wasn't that much to eat besides bananas, papayas, sour oranges, sweet passion fruit (granadilla), pineapple, watermelon and a few other items. Mangoes were just starting to be in season by the time I left, and all the ones we ate there were not the best.

Once I got back to Montreal, I visited my Italian market where I got most of my fruit. I was surprised to discover that the mangoes I could get in Montreal, imported all the way from Brazil, were amazing, better than the Costa Rican mangoes. Once in Quebec, I had access to better-quality fruits from all over the world, which made my recovery easier. I was also relieved to have my Vita-Mix again, and making a lot of smoothies was something I desperately needed to get enough calories to gain the weight back.

In spite of my weight loss, most people said I looked great after the fast. One Costa Rican, who was an amateur cyclist, was amazed when I told him my body fat was only 5%. He envied me, he said, and asked, "Quien eres, Lance Armstrong?" (Who are you, Lance Armstrong?). He tried to guess my age, and figured I must be around 18 or 19, judging from my looks. When I told him I was almost 29, he refused to believe me!

Even though I was skinny, I didn't scare anybody because I simply looked like a kid, not a concentration camp victim. My scrawniness wasn't associated with other signs of ill-health, so people just thought I was younger than I really was.

My Conclusions on the Fast

Although I experienced some challenges in my fast and I would certainly do it differently if I did it again, I don't regret my decision to fast. I just wish I had been more careful when breaking the fast, and I would have made different food choices after the fast. At the time, my understanding of low-fat raw vegan nutrition was not as complete as it is today. I'm confident I experienced many positive benefits from the fast, although they were not as apparent as for those people — older than me — who came to fast specifically because of health problems they had.

The main benefit from the fast was the incredible mental clarity and feelings of positivity and renewal that I experienced.

Fasting for Health

Fasting as spiritual purification is a tradition in many world religions. Likewise, many ancient philosophers, scientists and physicians saw fasting as an essential part of life and health. Socrates, Plato, Aristotle, Galen, Paracelsus and Hippocrates all believed in fasting as therapy.

But the reason Natural Hygienists use fasting is not because fasting itself is a cure for anything, but because the experience allows the body to rest from digestion and physical activity so all its energies can be directed towards healing.

After about three or four days of fasting, the body starts to feed on its own fat and convert it to ketones, an alternative energy source to glucose. Ketosis is the body's safety-mechanism, enabling us to survive for long periods of time without food.

Dr. Alan Goldhammer, who runs the *True North Health Center* in California, one of the few water-fasting centers in the world, writes:

> Throughout history, people have noticed that when they become acutely ill, they lose their appetites. The early Hygienic physicians reasoned that there must be some physiological reason for this loss of appetite. Through observation and experimentation, they discovered that fasting, the complete abstinence from all substances except pure water, in an environment of complete rest, allows the body to make a unique physiological adaptation.
>
> In the fasting state, the duration and intensity of the symptoms of illness, such as inflammation, mucus production, fever, diarrhea, etc., are often dramatically reduced. Fasting has been found to be the most efficient and powerful means available to facilitate self-healing.
>
> Further experimentation and observation found that fasting is also effective in the resolution of chronic disease. Chronic disease, including heart disease, diabetes, cancer, arthritis, respiratory illness, autoimmune disease, etc., can be the result of several different factors. These factors include inappropriate diet, such as the consumption of animal products and refined foods, the use of drugs, including tobacco, alcohol, coffee, etc., a lack of adequate sleep or exercise, or exposure to environmental stressors such as pollution, radiation, excess noise, etc., or excess psychological stress and hereditary factors.
>
> Fasting is an important tool in resolving the symptoms of acute illness and chronic disease, but its benefits are not limited to dealing with symptoms.[67]

There are a few types of fasting I have experimented with:

24-Hour Fast

The weekly 24-hour fast is a healthy, life-extending habit. Paul Bragg, one of the most influential authors of the natural health movement of the past century, wrote a lot about fasting. He claimed that he fasted 24 hours every week. The 24-hour fast is not a true fast but more a little digestive rest.

---

67   Do You Need to Fast? Dr. Alan Goldhammer. http://www.healthpromoting.com/ Articles/articles/need.htm

Skipping two meals and breaking that short "fast" with a light meal is a great way to give your digestion a chance to rest. I find it a really positive thing to do, and I often find myself fasting for 24 hours when I feel like it, especially when traveling, to combat jetlag.

3-4 Day Fast

The 3-4 day fast is not a true "fast," as the body barely has enough time to convert to ketosis completely. However, it is an extended digestive rest, and I find it a great way to get back on track when you've fallen off the wagon with your health program. Although I don't recommend the habit of "binging and fasting," sometimes circumstances in your health — such as great stress or the desire to break bad habits — may require a 3-4 day fast.

Long Fasts

A long fast is typically a fast that lasts anywhere from 7 to 40 days. Such a fast is a profound healing experience, but it should only be conducted under professional supervision.

Fasting is not something most people can undertake casually without supervision. While fasting for three or four days is rarely a problem for a healthy person, "It can be quite dangerous if you are not already eating a healthy diet, or if you've got liver or kidney problems, any kind of compromised immune system functioning, or are on medication," says Joel Fuhrman, MD, author of *Eat to Live: The Revolutionary Plan for Fast and Sustained Weight Loss* and *Fasting and Eating for Health* (Little, Brown and Company, 2005).

As with any therapy that has physiological effects, fasting has its hazards. The longer or more restrictive the fast is, the greater the potential for problems. A doctor or knowledgeable practitioner with significant experience with fasting and Natural Hygiene should supervise any long fast.

What Happened After

When I started writing this book, I just wanted to tell the story of my first few years on the raw food diet, and all the lessons I have learned since. As I continued writing the book, I realized there was more of my story to tell, and that all of my experiences and observations could be useful to other people.

However, I have to stop somewhere. Because my years after the fast were the busiest in my entire life (which was partly fueled by the mental clarity I got from the fast itself), it would literally take me another book to tell the rest of my life story up to now.

So what I'm going to do in this chapter is give you a brief overview of my life after the fast, and the lessons I have discovered since then. In the next chapter, I will talk about what I eat nowadays and how I see the raw food movement today.

After my fast, it took me a few months to find balance again. Once I did, my energy and motivation were literally through the roof. I accomplished more professionally in that one year than in the previous three years combined.

For many years, one aspect of my health that I always neglected was my fitness. Although I did lift some weights at that time, or did some jogging occasionally, I had a lot to learn in this area.

With Doug's influence, and after attending his *Health and Fitness Week*, I continued making dramatic progress in my fitness.

Although this is something that is still a weakness and that I constantly need to remind myself to work on more, over the last few years, I have made some important gains with my physical fitness.

In 2006, I continued on the path of the high-fruit, low-fat raw vegan diet, with great results. Although I did not always follow the diet 100%, I did my best to follow the basic principles and finally learned to eat enough fruit to get all the calories I needed to thrive, which was something I had failed to do in the years prior.

In a typical week, I would go to a giant fruit market in Montreal and come back with cases of fruits and vegetables (bananas, grapes, persimmons, whatever was in season), about $150 to $200 worth of it, and make myself giant fruit smoothies, salads and green smoothies.

I continued traveling the world, and even fulfilled a dream of mine and lived in Costa Rica for almost a year. I have since then moved back to Canada, although I do spend a few months of the winter in tropical countries such as Thailand, where there is a great abundance of fruits.

In all the years that have followed my fast in Costa Rica, I have continued preaching the same message: eat more fruit and reduce the fat. I've also stressed the importance of eating enough food to get all the calories and nutrients that are necessary for optimal health. This shouldn't be a starvation diet!

In 2006, I discovered the benefits of green smoothies through the work of Victoria Boutenko, and I have been spreading the word about them ever since.

Through my friend Roger Haeske, I've also become a big fan of Savory Veggie Stews (**www.veggiestews.com**), a kind of fat-free green soup that Roger eats almost every day, which I have found to be a great, satisfying, savory raw dinner meal.

During this time, I've had many periods of eating 100% raw, sometimes for months at a time. At times, I have fallen off the wagon, but I have always gone back to the same path of the low-fat raw vegan diet, because it's what I've found that works the best.

Sometimes people ask me, "Fred, why don't you eat 100% raw if you're so convinced of the benefits of raw foods?"

The truth is that something died in me the day that I stopped "believing" in the raw food diet. After my last "disastrous" visit to the dentist, I realized something: it is possible to strongly believe in something and be wrong, and making a small mistake in judgment can do a lot of harm over time.

When I first became a vegetarian, I used to laugh when people told me "Be careful! You have to really watch what you eat if you are vegetarian: otherwise, you can run into problems and deficiencies!"

I used to laugh, because this kind of advice implied that a Standard American Diet was perfectly adequate, yet a vegetarian diet somehow required special attention.

However, we all know some "junk food" vegetarians who think they can be healthy just by not eating meat, and stuff themselves all day with vegetarian junk foods, such as potato chips and fried tofu.

I now think that the advice,"You have to be very careful about what you eat when you eat raw: otherwise, you will run into problems" is absolutely true.

It's true because:

1. **Raw fruits and vegetables are nutrient-dense, but low in calories.**

   Therefore, their nutrients are diluted with a lot of fiber and water. That means you have to eat a LOT of them to get everything you need, and failure to do so will indeed create health problems — the most obvious ones being the inability to stick with the diet and cravings for bad foods.

2. **The raw food diet contains no complex carbs.**

   By removing the one calorie source that most cultures in the world eat the most of, we are left with only two possible sources of calories: fruit or fat. Eating enough fruit to meet our needs requires a lot more practice than most people think, and usually, it represents a lot more volume than people can imagine. At the same time, fruits can be low in some minerals, so special care is needed to ensure we get enough vegetables in the diet to compensate.

When I decided to get off the raw food diet completely back in 2004, I lost my raw food convictions that "this is the best way to live, no matter what, at any cost!"

There is nothing today that would convince me that eating steamed broccoli represents a health risk, or that having a massive amount of acidic, unripe pineapple would be better than eating a few cooked potatoes if I had the choice.

I simply no longer believe that everyone has to be 100% raw to be healthy.

However, I also continue to believe that it's possible to eat 100% raw and feel absolutely amazing and be healthy, as long as the diet is done properly.

In the raw food movement, I have seen the best results in people who follow the low-fat approach.

CHAPTER 20

Is Low-Fat, Cooked Better Than High-Fat, Raw?

In a boxing-ring contest between a cooked yam and a fatty raw lasagna, the yam will win hands-down, as far as how it will affect your health and energy.

Over the years since my interest in the raw food diet started, we've seen the raw food movement boom like crazy. Yet, when my book *Sunfood Cuisine* was published in 2002, there were only a few raw recipe books in print.

Now, you'll find row after row of raw recipe books, over 100 raw or "raw-friendly" restaurants in the USA, website after website on the subject, "superstores" on the Internet that sell raw foods by mail, and more books coming out every year than ever before.

Hundreds of thousands of people have tried this raw food diet "fad," and perhaps enjoyed eating their raw "burgers" and high-fat cacao smoothies for a while, but inevitably, they reverted back to their old diet.

Why? Because the high-fat raw diet is not a sustainable diet, and it's also one of the unhealthiest and most nutritionally unsound diets ever designed (next to Atkins).

By turning the concept of "raw" into a religion, with false and incorrect science to back it up and piles of recipe books that show you how to eat your nuts and your fat in hundreds of ways, the raw movement is not going in the right direction.

Why Do People Get Results?

If the raw food diet is such a fad, and the high-fat raw diet is so unhealthy, then why do people get such good results on it?

This is very simple to explain: on the high-fat raw vegan diet, people eliminate almost every single disease-producing food human beings can ever consume. The raw vegan diet avoids:

- All dairy products (a big step towards avoiding/healing heart disease, allergies, arthritis, fibromyalgia, etc.)

- All meat and animal products and fish, which often have hormones or mercury in them (which have been linked to so many diseases).

- All wheat and gluten products (to which a large proportion of the adult population is allergic or sensitive).

- All refined sugar, candies, pastries, cakes, sweets and sodas.

- Many grains and beans, which are acid-forming.

- All industrialized, processed, refined, fried and cancer-causing foods.

From that short list alone, it's easy to see why the raw vegan diet gives results. It's close to being the ideal diet. The only important things that are missing are:

- The raw vegan diet is too low in carbs.

- Not enough fruits are included to meet your needs for calories. The raw vegan diet is much, much too high in fat, with insane quantities of avocados, nuts, oils and fats.

People get results because of all the things they give up... not necessarily because the food they eat is raw. Since some very important nutritional mistakes are still being made, it's difficult to succeed with the diet in the long term, and ill health can often result.

In her book *Green for Life*, Victoria Boutenko describes the amazing health transformation her family experienced after following a high-fat raw vegan diet for many years. However, over the long term, this diet was not working anymore.

"After several years of being raw foodists, however, each one of us began to feel like we had reached a plateau where our healing process stopped and even somewhat began to go backwards. After approximately seven years on a completely raw diet, once in a while, more and more often, we started feeling discontent with our existing food program.

I began to have a heavy feeling in my stomach after eating almost any kind of raw food, especially a salad with dressing. Because of that, I started to eat fewer greens and more fruits and nuts. I began to gain weight. My husband started to develop a lot of gray hair.

My family members felt confused about our diet and often seemed to have the question, "What should we eat?"

There were odd times when we felt hungry but did not desire any foods that were "legal" for us to eat on a typical raw food diet: fruits, nuts, seeds, grains, or dried fruit. Salads (with dressings) were delicious, but made us tired and sleepy. We felt trapped. I remember Igor looking inside the fridge, saying over and over again, "I wish I wanted some of this stuff"... Such periods did not last.

We blamed it all on overeating and were able to refresh our appetites by fasts, exercise, hikes, or by working more. In my family, we strongly believe that raw food is the only way to go, and therefore, we encouraged each other to maintain our raw diet no matter what, always coming up with new tricks.

Many of my friends told me about similar experiences at which point they gave up being 100% raw and began to add cooked food back into their meals."

Later in the book, Victoria comes to the conclusion that the reason they were not succeeding on the raw food diet was because they were not eating enough greens.

Although I agree that greens are important and that eating green smoothies and vegetable soups is a great way to consume them, I no longer agree with Victoria that greens are the only "missing key" in the raw food diet.

I do not personally see the underconsumption of greens as the biggest problem in the raw food movement. The biggest problem is overconsumption of fat and underconsumption of carbohydrates.

When Victoria and her family switched to green smoothies, they automatically lowered the fat content in their diet dramatically and added more fruit. That's what made the major difference, not just the greens per se.

Almost every symptom she describes in the paragraph I quoted is very typical for raw foodists living on a high-fat diet without enough fruit.

Even though the traditional raw food diet composed of vegetables, avocados, nuts, oils and a little fruit is a big improvement over the toxic Standard American Diet, it's not nutritionally balanced and healthy enough to work in the long term and to be satisfying all the time.

Low-fat, high-carb cooked foods, such as potatoes, brown rice, corn, root vegetables, butternut squash, and so on, are better choices than all high-fat raw recipes. A diet based on these foods would be healthier in the long term than an extremely high-fat raw diet.

Many people find it is simpler and easier emotionally to stick to a 100% raw food diet, or close to it. That way, they know what to say "no" to and won't find themselves going from baked sweet potato to stir-fry, to spicy Indian food, to eventually eating sandwiches and junk food again.

There is a lot of value in knowing exactly what to do to be healthy, doing it 100%, and never looking back. If you can do it, and do it well, I can't argue against that.

Other people find it easier to eat mostly raw foods, but with some selected cooked foods that, through careful personal observation, they've noticed make them feel good overall and bring them more variety and enjoyment.

I know some people who eat a mostly raw diet, but a few times a week, they will have cooked sweet potato or squash. Albert Mosséri eats only three cooked meals per week (one every other day), usually of potatoes and vegetables.

Others can't live without eating some vegetarian Thai foods. A few times a month, they go out to their favorite restaurant.

My friend Wayne Gendel has been eating a raw diet for many years, and he eats around 90% raw foods. A few times a month, he'll have something cooked, such as air-popped popcorn with no oil.

In the context of a low-fat raw diet, occasionally eating high-fat recipes is not going to be unhealthy when you look at the overall health profile of the diet, and even eating something "bad" occasionally is not going to harm you, if you're careful the rest of the time.

What About "Moderate Fat, Moderate Fruit?"

I know some people will probably think I'm exaggerating the fat content in the typical raw food diet. They will imagine that it's possible to eat a "moderate fat, moderate fruit diet." This would be a diet that is 30-40% fat, perhaps half the fat content of the typical raw diet, and would also include more fruit.

For example, the diet could include a lot of fruit, possibly one or two avocados a day with a small handful of nuts, and maybe a tablespoon or two of olive oil over a salad. That would likely bring us to about 30-40% fat.

Is there anything wrong with that? From my personal experience, that kind of diet is a disaster. The reason is that the fat content in the diet is still too high, which means that a lot of fat will be in the bloodstream at all times. Combined with the sugar content of the diet (in fruit), health problems such as candidiasis, blood sugar swings and poor digestion can be expected.

It's best to stick with low-fat foods all the time, whether raw or cooked, rather than with a high-fruit diet that still contains too much fat. In any case, a low-fat raw diet is still the best.

This is why so many people think they feel better on a high-fat diet. They notice that they feel terrible when they start adding more fruit to their raw diet, yet they continue eating the same amounts of fat.

They blame the fruit, as it was the newest thing they added, and believe they can "run on" fat much better than on fruit. But the truth is, they don't even know that they could be feeling even better than they do now if they significantly reduced or cut out the fat completely and then tried a low-fat raw food diet.

Raw plant fats take a lot of time and energy to digest, and if you are experiencing detox-like symptoms long after going raw, you need to take a look at your diet and be honest with yourself about what is and is not working.

This also goes for high-fat cooked vegan diets and adding a lot of fruit to the diet. You will feel terrible, have gas and bloating, and feel lethargic. Fruit is not to blame here. It just does not mix well with unhealthy, oily, rich foods.

Aiming for low-fat foods is the best thing you can do to improve your health in a short amount of time, and eating enough fruit will stop your cravings and binging on high-fat recipes.

CHAPTER 21

What I Eat Now

Because I write a raw food blog, most people think I always eat 100% raw all of the time. They are naturally confused when they learn that I sometimes eat cooked foods.

My experience has shown me that it's better to keep an open mind and not necessarily be 100% strict with too many things if they bring negative stress and anxiety into your life.

My diet is fairly simple. When I'm at home, I will usually eat three meals a day, possibly with a snack. My breakfast is usually a large fruit smoothie or a green smoothie, but usually, I prefer fruits in season. (I love watermelon, melon, blueberries and pineapple.)

For lunch, I will often make a large smoothie containing one type of fruit that is richer and sweeter, such as banana or mango. To that, I might add another type of fruit. For example, a favorite smoothie of mine consists of several bananas with an entire papaya. If I'm not very active that day, then I might skip fruit for lunch and have a regular dinner meal for lunch instead (see below).

Dinner can be one of the following:

A low fat raw meal

My raw dinner meals are three-course meals. If I've been active enough during the day, I start with fruit. Then I follow it with a large raw veggie soup (my own creation or based on Roger Haeske's Savory Veggie Stews, **www.veggiestews.com**), and possibly a salad with fat-free dressing.

311

A dinner that includes cooked food

My favorite cooked foods are simple: root vegetables, such as potatoes or sweet potatoes, squash, green vegetables, beans or rice (I try to avoid wheat most of the time). Whenever I prepare cooked foods, I avoid all oils and added fats. With the cooked dinner, I try to have a salad, and there may be some nuts or seeds in the dressing.

A raw recipe

Occasionally (but quite rarely, I must admit) I have a raw recipe, such as creamy coleslaw, nori rolls with a nut pate, or guacamole. Even these fatty raw recipes are low in fat compared to traditional raw food recipes.

Just fruit

Occasionally but rarely, I have just fruit for dinner.

When I'm at home, near a juicer, I often drink 8 to 12 ounces of vegetable juice (celery, spinach, parsley, kale, etc.), sweetened with a little carrot or apple juice, and a touch of lime.

Vitamins B12 and D are the only supplements I currently take. When I travel, I take some barley grass powder to replace some of the vegetables I might not be getting enough of. I've experimented with a few other "superfoods," but at the moment, I do not take anything else.

When I'm at home, I try to follow a kind of menu. I only plan for dinners, because breakfasts and lunches are always the same and very easy to enjoy and adhere to.

About once a week, I have a cheat meal, or as some people like to call it, a "reward meal," when I throw some rules out the window. This may be a raw recipe that's fattier than usual or a night out at a restaurant. I still try to follow some basic principles and not go completely off the wagon, but I find that having one day a week where I'm less strict about my diet improves my soul and allows me to loosen up a bit. Then, I'm more motivated to eat a really good diet the rest of the week.

I like to eat mostly raw, but I don't like to be a purist. So sometimes what I do is eat simple raw foods, but I add a little bit of something that is cooked. For example, to flavor a salad, I might add a few tablespoons of store-bought organic salsa (that's cooked), instead of using lots of avocado or a fatty dressing.

When I travel, and eating enough fruit is difficult, I tend to eat less fruit and more low-fat cooked foods, such as rice, beans, vegetables and potatoes. However, my preference is to eat mostly raw and mostly fruit.

What's off-limits? Besides the obvious junk and industrialized foods, I generally don't eat animal products. I don't want to give a false impression that I've always been a perfect vegan. As I've related in this book, since I first started re-examining the raw food diet, I've experimented with animal products on several occasions, and even in the years after my fast in 2005, I've occasionally eaten some animal products, such as eggs, and even Costa Rican ceviche (a traditional dish made with raw fish marinated in lemon juice and flavored with vegetables, such as onion and red pepper). There were even times that I ate meat. Over time, I've found myself less and less attracted to animal foods.

I cannot say that I will never eat any animal foods again, but I can say that I have very little desire to do so. I might eat some honey on occasion in a recipe, but I don't eat it on its own because I find it too sweet and acidic, and it makes my teeth sensitive.

Research done on diets rich in animal products proves that eating a lot of animal protein is detrimental to health. However, if one eats a small quantity of "clean" animal products (equivalent to less than 3-4% of total calories), like our cousins the great apes do, there is no evidence that this would be a major detrimental force. The big question is: are there any benefits to doing so? I haven't concluded that there are any from my personal experience, but other people may disagree.

A vegan is someone who strictly avoids all animal products. My preference is still to (mostly) eat like a raw vegan. However, I'm no longer a strict vegan philosophically, and I will make no apology for it.[68]

The vegan diet encompasses an entire philosophy of life that I no longer subscribe to. I find that many vegans, in their drive and obsession to be kind to animals, have forgotten to care for the human animal: themselves.

For example, I wear merino wool shirts because I have found this material to be the best for traveling, since it dries quickly and never smells. I get these clothes from the company called **www.icebreaker. com**, which also cares for the ethical and sustainable treatment of their sheep.

I would much rather buy a t-shirt made with a material that I enjoy wearing, that has all the qualities that I seek, and that I can keep for a long time, even if it costs a little more and is not "vegan," instead of buying some kind of vegan "clothes" that I don't enjoy wearing (like hemp), that has none of the qualities that I seek (like cotton, that stretches and dries poorly for traveling), and that I will have to replace sooner.

Of course, because I've used the term "raw vegan" to describe the diet that I espouse, I've been criticized for not being a true vegan.

In reality, before 2001, the term "raw vegan" was nonexistent. I acquired the domain name **www.rawvegan.com** in 2000 when no one else was using that word. The term was coined by my editor, John McCabe, who

---

68 For you data freaks out there who want to know more about me and analyze my situation, I currently weigh 155 pounds. My height is 5 foot 10, and my body fat level around 13% (from the last time I checked in 2009). My blood type is A and I'm a "non-secretor" (meaning that I'm in the 20% of the population that does not secrete antigens to my blood type in my bodily fluids!). I wear glasses or contact lenses because I suffer from myopia. I have been nearsighted since I was 13, long before I decided to become a vegetarian or raw foodist. In the last 10 years, my vision has remained more or less stable. I once got rid of my glasses for an entire year when I was in California (this is a story I did not tell), and only experienced a slight improvement in my vision. I also ended up in an accident because of it, so that's why I wear glasses again. The last blood test I took was in 2004, so I'm due for another one.

first used it in my magazine *Just Eat an Apple*. He started using the term to differentiate the raw food diet we promoted from other kinds of raw food diets that included raw animal products. After we started using the term in the magazine and on the Internet, it spread, and now it is a very common term in this field.

I use the term "low-fat raw vegan" because "raw foodist" can mean eating anything raw, including raw beef or raw bear. Raw "vegan" specifies that no animal foods be eaten. "Low-fat" specifies that this diet be based on fruit for sufficient carbohydrate consumption.

In reality, the term "vegetarian" initially referred to a vegan diet composed of plants. When vegetarians started using eggs and dairy products, someone had to invent a term to specify that their diet did not contain any dairy products. The term "vegan" was coined by Donald Watson in 1944, from the first three and last two letters of the word "vegetarian," to describe a "non-dairy vegetarian."

Since then, the term "vegan" has come to connote an entire philosophy of life, where one avoids all foods and products made from animals. This includes honey, wool, leather, gelatin and even car tires (which contain some animal byproducts.).

Ultimately, becoming a pure vegan is a fantasy, since the very nature of our existence means that we use other lives to sustain our own. To take the vegan philosophy to the extreme would be to live like followers of the religious cult of Jainism, who avoid eating root vegetables (because of the tiny life forms that may live on them), foods that have been stored overnight (because of the microorganisms again), fermented foods, and may even walk around with a mask to avoid breathing in bacteria and killing them!

I have absolutely zero desire to live like this…

The words for "vegetarian" and "vegan" do not exist in many languages. For example, there is no word for "vegetarian" or "vegan" in Thai. The only term that approximates it is "Jay," which is related to the word for

"Jain," and it is seen more as a religious asceticism practice that includes the avoidance of all animal products. The concept of vegetarianism for health has not yet made it to that country, nor to most countries where vegetarianism is a religious choice.

What About 100% Raw?

I think people get caught up in these terms, such as "raw foodist" or "raw vegan," which have become semantic traps rather than useful descriptions. This is similar to what is done in politics when someone is labeled as "right-wing" or "left-wing" and ultimately judged on this position alone.

For example, let's imagine that someone has not eaten meat for 10 years, but then eats some. Then, after eating the meat, that person goes back to being vegetarian. Does he stop being vegetarian the day he eats meat? Then, after the incident, how long does it take for him to be considered a vegetarian again? One week? One year? One day?

Is a raw foodist still a raw foodist if they eat something that is slightly cooked, such as maple syrup, but everything else is raw? I know that most gurus who claim to be 100% have eaten such things over the years and either conveniently "forget" or simply omit mention of the incident to retain their credibility among raw health seekers.

Is a vegan still a vegan even though they drive a car that has some leather detailing in it?

Although I don't view myself as a raw foodist in the strictest sense of the term (which would be someone who eats only raw foods), I have enough experience and accumulated knowledge to give advice on the raw food diet, whether it is a 100% raw diet or an 80% raw diet.[69]

---

69 I do agree, however, that you should get advice from people who are getting the results you desire. Therefore, if your goal is truly to succeed on a 100% raw vegan diet with no exceptions, you might seek other role models than myself.

And since there is no term that currently exists to describe someone that "eats mostly raw fruits and vegetables, with some cooked vegetables and low-fat vegan foods on occasion, while avoiding oil, dairy products and wheat," I will stick to the term "raw vegan." And, if someone has a problem with that, they can just say that I'm not a strict raw vegan, while some other people are.

Some people think that everyone and everything needs a label. "100% raw," "Truly Raw," "100% vegan," "80/10/10," "Paleo," etc. If you feel you need to be defined by a label to be a raw foodist, ok, but not everyone else feels the same.

I want to eat the healthiest diet possible that I can maintain without being confined by dogmatic beliefs against which I struggle, to my own detriment.

It's just food, and if it's not making our lives better in every sense, can we really consider ourselves to be informed health foodists?

Another interesting note: I have noticed that the longer a person is a "raw foodist," the less they care about labels and proclaiming their "rawness" to the world. Every raw foodist has friends and family members who are not raw and who don't really care how raw they are or what they eat anymore. Eventually, many people realize that the people you love and care about are not concerned with how raw you are — they just want you to be happy and healthy.

It seems like the raw food movement is currently fueled by newly converted, overzealous raw enthusiasts who prefer to "take sides" and band together to feel like they are fighting some kind of raw war against cooked foods or even meat-eaters in general.

Many people I have met who have been into raw foods for a long time are not obsessed about their diet anymore and are at peace, whether they are 80%, 90%, or even 100% raw, and that's just great.

100% Raw or 80% Raw: Which One Is Best?

Because there are absolutely no scientific studies to compare the two approaches, we have to rely on anecdotal evidence to decide which one is best.

Based on my experience and observations, I believe it is possible to establish some pros and cons of eating 100% raw versus eating a mostly raw diet.

So to compare the diets properly, I'd like to show the differences between an ideal low-fat raw vegan diet, where one eats enough fruits, enough greens and low fat, to a similar diet that includes a little less fruit, but some low-fat cooked foods, such as steamed vegetables, potatoes, beans, and brown rice.

What is Cooked?

What I hate about certain raw foodists is their lack of distinctions. They will claim that "cooked food is toxic," as if cooked food is one big category, where steamed asparagus stands toe to toe with a Bacon Double Cheeseburger.

All raw foodists, with a bit of knowledge, will agree that all raw foods are not created equal either.

Eating a head of lettuce will not give you the same results as eating a cup of coconut oil mixed with honey, and eating 5 bananas will not give you the same results as eating a jar of raw almond butter.

Cooked foods are also not created equal. Barbecued meat might be the worst culprit, while a lightly steamed vegetable would be on the other end of the spectrum, as rather inoffensive.

There's strong evidence to show that certain cooked foods are indeed toxic. The carcinogens found in grilled meat are a reality.[70]

On the other hand, I haven't seen any scientific evidence that could prove that eating steamed vegetables could somehow damage your health in a measurable way.

70 Gross, G., Turesky, R., Fay, L., Stillwell, W., Skipper, P., & Tannenbaum, S. (1993). Heterocyclic aromatic amine formation in grilled bacon, beef and fish and in grill scrapings. *Carcinogenesis, 14*(11), 2313-2318.

CHAPTER 22

Pros and Cons of Eating 100% Raw

PROS of 100% Raw

By not eating cooked foods, you've already eliminated 99% of common culprits that damage health, such as:

- Fried foods

- Excess animal protein and fat

- Grains

- Wheat and gluten

- Refined soy products

- MSG

- Preservatives and excitotoxins

Therefore, most of the benefits of the raw food diet come from the avoidance of these products and not from the fact that the food eaten is raw. However, there are a few benefits that are specific to the "rawness" of the diet. There is no science to back it up, but the experience of raw foodists all around the world shows it's true to some degree.

Increased Energy

The main pro of the 100% low-fat raw vegan diet is a greater sense of vitality. Most people report increased energy and a better mood, with fewer ups and downs. You'll wake up feeling better in the morning, without needing to drink a cup of coffee to lift you up. You'll feel lighter after a meal and ready to get going, without needing to rest to digest.

Easier to Stay Consistent

Another benefit of eating 100% raw is that it makes it easier to avoid going off the wagon completely. If you eat mostly raw, but allow yourself cooked vegetables, you might quickly escalate to more "dangerous" cooked food, and pretty soon, you're no longer eating raw. A lot of people report that mentally it's a lot easier to eat 100% raw, because they don't have to constantly make compromises and choose the lesser of two evils. By sticking to 100% raw foods with no exception, the answer to the question "What to eat for dinner?" is pretty straightforward.

Better for Those with an Active Lifestyle

My experience eating this way is also that it is the best diet when you are very active. The stable blood sugar and high energy provided by fruit is great for endurance sports, such as running and cycling.

Better for Weight Loss

It is easier to reach your ideal weight on 100% raw than on a mostly raw diet because the foods eaten are low in caloric density.

Requires Less Sleep

Raw foods often require less energy to digest than cooked foods. Also, raw foodists tend to eat fewer total calories. I believe that this is the reason that many people eating a 100% raw diet report needing less sleep, on average 1-2 hours less per day.

CONS of 100% Raw

What are some of the negative aspects of the 100% raw vegan lifestyle? Let's take a look.

Social Isolation

The social isolation brought about by a strict 100% raw diet is by far the most important negative aspect of this lifestyle. On a 100% raw diet, you can't fully participate in normal socializing society (and if you do, you'll probably get sick). Even though some restaurants will cater to raw foodists, the food they generally serve is not healthy (and certainly not healthier than a lot of cooked foods). In most other restaurants, it's possible to get a salad, but it will rarely be one that meets your standards. Other types of invitations involving food are also difficult. For this reason, most people I know who have children and raised them as raw foodists eventually let them eat some cooked foods so that they could be part of the social network. For adults, there are many creative ways around these social obstacles, which can mean more for certain people and less for others.

Quantity of Food Needed

Another important negative aspect of this lifestyle is the quantity of food that must be consumed on a daily basis, namely, fruit. This makes traveling difficult or impossible if you don't know where to buy produce. Some trips are impossible to make as a low-fat raw vegan (unless you had a camel to carry all your fruit!) Most low-fat vegans just avoid traveling, only go to certain places they know will have fruits for long periods of time, or compromise when they travel. Living in an area where there is an adequate availability of good quality, affordable fruits and vegetables makes it easier.

Increased Cost of Food

A raw food diet costs more than other diets. In recent years, food costs have risen substantially. I now pay 50% more for a case of bananas than I used to a few years ago. Growing your own vegetables and having some fruit trees can help you save a bundle, but the most important trick to save money is to buy in bulk. For more information, please refer to an important special report on raw bulk food costs and best value per calorie available as part of the **Raw Vegan Mentor Club. (http://www. fredericpatenaude.com/mentorclub.html)**

On the other hand, you will save a lot in restaurant bills and, of course, on your health costs.

Body Sensitivity

The more pure your diet is, the more sensitive your body becomes. I've already talked about this interesting phenomenon of the Law of Vital Accommodation, or "the raw curse." It's usually not a problem if you can stick with the diet 100% without any exception, but going back and forth between 100% raw and eating some cooked food usually creates a lot of problems. Even eating raw with no salt and oils can make you sensitive if you unknowingly eat them at a raw potluck.

Detrimental Dental Health

A fruit diet may be more cariogenic than many other diets. As mentioned previously, the main way to avoid that problem is to eat less often (not snacking all day), and have a strict dental hygiene routine. There is also an issue with exposure to acidic foods. One German study found that raw foodists have more enamel erosion than most people, a fact I have confirmed in surveying raw food groups over the years. Again, this is caused by the frequency of exposure to acidic and sweet foods.

Tired of Sugar

It's fairly easy to eat fruit for breakfast and even for lunch. But to have fruit for breakfast, lunch and dinner (before a large salad or vegetable dish) is a lot of work, and sometimes, you get tired of eating sweet foods all day and crave something more.

However, despite these difficulties, many people find a way to make it work in their lives, because the benefits far outweigh the negatives.

CHAPTER 23

Pros and Cons of Eating Mostly Raw

If nobody found any benefit to eating cooked food, everyone would invariably be 100% raw.

The main reason raw foodists cannot thrive on a 100% raw food diet is because they are following a program that is not sustainable. Inevitably, the body will give enough signals for these people to listen and stop their high-fat raw food diet to try something else.

However, even people who are aware of the low-fat raw food diet might still eat cooked foods, for these and other reasons:

- Not able to get enough calories. They haven't learned to get enough calories from fruit, so it's easier to make an extra meal from cooked starches like potatoes.

- Desire to go out with friends, be more social, etc.

- Living with a family that is not raw and the temptation of trying other foods

- Lack of variety of fresh fruits

- Not able to chew vegetables well and not wanting to eat blended foods all the time

- Lesser of two evils: finding it easier and healthier to eat steamed vegetables rather than big salads that require a fatty dressing to be tasty

- Tired of eating sugar all day (in fruit)

- Actually enjoying some cooked foods rather than always eating raw

We will call this other path "mostly raw", which is generally what most people end up following. To qualify as "mostly raw", the diet should be at least 80% raw by volume and at least 70% raw by calories. The best applications of this lifestyle I have seen are:

- Eating raw all week, but allowing one day a week of "cheating" or a few times a month eating something cooked

- Eating raw every other day, with the second day including one cooked meal

- Eating a small cooked meal every evening, but eating some raw ingredients along with it too (such as adding some cooked ingredients to a salad or steamed vegetables)

In order to work, this "mostly raw" lifestyle should:

- Be low in fat (not more than 15% of total calories)

- Contain a lot of greens (cooked and raw)

- Contain a sufficient amount of calories, especially coming from fruit and other carbohydrates

- Avoid most grains (especially gluten-containing ones, like wheat and processed flours). Instead, cooked carbohydrate sources can be sweet potatoes, squash, white potato, fresh corn, and "super-grains," like amaranth and quinoa (which are more akin to seeds and grains, nutritionally speaking). Brown or white rice is also easy to digest.

- Include one source of essential fatty acids (such as hemp seeds or walnuts)

- Be low in sodium

- Avoid excessive amounts of animal protein (a vegan diet is best, but if animal products are consumed, they should not constitute more than 5% of total calories)

Depending on your needs, breakfast and lunch are usually fruit or fruit and greens (such as green smoothies). Dinner can start with fruit or a large salad, along with some well-proportioned amounts of cooked, low-fat, vegan foods, up to a few times a week.

These foods can be things like steamed vegetables, sweet potato with some herbs or salsa, brown rice or quinoa, beans, vegetables in tomato sauce, low-fat vegetable soups, and other similar low-fat items.

Some people find that after making the "mostly raw" plan work for a while, they feel ready to jump to 100% raw. This is great, because if you ever fall off the wagon, you are likely to revert to the last thing you learned, which is healthy low-fat vegan food. This is much better than going back to SAD junk food.

PROS of Mostly Raw

What are some of the benefits of this "mostly raw" lifestyle versus 100% raw?

More Flexibility

Having the flexibility to eat some cooked foods can be useful for social reasons. For some people, the desire to socialize and eat cooked foods on occasion might be more important than the desire to be 100% pure.

Less Sensitivity

One of the side effects of being less pure may be a hidden benefit. Being less sensitive to foods means you're less likely to get sick if you eat something bad for you or if you are treated with certain drugs in an emergency.

More Variety

Some research shows that having a combination of both raw and cooked vegetables is best for overall nutritional balance. Some nutrients are better preserved in raw foods, while others are more accessible after cooking.

Less Fruit Sugar

Although cooked carbohydrates are ultimately converted into simple sugars by the body, having less reliance on fruit sugar at every meal may be a benefit for some people still battling with blood sugar issues, such as candidiasis, or dental problems.

Easier to Chew

Some people have difficulty chewing raw vegetables, due to a poor bite or lost teeth. Blending vegetables can solve this problem, but so can steaming them, which breaks down their fiber.

Easier in the Winter

Long and cold winters are one of the main reasons why raw foodists might not stick to their diet year-round. Having the possibility of eating something warm in the winter is comforting and emotionally helpful.

Longevity and Health

For longevity, there is no evidence that eating a 100% raw diet is more beneficial than eating a mostly raw diet or even a healthy low-fat, mostly vegan diet.

CONS of "Mostly Raw"

From my perspective, the negatives of the "mostly raw" lifestyle versus the 100% raw ones are the following:

"The Open Gate to Hell"

The main problem of this way of eating is the fact that it may be hard to limit yourself to healthy cooked foods. As I experienced many times going back to cooked foods, adding steamed vegetables and cooked greens often led me to food choices that made me feel worse instead of better. I've noticed that this seems to be a common phenomenon among people who have emotional connections to food.

Less Peppy

There is a certain lightness of being that only seems to be possible on a 100% raw diet. Digesting most cooked foods will make one feel more tired than digesting most raw foods. I've noticed that the 100% raw food diet is better at lifting mood and making one feel energetic, but also, that this feeling is lost when eating a high-fat, raw diet.

Overall, the 100% raw food diet, when done properly, is the best diet to increase your sense of vitality and bring you health.

Based on this analysis, I have chosen, at the moment, to remain mostly raw, although this may change in the future. I believe it's possible for anyone to make a rational choice without having to fall for the hype of either camp.

The Benefits I Have Experience From Eating This Way

Throughout this book, I have discussed the many mistakes I made eating raw. I touched a little on the benefits that I experienced, but as my story shows, my first few years on the diet brought me more negatives than positives.

Even though I do not eat strictly raw or strictly vegan, the way I currently eat has brought me many benefits, including:

Stable Blood Sugar

When I eat fruit with little fat, my blood sugar is very stable. In the summer of 2009, I trained for a marathon, and during that time, I could easily tell how foods affected me. I got the best results eating large quantities of fruit and drinking watermelon juice during my races. In spite of all the sugar in the fruit, my blood sugar remained remarkably stable.

Better Energy

As I explained in the book, lack of energy was my main problem for many years. Now, those days feel like a distant memory. Eating more fruit and less fat, my energy is higher and much more stable, with fewer ups and downs.

No Dental Decay

The rampant dental decay I suffered from has stopped. My last checkups have been very positive, although due to the large number of fillings I have, one of them has to be replaced occasionally. I also have to be extra careful because I'm now more prone to cavities, which can creep up behind fillings. In spite of that, my teeth have been doing great. I'm lucky the decay has never been bad enough to require major intervention, such as root canals.

Better Endurance

One of the surprising results of the fruit-based, low-fat diet is improved endurance. In the past, I could only do about 35 to 40 pushups in a row. Now I can do 50 pushups in a row in the first ten minutes after waking up in the morning, without even warming up. The more fruit and the less fat that I eat, the better my endurance is.

More Youthful Appearance

When I went back to eating a lot of cooked foods, I gained weight, and at some point, I even reached the weight of 172 lbs, the most I've ever weighed in my life. I no longer looked youthful. Ever since I have been mostly raw, I remain at a stable weight and look and feel younger. In spite of some graying hair (which started when I was 18), most people think I'm a little younger than my age.

Great Concentration

When I was eating high-fat raw foods, I would crash in the afternoon and could barely concentrate after meals. Ever since I changed my diet to include more fruit and less fat, I've unleashed a monster of productivity. Since 2005, I've written millions of words, and I credit that partly to being able to focus more clearly on the task at hand.

What About You?

After reading my strange and surprising tales, you're probably wondering "what now"?

Is 100% raw bad?

Is 100% raw achievable?

Is cooked food really all that bad for me?

The point I want to get across to people is that yes, we are all different, but we are all a lot more alike than we think. I don't subscribe to the "metabolic typing" diet, but I do think that our diet must fit our individual circumstances and, often, our physical weaknesses. In this sense, there is truly no right diet for everybody.

In most cases, the changes to make to individualize the diet will be fairly minor, but nonetheless important.

The major differences are in caloric needs between men and women and fat and protein needs between children and adults. On average, men need 600 more calories per day than women.

It's important to determine the amount of calories you need to consume on a daily basis to maintain your weight and energy levels.[71]

What about you, the reader?

Not knowing you personally, I don't have all the answers. But I've learned a fair bit through extensive trial and error and through reading nutrition books and scientific studies, as well as keeping in touch with raw foodists from around the world.

A 100% raw, low-fat, vegan diet (or close to it) works wonderfully for a lot of people. On the physical level, most people usually feel their best eating this way. It may, however, be too difficult for some on other levels, which leads me to say that 100% raw will not work for everyone, and no, eating some cooked food will not kill you.

When I say 100% is not for everyone, I mean that some people are not comfortable with the idea of forcing themselves to live such a strict and regimented life.

You can be successful on a 100% raw, low-fat, vegan diet. I see it all the time, but then you can also be unsuccessful when you eat too much, eat too little, or don't exercise enough or at all. Eating a high-fruit diet, snacking on fruit all day and not exercising is not the worst thing you can do for your health, but it's far from being the best.

There is nothing wrong with you; it's just your application of the diet that is incorrect and not working for you. Eating raw is a trained skill, not an innate skill you were born with. It takes practice to achieve your goals.

---

71   I've always used a rough formula, which is to multiply your ideal body weight by 10 to get the absolute minimum number of calories you should not go below. To that, you'll need to add enough for your daily activities and your level of activity.

When I say cooked food will not kill you, I'm referring to whole, lightly cooked, barely processed foods, like greens, vegetables and root vegetables.

I don't believe that you need to eat cooked food to be healthy, but perhaps you may need it at certain times when you fall off the wagon, aren't getting enough calories from quality fruit, or in social situations when there's literally nothing else to eat.

One problem I experienced when I first went raw was that my main aspiration was to be a 100% raw foodist, and I believed that all I needed to do to be successful was willpower and discipline. I see many people today in the same boat. Even some raw food teachers preach this and convince people to go 100% overnight, no looking back, and with few, if any, skills with raw food to start with. What a recipe for disaster for the majority of us…

These people convince themselves they not only can, but *must* do it, for fear of being berated by their peers, questioned by their family members, or to become the ultimate raw food puritan, where no illness or disease can ever touch them (thereby forever proving any naysayers about their diet wrong).

If you feel inspired to go 100% raw, do it! But your journey doesn't stop there. I implore you to learn about calories, learn how to make delicious, low-fat foods, be aware of the fat content of your food, teach yourself to be able to eyeball quantities of fruit to know how much food you need for each meal, and so on. I will review some important principles in the next chapters.

Make sure you are still able to think outside the box and not just wash your hands of all responsibility for your success and health because you are a "100% raw foodist," who is now somehow superhuman and above everyone else.

If you just can't commit to 100% raw, but you still want to do something positive for your health, then perhaps you would do better on what I call a "mostly raw" diet plan.

This is not a "just eat some fruit and whatever other junk you want to eat too when you feel like it" diet. It's still carefully planned and selective of the best quality foods, but it might give you a little legroom from the stress of being 100% perfect all the time and the ability to still feel comfortable in social situations where food is served without feeling guilty about it. It's also something that is a little more family friendly, and you can generally make the same meals for yourself as your family and enjoy a pleasant meal together at dinner.

I want you to set yourself up for success. So, regardless of which route you choose, you need to make sure that you have a handle on buying enough food for yourself and your family, bringing prepared foods when going to work, eating something before going out to dinner with friends so that you are less tempted to eat unhealthy foods, practicing making healthy recipes that are not laden with nuts and oils, and actually enjoying the food you make. If you fail at some of these basic necessities, it won't be long before you fall off the wagon, feel bad about it, become frustrated with the diet, and possibly give up altogether.

The last thing I want is for you to give up on the low-fat raw vegan diet or vegan lifestyle completely because you were unable to master it properly and comfortably for the rest of your life. I almost did that on several occasions, just because I didn't know how to make the diet work.

If you'd like to get more valuable information on how to make this diet work in the real world with real-life examples and recipes, I suggest that you check out the bonus DVD that is offered with this book, called *Raw Food Nutrition Explained*. If you don't have it already, make sure you get it at a discount by going to

www.rawcontroversies.com/dvds

CHAPTER 24

Tips for Success on the Raw Food Diet

I would like to end this book with a summary of the numerous "raw food mistakes" one can make, as well as my best pieces of advice I have learned over the years. I have made many of these mistakes myself and seen others make the rest. Now you can be well prepared and avoid painful years of trial and errors.

Calories: Not Getting Enough

This is by far the most common mistake that leads raw foodists to endure strong cravings for cooked foods, and then fall off the wagon or give up the diet completely. The few intrepid souls who are motivated enough to stay in for the long term are going to get even worse problems.

When going raw initially, this deficit in calories is going to cause a massive weight loss, which is usually embraced. Over time, if this deficit is not corrected, the person is going to start feeling the real effects of not giving the body everything it needs: lack of energy, deficiencies and failure to thrive.

Not Eating Enough Carbs

It is possible to manage to get enough energy (calories) on the raw food diet, but still experience all the problems mentioned above. This occurs when a significant proportion of the calories come from fat instead of carbohydrates (fruit). Carbohydrates play a very important role in the human body. The first symptom of not getting enough carbs is lack of energy. The second consequence is consuming too much fat, which causes the problems listed below.

Eating Too Much Fat

Eating too much fat is generally an after-effect of not eating enough carbohydrates. The body needs to get its energy from somewhere, and if it can't get it from carbohydrates or protein, then it will get it from fat.

Eating too much fat is a major cause of type-2 diabetes and other blood sugar problems, which are incorrectly attributed to sugar itself. Candidiasis can also be caused by eating too much fat, which can also lead to a wide range of other health problems, such as chronic fatigue, failure to thrive, lack of energy, depression, skin problems, and more.

Not Eating Enough Fruit

Because the only real source of carbohydrates in the raw food diet is fruit (besides some other items like honey, which could never be a primary source of calories), a deficit in carbohydrates and energy automatically means not eating enough fruit.

So how much fruit should you eat? It really depends on caloric needs. On a totally raw diet with some physical activity, the minimum number of necessary calories to consume would be approximately 2000 for women and 3000 for men. Of course if you're in your 60s or 70s you might require less than these amounts.

For men who are training with weights to gain muscle mass, the minimum number of calories to consume in fruits and vegetables is 3500 calories (or 3000 for women) to see any results.

The reason it took me so long to recover from my water fast is that I was aiming at getting 2500 calories a day, but I was usually failing. At the same time, I was burning more calories in daily activities.

Because it's difficult to gain weight on a completely raw diet, while eating fruit as a main source of calories and with little added fat, it's probably better to err on the side of eating "too much" fruit rather than not enough (but not snacking on it all day, to prevent dental problems)

Not Counting Your Calories

The raw food diet is probably the only diet in the world where it's easier to eat too little than to eat too much!

For that reason, it's important to count calories, at least in the beginning stages.

Many experienced raw foodists count calories using online software. Here are a few that I recommend:

www.sparkpeople.com (because you can create a recipe database if you frequently eat the same meals)

www.fitday.com

www.nutridiary.com

If you own an iPhone or iPod Touch, you may want to try the apps *Absolute Fitness* or *MyNetDiary*.

Eating Lots of Fat, Nuts, Seeds and Avocados

Eating too much fat in the raw food diet can only mean one thing: eating too many nuts, seeds, avocado or oil. To that category, we can also add durian and coconuts.

We tend to revert to what we know. On a Standard American Diet, what we know are heavy and dense foods. We all know that a cheeseburger is extremely fatty and can pack in a lot of calories in a small amount of space. Here's a big surprise: even a McDonald's Big Mac with a large order of French fries is still lower in fat than many gourmet raw food recipes!

	Big Mac	Big Mac w/ Large Fries	Raw Taco*
Calories	570 calories	1040 calories	1500 calories
Fat	34 grams	54 grams	142 grams
Protein	24 grams	31 grams	30 grams
Carbs	47 grams	108 grams	57 grams
Sodium	1070 mg	1394	1700 mg

*For the Raw Taco recipe, I used a recipe found at: **http://www.live-green-smoothie-diet. com/2009/04/genuinely-meaty-raw-taco-meatwith-chunky-guacamole-and-fresh-cherry-tomato-jalapeno-salsa/**. It is made with mushrooms, walnuts, olive oil, raw cacao, tomatoes, avocado, pine nuts and a few other seasonings.

My point is not that a Big Mac with Fries is better for health than a Raw Taco, but rather that a Raw Taco (as well as many other raw recipes) is not necessarily better in many ways than some of the worst junk food. Of course, the Raw Taco will have more vitamins and minerals and none of the chemicals of the Big Mac and Fries, but the McDonald's meal has the advantage of being lower in fat and surprisingly, lower in sodium too. Also, the Raw Taco is lower in carbs and higher in fat than the Big Mac and fries. That means that you'll be less satisfied eating it than eating a Big Mac and fries, even though it's higher in calories.

The popularity of raw food recipes containing avocado, coconut and durian in the raw food world can be explained by the fact that most people are struggling to get enough calories on this diet. Because they haven't learned to eat enough fruit, they naturally revert to the one thing that's heavy and dense they can eat: nuts, seeds, oil, avocado and durian.

The fact that raw foodists revere the durian is a good indication of the nature of the problem. The durian is a big, spiky, tropical fruit found in Southeast Asia. It often smells bad, but its taste is unique. It's very creamy and sweet, being rich in both fat and sugar. Eating an entire durian can represent almost 1000 calories! For puny raw foodists who struggle to pack in 400 calories in a smoothie, eating a big durian is a big caloric reward. Their bodies are thanking them for giving them enough food at once, and they crave more, like a dehydrated man in the desert who finally gets a sip of water.

Craving fatty foods is always an indication that one is not eating enough fruit. Every time that I thought I was craving something fatty, I realized that the craving mysteriously disappeared after I ate more fruit! I wasn't craving fat... I was just hungry!

Using Oil

Because we want to stick to a low-fat diet, using any kind of oil will inevitably mean getting too much fat. One tablespoon of oil is over 120 calories. Also, by consuming certain types of vegetable oils (such as sesame or sunflower), we risk getting too many omega-6 fatty acids, which will create a deficiency in omega-3 fatty acids.

There's really no reason to use oil — a refined food — when you can get all the fat you need from whole foods, such as nuts, seeds and avocado, used sparingly. Even a dressing can be made creamy by blending in some hemp seeds or avocado.

Not Eating Any Fat At All

Some people in the low-fat raw vegan crowd seem to think that because too much fat is bad for you, the best diet must be a completely fat-free diet. While it's true that fruits and vegetables contain a small percentage of essential fatty acids (generally around 3-5%), relying on those foods alone for our essential fatty acid needs can be problematic. Some people even shoot for a *90/5/5* diet, with just 5% of calories, or even less, coming from fat. Many men who eliminate all overt fat sources from their diet report a very low libido, which could be an indication they are lacking certain important elements found in nuts and seeds. Some women report loss of menstruation, and other hormonal problems.

I recommend eating some nuts and seeds a few times a week. I favor the nuts and seeds that are rich in omega-3 fatty acids, which are generally lacking in most people's diets. These nuts and seeds include: walnuts, and hemp seeds. Avocado is a good source of fat, as well as coconuts. However, we should be aware that coconuts are rich in saturated fats, and they must be consumed in moderation.

Not Eating Greens

Fruits are great for calories and many vitamins, but they tend to lack certain nutrients, particularly alkaline and acidic minerals, such as calcium and phosphorus. Although it's possible to live on fruit alone for a while (I have done it many times while traveling), for long-term health, you should eat your greens.

Green vegetables include: lettuce, celery, spinach, cabbage (all types), broccoli, kale, collard greens and parsley.

It's not necessary to force yourself to eat greens that are bitter and unpleasant to the taste, such as dandelion greens or even raw kale. Just getting a variety of lettuces and celery is enough for basic needs. Curiously, one of the best vegetables, nutritionally speaking, is common cabbage.

How much to eat? Usually, one pound of greens per day is what you need. Dr. Fuhrman recommends one pound of raw vegetables (in salads or blended salads) and one pound of cooked vegetables (such as broccoli, spinach, kale, collard greens, snow peas, etc.). If you're going to eat any cooked foods at all, make sure that cooked greens are on the menu. Of all raw and cooked foods, they're the most nutrient-dense.

Eating Too Often

I've already mentioned the problems related to eating too often during the day. Constant exposure to sugar will cause dental problems more quickly than high quantities of sugar in the diet overall.

It may be difficult to stop snacking because we're used to eating a certain quantity of food we think of as "normal." However, we have to look at real-life results. After a meal, how long does it take for you to be hungry again? If you're hungry again after an hour, you haven't eaten enough.

Ideally, you want to eat enough at a meal to power you for at least 3 hours after breakfast, and 4-5 hours after lunch and dinner. In general, that means eating a lot more food than you're used to.

For example, a few years ago, I was training for a marathon, and I realized that I needed to increase my food intake at lunch in order to be satisfied until dinner. I resisted doing this, and for a while, my performance during the runs was inadequate. Reluctantly, I decided to increase my food intake for lunch to 1500 calories, which meant about 15 bananas or the equivalent in other fruits, and my energy came back, my performance was up, and I was satisfied for hours until dinner time.

Finding the optimal amount of fruit to eat at a sitting is a matter of personal experimentation. Too often, I see people consuming a smoothie of an apple, a pear and some greens (175 calories if you're lucky) for breakfast and wondering why they're hungry after an hour. They forget that in their previous life before raw, they probably ate at least 600 calories for breakfast![72]

Eating a Lot of Sweet Fruit While Being Sedentary

One mistake that is not often talked about, but one that I've personally made as well, is to try this high-fruit diet while being sedentary.

---

[72] It's possible that some people may feel very uncomfortable eating a large quantity of fruit at one time. This can be alleviated by consuming mono-meals (only one kind of fruit at a time), and a gentle transition towards a diet with more volume. I do not recommend eating to the point of physical discomfort. When I eat 100% raw, I find that I have to eat tremendous quantities of fruit to be satisfied. Now that I include some cooked carbohydrates in my diet, I find I do not have to eat as much fruit as before, which makes it easier to eat fewer meals.

Fruit is premium-quality fuel. It burns clean. It can power you quickly, but it can also last you for hours. Eating a lot of it while being sedentary is like putting premium fuel or diesel fuel in a car that is not designed to receive it.

While eating too much fruit and being sedentary is not as bad as eating a lot of fat AND fruit while being sedentary, you can still expect negative consequences.

All that sugar that you're eating in fruit needs to be burned!

I've often fooled myself into thinking I was active because I was going to the gym three times a week.

We need exercise on a daily basis. The strict minimum would be about half an hour of relatively intense physical activity every day, but ideally, we want to shoot for 45 minutes or longer.

If, for some reason, you're not exercising that much, then you should decrease the amount of fruit that you're eating and eat more vegetables instead.

At the bare minimum, try to at least get a few minutes of exercise every day, even if it's only 5 to 15 minutes.

Raw Cacao and Raw Drugs

I've discussed this extensively in my other books *The Raw Secrets* and *The Raw Vegan Coach*, as well as on my website **www.fredericpatenaude. com**

Over the years, I've seen people looking for the "magic potion" and superfood that will solve all of their health problems. Every year, it's a different thing. One year, the craze was noni juice, the next, it was raw cacao. While some of these superfoods can have value, a few of them are clearly stimulants that have no place in the diet. Raw cacao belongs to that category. The negative aspects of cacao far outweigh any benefits from consuming it regularly, as a two-ounce piece of raw cacao has the same stimulative power as a cup of coffee. [73]

Feeding This Diet to Children

Let's be clear that everything that I've discussed in this book applies to grown adults. One should not extrapolate these ideas and apply them to feeding growing children.

The needs of growing children are different and delicate. We know, for example, that mother's milk is over 50% fat by calories (not by weight, as all milk products are advertised). It also contains more sugar than the milk of most mammals.

I do not have children myself, and I have little experience in this area. All I can relate is third-party experience.

I've known some successful 100% raw foodists, such as Solange Rodrigue, the only French-Canadian raw foodist I had heard of when I first went raw in 1997, who has raised entire families on a 100% raw diet, but they included raw dairy products in their menu.[74]

Other Natural Hygienists include potatoes, beans, and other starchy foods, and some of them even include eggs.

One controversial article was published by Dr. Stanley Bass on "Three Generations of Vegetarian Hygienists." It followed the story of raw food families following Natural Hygiene principles.

Dr. Bass' conclusion was that this diet worked for the first generation, but after a few generations, there were problems, such as improper development.

Quoting from this article:

---

73   80 milligrams of caffeine. Value obtained by combining the caffeine and theobromine content of chocolate, from the book *Caffeine Blues*. Content may vary in raw cacao.
74   http://www.fredericpatenaude.com/articles/interview-solange.html

"I noticed in the beginning of the third generation, some of them that were born—this is where I noticed the nearsightedness, the hydroceles, and the abnormalities. Then I made my shift into more green stuff, blended salads early, cut out the orange juice — like I'd give the child the milk and I'd use the vegetable juice. Then I saw the difference. The children were better — were more sturdy. Instead of pigeon-chested or chicken-chested, they were fine-chested.

Their diet would be predominantly fruit, nut proteins, and a relatively small amount of salad compared to what they get now — they used to get one salad a day. They'd have a fruit meal in the morning, a fruit meal at noon, and a salad at night. In the morning, they'd have just fruit; at noon they'd have the fruit and nuts, and at night they'd have the salad, sometimes with nuts and sometimes with vegetables — but on this kind of a setup, I've been noticing the inadequacies in these children. Then I made the drastic changes! First, I noticed the hydroceles, nearsightedness, and the skeletal development. And the musculature was not developed in these children.

But, at any rate, I started to think it was only after adding green stuff that I started to see in the pregnancies that followed, and also in the children that were grown, that came from these pregnancies, the difference. Round heads instead of pear-shaped heads, better-formed teeth. And all the aberrations I had noticed — the nearsightedness, the hernias, the hydroceles, and the musculature that was weak — that all disappeared. There was never another case after this. I was also able to witness an increase, for example, in the blood chemistries, the improvements in the mothers and in the adults, who were put on this kind of a setup. Hemoglobin — where they had microcytic anemia or macrocytic anemia, the nutritional anemias — they cleared up. Now, this was with the addition of the salads, but even so, I was not satisfied. In trying to evaluate the absolute amount of every nutrient, I found it was inadequate. They couldn't eat that amount, and they didn't have the time to eat that amount.

Dr. Bass: The salad?

Dr. Cursio: Hence the blended salad. To ensure the proper impact, the proper intake in sufficient amounts with minimal expenditure of energy, especially in the ill, so that we had the assimilation, and we had the utilization with the minimal usage of vital power, and leaving sufficient energy, you know, for reparative and healing and restorative purposes."

Although I don't find that this article quoted above answered everything, some ideas in it were interesting.[75]

This definitely points towards the importance of incorporating blended salads, green smoothies and veggie stews in the diet.

In the same article, Dr. Cursio also talks about his use of egg yolk and a certain type of raw cheese (never cooked) in the children's diet and for people who need to overcome certain health problems.

Now, we do not know if the generation of hygienists with all these problems was using unripe fruit, not consuming enough calories, or how long they were breastfed. But it seems certain that they were not consuming enough vegetable matter.

A few observations:

Getting enough food is a big concern.

Most of the disaster stories I have heard from raw vegan parents feeding their children inadequate diets were in households that restricted some kind of food category: fruit, fat, nuts, etc. The raw vegan children I've seen thrive ate very large amounts of fruits and vegetables and generous servings of nuts and seeds with other fatty foods.

Low-fat is out of the question.

Dr. Doug Graham reasons that because our ancestors used to breastfeed children for longer periods of time out of necessity, sometimes as long as 5 to 6 years, growing children have an increased need for fat. They simply cannot get all the calories they need from just fruit. At some point, before puberty, they can transition towards a lower fat diet and eat like adults. It is possible that if children were fed some cooked carbohydrates, getting enough calories would be possible without using

---

75   http://www.drbass.com/freedownload/files/drbass04.pdf

as much fat. We would have to see what the vegan doctors say about child nutrition on this topic.

Getting Enough Greens is Critical

Most fruitarian diets simply cannot supply enough minerals for the health of growing children. But because children are generally not attracted to salads and raw vegetables (it seems to be a widespread phenomenon), finding creative tricks to get children to eat their greens is important. This may mean making green smoothies they like, or even a special soup made by blending cooked greens.

There is a controversy about feeding children a vegan diet.

I've seen an unusual number of raw foodists notice that their growing children were not doing so well on a vegan diet, and they introduced some animal foods in their diet, such as eggs and raw dairy products, with great benefits. Surprisingly, many of these parents are prominent raw foodists, but very few went public with this information. To respect their privacy, I won't name names, but let's say that these are some well-known people in the raw world. Most of these people continued with the raw vegan diet themselves, but let their kids eat some animal foods.

It could be simply that with the raw vegan diet, their caloric needs were not being met. It's quite common that even SAD children are not getting their caloric needs met. It could also be that there are certain nutrients in animal foods that are important for children and hard to get in the raw vegan diet.

One author who went public with her child-raising experience is Shazzie, who, incidentally, promotes quite a different diet than I do, but her experience is nonetheless interesting:

> "Since 2000, I've had the opportunity to meet thousands of raw foodists. I've also met hundreds of raw children in that time. By far, the children who are vegetarian seem healthier than the vegan children.

These observations led me to research from the ground up childhood nutrition, vegan nutrition, and raw food nutrition. I had a very good reason to get it right -- my daughter Evie. I wanted her to be raw for health reasons. I wanted her to be vegan, because I'd been vegan for so long.

However, all the while I was researching this information, I saw huge amounts of misinformation being fed to the raw food community. I also saw children with very damaged teeth, stunted growth, and developmental problems.

Worryingly, the children of some of those who actively promoted raw food had experienced the worst symptoms. If these children were put on a raw or cooked vegetarian (not vegan) diet, and were given supplements, they caught up. Those who are still raw vegan are still experiencing development and growth issues.

I was most concerned that these "raw food promoters" never, not once, publicly stated what had happened to their children. In fact, when other raw parents were having issues with the development of their children, these very same raw food promoters and coaches told them to keep on doing what they were doing. This caused the raw food community to remain oblivious to the dangers of raising children raw. It all added up to a cover up in the raw food community spanning years.

These parents clearly love their children. And I can't believe for one second they would wish their traumas on other families, so why haven't they spoken publicly? FEAR. Fear at being judged, fear at being seen as failures, fear at ruining their careers, fear of the small, yet vocal hard line fruitarian-types, saying they'd got it wrong, because they weren't following their dogmatic diet.

Parents who have had the courage to speak up have been hounded and slated, ostracized and ridiculed. Their experiences have been dismissed, and they haven't been listened to. Their experiences certainly haven't been welcomed as something for the raw food community to embrace.

Even worse are the lies in this cover-up.

Take these examples:

One mother experienced severe growth defects in her children on the raw vegan unsupplemented diet and resorted to feeding them large quantities of dairy and meat. She has since stood shoulder to shoulder with the other raw vegan dogmatists and writes on raw food forums pretending to be someone else! She says that she has been successful in raising her children raw vegan, yet she clearly hasn't.

The raw vegan child who was severely behind his development schedule and had fluorosis. His mother, a "raw food coach" altered his diet (to cooked vegetarian plus supplements, plus some fish in the early days), and he eventually began to sit, crawl, and catch up. Even after this harrowing experience, this coach continued to tell mothers of children that weren't thriving on the raw vegan diet that raw vegan is OK and to eat more fruit. She has never made a public statement about this experience and continues to be vague about what makes a healthy raw food diet for adults and children.

The raw vegan family in the USA who has several children. The last child wasn't even sitting up by the age of two. All the children are extremely thin and "bird like".

The raw vegan fruit promoter who says all non-vegan children are too tall, and so vegan children are supposed to be small.

The tiny raw girl on YouTube who has hardly any top teeth due to visible decay.

In fact, I've scoured the world and asked and asked. And this is the truth: no-one has yet come forward with a child who has been raised 100% raw vegan unsupplemented who is the correct weight and height for their age and is beyond breastfeeding years.

Why?

Because it's impossible to grow a child healthily on that kind of diet.

Why do seemingly intelligent people say it's possible?

Indoctrination and dogmatism. These people are so tied in to a belief system that nothing, not even the visible deteriorating health of their child, can bring them out of their hypnotic state.

The truth is, though I'd love to see it, I have never once seen a 100% raw 100% vegan 100% unsupplemented child beyond breastfeeding age who has no tooth decay and is the correct weight and height for their age. Not one. Ever.

On the other hand, I have, since 2001, seen countless raw vegan unsupplemented children spanning several countries (including the USA) with growth, teeth, and mental disorders.[76]

We can really feel the passion that Shazzie has with this issue. Unfortunately, there's not a whole lot of evidence to support either claim (that a raw vegan diet is best for children or that it could be extremely damaging).

I've heard of some successful raw vegan children. There's the Talifero family, but I do not know them personally.[77] The Taliferos don't feed their kids a low-fat diet, and I believe they use some supplements and superfoods.

My friend Karen Ranzi has just released a very well-written and extensive book called *Creating Healthy Children*, which advocates a raw vegan diet for children and lists stories of many raw vegan and raw food families in her book.

I have met a few raw vegan families, but in most cases, the parents eventually re-introduced some cooked foods and sometimes animal foods in the diet, often because of a combination of fear of nutritional inadequacy and social pressures that make it difficult for children to stay raw.

I know some people who claim to raise their children 100% raw, but unfortunately, they have remained very silent regarding the specifics of the children's diets. Due to fears of being accused of child abuse, raw vegan parents don't often share their experience, whether it's a positive one or a negative one.

Like Shazzie, I have seen some disturbing cases of raw vegan children that were suffering from obvious nutritional deficiencies caused by an inadequate diet. Relating them would add nothing more than weak anecdotal evidence, so until I come to definite conclusions about this

76 http://www.shazzie.com/life/articles/raw_vegan_children.shtml
77 http://www.thegardendiet.com

issue, I will continue stating that this is a delicate topic that must be carefully looked at by any prospective parents who intend to raise their children as raw vegans.

What About Organic Food?

The organic food movement is an important part of building a healthy future for our planet and our health. I try to buy organic food whenever possible. However, I don't think it's necessary to eat only 100% organic food to be healthy. I buy organic food when the produce is fresh, ripe and of high quality.

If you are sensitive and get sick eating produce that is not 100% organic, then by all means continue to eat all-organic. A small percentage of people fall into this category.

It's important to keep things in perspective and realize that "certified organic" is not the only criterion. I would prefer to eat a very fresh, conventionally-grown carrot from a small local farmer than a bag of mass-produced, organic carrots that have been picked months ago.

Sometimes, commercially-grown produce is of better quality than organic, and a lot of the time, organic is better. What is certain is that eating only organic foods is not enough to do much to improve your health. Therefore, it's not a priority as important as the others I mentioned previously.

Overall, organic food is more nutritious and healthier than conventional food. It is more nutritious because it tends to have more minerals (overall: there may be exceptions) and vitamins, and be healthier because there are fewer pesticides and other toxic residues.

CHAPTER 25

The Supplements Controversy

Are there supplements that are beneficial to take on the raw vegan diet? Are there some that should be avoided?

It's easier to answer the latter than the former. Studies have shown that the vast majority of supplements do more harm than good.[78] The supplements that have been shown to be dangerous to take include:

- Iron[79]

- Vitamin A[80]

- Folic acid (not folate found in food)[81]

- Vitamin D (in amounts beyond what one could normally synthesize from sunshine exposure)[82]

- Copper[83]

- Vitamin E[84, 85]

---

78 See "Just to be on the safe side, don't take vitamins" **http://www.drmcdougall.com/ misc/2010nl/may/vitamins.htm**

79 Daram, S., &Havashi, P. (2005).Acute Liver Failure Due to Iron Overdose in an Adult.*Southern Medical Journal, 98*(2), 241-244.

80 Leithead, J., Simpson, K., &MacGilchrist, A. (2009). Fulminant hepatic failure following overdose of the vitamin A metabolite acitretin.*European Journal of Gastroenterology &Hepatology, 21*(2), 230-232

81 Evans, C., & Lacey, J. (1986). Toxicity of vitamins: complications of a health movement. *British Medical Journal, 292*(6519), 509-510.

82 (2008). Vitamin D overdose.*Reactions Weekly,* (1188), 22-23.

83 Kasama, T., & Tanaka, H. (1988).Effects of copper administration on fetal and neonatal mice. *Journal Of Nutritional Science And Vitaminology, 34*(6), 595-605.

84 Smith, I. (2000). Vitamin Overdose. *Time, 155*(16), 89.

85 L.B. (2005).Vitamin E Media Coverage Misleading.,*Natural Grocery Buyer, 4*(1), 5. In this study, Researchers reviewed 19 previous studies on the effects of high-dose vitamin E supplementation and they concluded that people who take more than 400 international units daily of vitamin E have a 5 percent greater risk of death than those who don't supplement.

Supplements that contain nutrients in doses that are much beyond what one could realistically get from food can also create nutritional imbalances.For example, even though Vitamin D normally protects you from some cancers, high doses of many other vitamins can have the opposite effect.[86]

Even without scientific studies, it's simple common sense that man-made vitamins are not as good as real vitamins found in food. However, we also know that in certain cases, some supplements, when taken appropriately, can be very useful. One example is in the case of Vitamin B12 deficiencies causing nervous system degeneration. This can be reversed by injections of Vitamin B12.[87]

The nutritional profile of a raw vegan diet can also be surprisingly high. Here's the typical nutritional profile of an active man eating 3000 calories in a day, coming mostly from fruit (watermelon, mango and banana), including two bunches of greens (spinach and lettuce), some celery, several tomatoes and cucumbers and one and half ounces of almonds.

Nutrient	Raw Vegan Diet	SAD Recommended Levels	% of Recommended Level
Protein	73 grams	57 grams	128%
Vitamin A	3,534.7 mcg	900	392%
Vitamin B6	8.5 mg	1.3	655%
Vitamin B12	0 mcg	2.4	0
Vitamin C	873.2 mg	90	970%
Vitamin D	0	1000 iu	0
Vitamin E	40.1 mg	15	268%
Calcium	1,239.3 mg	1000	124%

86 Giovannucci, E., & Chan, A. (2010). Role of vitamin and mineral supplementation and aspirin use in cancer survivors. *Journal of Clinical Oncology, 28*(26), 4081-4085.
87 Ahmed, A., & Kothari, M. (2010). Recovery of neurologic dysfunction with early intervention of vitamin B12. *Journal Of Clinical Neuromuscular Disease, 11*(4), 198-202.

Nutrient	Raw Vegan Diet	SAD Recommended Levels	% of Recommended Level
Copper	5.3 mg	0.9	587%
Iron	29.4 mg	0.9	367%
Magnesium	1,282 mg	430	305%
Manganese	10.9 mg	2.3	476%
Niacin	30 mg	16	187%
Phosphorus	1,601.5 mg	700	229%
Potassium	15,530.5	4700	330%
Riboflavin	3.6 mg	1.3	274%
Selenium	33.7 mcg	55	61%
Sodium	726.2 mg	1500	48%
Thiamin	3.1 mg	1.2	260%
Zinc	12.2	11.0	111%

From the chart above, we can clearly see that as long as enough greens are consumed on a low-fat raw vegan diet, together with plenty of fruit and some nuts and seeds, it provides a tremendous amount of nutrients. The raw vegan diet blows through the recommended values for most vitamins and minerals by a wide and safe margin.

However, it seems to fall short in some categories. Let's take a look at them:

Vitamin B12

B12 is a water-soluble vitamin that is essential for proper functioning of the brain and nervous system and blood formation. Only bacteria and algae can synthesize this vitamin. For this reason, B12 is not normally found in a vegan diet, but is found in animal foods. It is possible that the human body can synthesize all the Vitamin B12 it needs, but the balance of this vitamin's production and delivery system is very delicate.

Lack of the "intrinsic factor," an element crucial for the absorption of Vitamin B12, can cause a Vitamin B12 deficiency. This intrinsic factor can be affected or destroyed by a wide range of conditions, and this may be why Vitamin B12 deficiencies are relatively common.

In the animal world, many herbivorous animals obtain their Vitamin B12 by eating their feces. Because pure veganism is a modern invention of humans, it is possible that throughout history, the main source of Vitamin B12 for humans was the consumption of some animal products. Vitamin B12 is found in animal flesh, fish, milk and eggs (although eggs contain a factor that can block the absorption of B12).

Vegan foods that have been reputed to contain B12, such as seaweed, barley grass, nutritional yeast, spirulina and micro-algae have been shown to contain an an analog form of Vitamin B12, which competes with real B12 for absorption and thus increases our need for it.[88]

Most vegetarians and vegans, as well as the rest of the population, get most of their Vitamin B12 from fortified foods, such as soy milk, breakfast cereals, energy bars, fortified nutritional yeast, fortified orange juice, etc.

Because raw foodists take none of these foods, they are at risk for a Vitamin B12 deficiency.

The recommended intake for B12 is 2 to 4 mcg per day. It's possible that not all the Vitamin B12 is absorbed in a supplement, so the Vegetarian Resource Group recommends 5 to 10 micrograms per day or a weekly B12 supplement of 2000 micrograms.[89]

---

88 The Importance of Vitamin B12 - Gabriel Cousens, **http://www.fredericpatenaude. com/blog/?p=862**

89 See, "Vitamin B12 in the Vegan Diet" **http://www.vrg.org/nutrition/b12.htm**

Vitamin B12 is stored in the liver and other parts of the body. Our stores of Vitamin B12 can be depleted, depending on how much we can absorb, how much is present in the diet, and how much is secreted or used up every day.

What Are the Symptoms of Vitamin B12 Deficiency?

- Vitamin B12 deficiency can cause damage to the brain and nervous system.[90, 91]

- Low levels of Vitamin B12 can cause fatigue, depression and poor memory.[92, 93, 94, 95, 96]

- Vitamin B12 deficiencies can lead to increased blood homocysteine (an amino acid). Studies have shown that elevated homocysteine levels are related to an increased risk of coronary heart disease, stroke, and peripheral vascular disease.[97]

90 Zhuo, J., &Praticò, D. (2010). Acceleration of brain amyloidosis in an Alzheimer's disease mouse model by a folate, Vitamin B6 and B12-deficient diet.*Experimental Gerontology*, *45*(3), 195-201.

91 Black, M. (2008). Effects of vitamin B12 and folate deficiency on brain development in children.*Food And Nutrition Bulletin*, *29*(2 Suppl), S126-S131.

92 Engels, A., Schröer, U., &Schremmer, D. (2008). [Efficacy of a combination therapy with vitamins B6, B12 and folic acid for general feeling of ill-health. Results of a non-interventional post-marketing surveillance study].*MMW Fortschritte Der Medizin*, *149 Suppl 4*162-166.

93 Pontes, H., Neto, N., Ferreira, K., Fonseca, F., Vallinoto, G., Pontes, F., et al. (2009). Oral manifestations of vitamin B12 deficiency: a case report. *Journal (Canadian Dental Association)*, *75*(7), 533-537.

94 Karakuła, H., Opolska, A., Kowal, A., Domański, M., Płotka, A., &Perzyński, J. (2009). [Does diet affect our mood? The significance of folic acid and homocysteine]. *PolskiMerkuriuszLekarski: Organ PolskiegoTowarzystwaLekarskiego*, *26*(152), 136-141.

95 Barghouti, F., Younes, N., Halaseh, L., Said, T., &Ghraiz, S. (2009).High frequency of low serum levels of vitamin B12 among patients attending Jordan University Hospital.*Eastern Mediterranean Health Journal*, *15*(4), 853-860.

96 Hin, H., Clarke, R., Sherliker, P., Atoyebi, W., Emmens, K., Birks, J., et al. (2006). Clinical relevance of low serum vitamin B12 concentrations in older people: the Banbury B12 study. *Age And Ageing*, *35*(4), 416-422.

97 Elmadfa, I., & Singer, I. (2009). Vitamin B-12 and homocysteine status among vegetarians: a global perspective. *American Journal of Clinical Nutrition*, *89*(5S),1693S-1698.

The symptoms of a deficiency may include:

- Itchy or tingling tongue. The tongue suddenly itches from time to time without warning.[98]

- Hyperpigmentation of the skin and nails, and premature white hair (in which patches of skin become darker in color than the normal surrounding skin)[99]

- Oral ulcers[100]

- Shortness of breath, but without chest pain. This can occur when walking just a few yards.[101]

- Tingling along the back of one or both thighs, starting at the hips and shooting downward.[102]

- Memory loss and/or disorientation.

- Migraine headaches.[103]

- Irritability and/or depression and/or personality changes.

Vitamin B12 Content of Animal Foods

Some people might not like the idea of taking a supplement, and think that they can get all the Vitamin B12 they need by eating a small amount of animal products once in a while, such as a bit of yogurt once a week or a few eggs in a smoothie occasionally.

---

98 Güney, F., Kozak, H., Genç, E., Kıreşi, D., Keleş, B., & Toy, H. (2008).B12 vitamin eksikliğiilebirliktegörülenamyotrofik lateral sklerozis (Olgusunumu).*Genel Tip Dergisi*, *18*(2), 85-88.

99 Noppakun, N., &Swasdikul, D. (1986). Reversible hyperpigmentation of skin and nails with white hair due to vitamin B12 deficiency.*Archives Of Dermatology, 122*(8), 896-899.

100 Pontes, H., Neto, N., Ferreira, K., Fonseca, F., Vallinoto, G., Pontes, F., et al. (2009). Oral manifestations of vitamin B12 deficiency: a case report. *Journal (Canadian Dental Association), 75*(7), 533-537.

101 Pontes, H., Neto, N., Ferreira, K., Fonseca, F., Vallinoto, G., Pontes, F., et al. (2009). Oral manifestations of vitamin B12 deficiency: a case report. *Journal (Canadian Dental Association), 75*(7), 533-537.

102 Henchcliffe, C. (2008). Painful Legs and Moving Toes: How to Diagnose and What to Do? (Cover story).*Neurology Alert, 27*(4), 25-26.

103 2009). "Functional" Vitamin B12 Deficiency Common in Migraines.*Alternative & Complementary Therapies, 15*(2), 92.

Our daily needs are estimated at 2.4 micrograms a day. Like some of the other recommended daily allowances (RDA's), this may contain a generous margin of safety. But let's keep this official number in mind.

If we look at the table below, we'll find that eating small amounts of most animal products (except fish) does not provide enough Vitamin B12. Even eating one egg per day would only cover about 25% of our needs. It's possible that these numbers would be higher if they came from organic or "grass-fed" products, but this is the data that's available.

Even though one could get some Vitamin B12 from the addition of some animal products to the diet, there are also negative consequences to doing so, from the added saturated fat, cholesterol, animal protein and contaminants (especially in fish).

So, to be safer, take a supplement.

Food	Vitamin B12 Content	% of Daily Need
1 egg (large, raw)	0.65 mcg	27%
1 egg (large, boiled)	0.55 mcg	23%
Salmon, raw, 3 ounces	3.5 mcg	148%
Salmon, cooked, 3 ounces	4.3 mcg	177%
Yogurt, plain, whole milk, 1 cup	0.91 mcg	38%
Cheese, goat, 3 ounces	0.15 mcg	6%
Chicken, roasted, 4 ounces	0.36 mcg	15%
Beef, cooked, 4 ounces	1.8 mcg	85%

Vitamin D

We all know that Vitamin D is different than other vitamins, in the sense that it's a fat-soluble vitamin that animals (including humans) produce after exposure to sunshine. Vitamin D acts more like a hormone than a vitamin. It promotes calcium absorption, and it is important for bone health. When living in areas of the world with less sunshine and long winters, it's possible to become deficient in Vitamin D. Vitamin D can be found in the fat of some types of fish, as they may have accumulated this vitamin in their tissues. Some recent studies are linking Vitamin D deficiencies to certain diseases, such as depression,[104] cancer, asthma,[105] diabetes,[106] auto-immune diseases[107,108] and bone problems.[109]

Getting enough sunshine for Vitamin D is a double-edged sword. On the one hand, it may be effective to get enough Vitamin D, but on the other hand, too much sun exposure ages the skin.

Those who tan to look good and to get enough Vitamin D should realize that *there is no such thing as a safe tan!* If you're staying in the sun for long enough for your skin to appreciably tan, then you are causing DNA damage (which we visibly recognize as aging of the skin).[110,111]

I do not believe that this will cause skin cancer if your diet is rich in antioxidants and if you are vegan (I have never heard of any raw vegan or vegan with skin cancer), but it will still cause aging and wrinkling of the skin.

104 Penckofer, S., Kouba, J., Byrn, M., & Estwing Ferrans, C. (2010). Vitamin D and depression: where is all the sunshine? *Issues in Mental Health Nursing, 31*(6), 385-393.
105 Ray, J., &Meikle, A. (2010). D-Light: Vitamin D and good health. *MLO: Medical Laboratory Observer, 42*(5), 32-38.
106 Sabherwal, S., Bravis, V., & Devendra, D. (2010). Effect of oral vitamin D and calcium replacement on glycaemic control in South Asian patients with type 2 diabetes. *International Journal of Clinical Practice, 64*(8), 1084-1089.
107 Pelajo, C., Lopez-Benitez, J., & Miller, L. (2010). Vitamin D and autoimmune rheumatologic disorders.*Autoimmunity Reviews, 9*(7), 507-510.
108 Maruotti, N., & Cantatore, F. (2010). Vitamin D and the immune system.*Journal of Rheumatology, 37*(3), 491-495.
109 Lanham-New, S., Thompson, R., More, J., Brooke-Wavell, K., Hunking, P., & Medici, E. (2007). Importance of vitamin D, calcium and exercise to bone health with specific reference to children and adolescents.*Nutrition Bulletin, 32*(4), 364-377.
110 Harbottle, A., Maki, J., Reguly, B., Wittock, R., Robinson, K., Parr, R., et al. (2010). Real-time polymerase chain reaction analysis of a 3895-bp mitochondrial DNA deletion in epithelial swabs and its use as a quantitative marker for sunlight exposure in human skin A. Harbottle et al. Measure of acute UV damage in human skin.*British Journal of Dermatology, 163*(6), 1291-1295.
111 Steinberg, M., Hubbard, K., Utti, C., Clas, B., Hwang, B., Hill, H., et al. (2009). Patterns of Persistent DNA Damage Associated with Sun Exposure and the Glutathione S-transferase M1 Genotype in Melanoma Patients.*Photochemistry & Photobiology, 85*(1), 379-386.

I have known many raw vegan gurus who are sun-worshippers, exposing their skin with no sunscreen or sunglasses at the time of day when the sun is strongest, hoping to get maximum benefits from sunshine and thinking that, since they were already tanned, their skin was protected. They might have been getting enough Vitamin D, but now their skin looks old. Their appearance is wrongly attributed to the effects of their diet when it's the exposure to sunshine that should be blamed.

For many years, I also believed that getting lots of sunshine whenever possible was a great idea. At the age of 34, I can already see that I've done some damage to my skin (mostly visible as wrinkles on the corners of my eyes) by getting too much sun at times when I was younger.

I have spent most of the last winters in sunny and tropical environments, but in spite of this I have started taking supplemental vitamin D.

I'm now more careful with sunshine exposure, without being paranoid. I avoid sunshine exposure when the sun is at its strongest (usually between 10 a.m. and 3 p.m.) There are many benefits to regular sunshine exposure,[112] but remember that if you're staying long enough to tan, you're causing DNA damage, and your skin will age faster.

Unfortunately, exposing our skin outside of these hours and for a duration insufficient to cause appreciable tanning of the skin is likely to also not produce that much Vitamin D. Therefore, taking supplemental Vitamin D is also advisable.

The recommended intake in supplemental form is between 1000 and 3000 *iu* a day, although intakes up to 10,000 *iu* have been shown to be safe. It's important not to take more than the amount that could realistically be produced by the body through sunshine exposure.[113]

---

112 Sivamani, R., Crane, L., &Dellavalle, R. (2009). The benefits and risks of ultraviolet tanning and its alternatives: the role of prudent sun exposure. *Dermatologic Clinics*, 27(2), 149.

113 Michael, H. (2009). Vitamin D and Health: Evolution, Biologic Functions, and Recommended Dietary Intakes for Vitamin D. *Clinical Reviews in Bone & Mineral Metabolism*, 7(1), 2-19.

I therefore recommend that you get your levels of Vitamin D checked or supplement with the recommended amounts if in doubt. Dr. Fuhrman sells a Vitamin D and B12 supplement formulated for vegans. Other brands are widely available as well.

Selenium

Levels of selenium can be a little low in some raw vegan menus. However, there are plenty of sources, the best one being Brazil nuts. Just eating a few Brazil nuts once in a while is a great way to obtain extra selenium. Other than that, I don't think it's necessary to supplement with selenium.

Sodium

If salt is not added to the diet, sodium levels will be low, but adequate — and that's good. Keep in mind that the recommended 1500mg constitutes an upper limit, not a minimum! Many health organizations have lowered the upper limit for sodium intake from 2300 mg to 1500 mg.[114] Therefore, the levels of sodium naturally found in a raw vegan diet that includes sufficient greens (usually between 300 and 500 mg) are perfectly adequate. Eating some foods containing a little sodium (such as tomato salsa) is no cause for alarm, as a few tablespoons of salsa might increase your sodium intake to 1000 mg, which is still a healthy level. However, adding too much salt to your food will inevitably bring you into the unhealthy range for sodium intake.

---

114 CDC. "CDC Features - Most Americans Should Consume Less Sodium (1,500 mg/ Day or Less)." *Centers for Disease Control and Prevention*.N.p., n.d. Web. 13 Dec. 2010. **http://www.cdc.gov/features/sodium/**

Is Sea Salt Any Better?

Although raw food chefs shun table salt and go for exotic types of salt like Himalayan Salt, Celtic sea salt, and Nama Shoyu, there is no evidence that these salts are any better than table salt. According to *Nutrition Health Review, Fall, 1990*:

Sea salt is not more healthful than regular salt. Salt is sodium chloride, no matter from what its derivation.

Sea salt is essentially sodium chloride, and unrefined salt, obtained from the sea, has little nutritional advantage.

Sea salt does contain some minerals not present in ordinary table salt such as magnesium, sulfur, calcium and potassium, but the amount of these trace minerals is practically undetectable.

Nutrition Health Review, Fall, 1990

There are different kinds of salt touted as "healthy" in the raw food movement. Here's what's important to know:

Type of Salt	% Sodium Chloride	Other Elements Present
Table Salt	99%	Anti-caking agents (such as sodium silicoaluminate or magnesium carbonate), supplemental iodine
Himalayan Salt	98%	10 other minerals
Celtic Sea Salt	83%	14.3% moisture 1.8% trace elements (about 60)
Fleur de Sel	85%+	10%+ moisture About 10 other minerals Impurities

As we can see from the table above, all of the special salts are not so special at all. They are composed mostly of sodium chloride, just like table salt. In some cases, when the salt is moist, it may appear to be lower in sodium.

But once you take the water out of the equation, the 85% sodium of the "fleur de sel" quickly becomes a good 95%. It's the same for Celtic sea salt.

As for the trace minerals found in those salts, there is simply no reason to consume them in the form of salt. Would you trade a product that was 98% sodium chloride in exchange for a few minerals you could find easily in fruits and vegetables?

DHA

In the past few years, there's been a lot of discussion about essential fatty acids. The science of fatty acids can be quite complicated, and I think that's partly why there is so much confusion in this field.

Let's try to keep it simple.

Fat can be found in a variety of forms:

Saturated fat, which is solid at room temperature and mainly found in meat and coconuts. Saturated fats are called "saturated" because the carbon chains are saturated with hydrogen atoms.

Cholesterol is also a fat found in animal products and fish.

Monounsaturated fats are found in olive oil, peanuts, avocados, nuts and seeds. It's called monounsaturated fat because of a single double bond between two carbon atoms.

Trans fat is a man-made fat produced by hydrogenating vegetable oil, so the oil becomes solid at room temperature and acts more like a saturated fat.

Polyunsaturated fats are found in vegetable oils (sunflower, corn, safflower, cottonseed), and in nuts and seeds. They are called polyunsaturated fats because they have at least two double bonds between carbon atoms. In this category, we find the omega-6 and omega-3 fats.

We also know that there are certain types of fat that are *essential* because our bodies cannot manufacture them. As we'll see, the human body can literally create certain fats from other types of fat it consumes, or even from sugar, but certain fatty acids are essential and must be consumed in food. That's why they're called *essential* fatty acids or EFA's. EFA deficiencies are common in the general population.[115]

The two types of fat that are essential are ALA (or alpha linoleic acid) and LA (linoleic acid).

The first one, ALA, is an omega-3 fat.

LA is an omega-6 fat.

The relationship between these two fatty acids is at the heart of all the debates about fat. Why? Because these essential fatty acids can be converted by the human body into other necessary fats.

ALA can be converted into EPA, which is then in turn converted into DHA, an extremely valuable fat that is vital for brain function and hormone regulation.

It's been found that in most societies eating a very healthy diet, close to nature and in superior health, the ratio of omega-6 to omega-3 in the diet was between 1:1 and 4:1.[116] That means they either got the same quantities of omega-3 fats in the diet as omega-6, or maybe twice as many omega-6, and up to four times as much.

However, the modern American Diet is extremely unbalanced in essential fatty acids, containing a very unhealthy ratio, high in omega-6 fatty acids, but low in omega-3.

---

115 Di Pasquale, M. (2009). The essentials of essential fatty acids. *Journal of Dietary Supplements*, 6(2), 143-161.
116 The importance of the ratio of omega-6/omega-3 essential fatty acids. **http://www. ncbi.nlm.nih.gov/pubmed/12442909**

Food	Omega 6-3 Ratio
Flax	1:4
Hemp	4:1
Walnuts	7:1
Avocado	15:1
Average American Diet	20:1

LA is found in high quantities and ratios in a lot of vegetable oils, such as corn, sesame, cottonseed and sunflower.

ALA is found in high quantities and ratio to LA in leafy greens, fruits and vegetables, canola oil, flax, soy, hemp and walnuts. (The ratio will vary from food to food.)

It's been estimated that we need approximately 2 grams of ALA per day.[117] So where can we find this on a raw food diet?

Food	Quantity	ALA content
Greens	125 calories (2 heads of lettuce)	1 gram
Fruits and vegetables	1000 calories	1 gram
Flax seeds	1 1/2 TBS	2 grams

As we can see from the table above, if someone only ate fruits and vegetables, providing they ate enough to meet their caloric needs, and also included a good amount of greens, they could theoretically get the essential fatty acids from those foods, without needing to add fatty foods to the diet.

---

117 Omega-3 fatty acids. (2010). *University of Maryland Medical Center.* Retrieved December 13, 2010, from **http://www.umm.edu/altmed/articles/omega-3-000316. htm**

It's possible that we don't digest all the minute quantities of fat in fruits and vegetables, so it's advisable to also add to the diet a few good sources of fats that will provide additional essential fatty acids in the appropriate ratio.

Selectively choosing your fat sources to be those that have a better omega-3 to omega-6 ratio (such as hemp or flax) will help balance things out.

DHA

Finally, we have the question of DHA. We know that DHA is a very important fat that could account for as much as half the fat content of the human brain. It's essential for hormone production and brain function, and it is a critical fat for pregnant women.

DHA deficiencies have been linked to depression and even Parkinson's disease. In one article, Dr. Fuhrman analyses the deaths of some Natural Hygienists and raw vegans from Parkinson's disease, and asks this question:

> Was it a coincidence, that these leaders in the natural food, vegetarian movement, who ate a very healthy vegan diet and no junk food, would both develop Parkinson's? I thought to myself--could it be that deficiencies in DHA predispose them? Why does Parkinson's affect more men than women? Is there evidence to suggest that DHA deficiencies lead to later life neurologic problems? Are there primate studies to show DHA deficiencies in monkeys lead to Parkinson's? The answer to all of these questions is a resounding, yes.

> Recent scientific findings show diets rich in omega-3 fatty acids, in particular DHA (docosahexaenoic acid), have a protective effect on this type of neurodegenerative disease. Studies in animals clearly show that supplementation of DHA can alter brain DHA concentrations and thereby modify brain functions leading to reduced risk of neurodegenerative diseases like Alzheimer's and Parkinson's.

A recent study examined mice which were exposed to two diets; one group was fed a diet with DHA and other omega-3 fatty acids; while the other group was given ordinary food, lacking DHA. After a period of time, they were given a dose of a chemical that causes the same damage to the brain as Parkinson's disease. The mice on the DHA diet seemed to be immune to the effects of the chemical, whereas the mice that ate ordinary food developed symptoms of the disease.

According to the researchers, among the mice that had been given omega-3 supplementation - in particular DHA - omega-3 fatty acids replaced the omega-6 fatty acids in their brains. Due to the fact that concentrations of other omega-3s (LNA and EPA) had maintained levels in both groups of mice, the researchers suggested that the protective effect against Parkinson's indeed came from DHA.

Another conclusion drawn from this finding is that a brain containing a lot of omega-6 fatty acids may create a fertile ground for developing Parkinson's disease. These fatty acids are abundant in foods rich in either vegetable oil or animal fat, which we already know contribute negatively to our health.

Another study observed the effect of DHA on monkeys treated with MPTP, a drug that induces Parkinson's-like symptoms, and the results suggested that DHA can reduce the severity of, or delay the development of, these drug-induced symptoms and, therefore, can offer therapeutic benefits in the treatment of Parkinson's.

Overall, this research provides evidence that DHA deficiencies can leave us vulnerable to developing diseases like Parkinson's and Alzheimer's. If you are a nutritarian, flexitarian, vegan, or vegetarian, and you are not taking DHA or confirming your levels are adequate with blood work, you are being negligent and potentially increasing your risk of such a disease in later life. All the good efforts on proper nutrition can be undone with one deficiency, such as Vitamin D, B12, or DHA. I see this every week in my practice.[118]

We know that cold-water fish contains EPA and DHA (fish such as salmon and trout), and that's why fish oils are so popular as a nutritional supplement.

---

118 http://www.diseaseproof.com/archives/healthy-food-leaders-of-the-vegan-movement-develop-parkinsons-case-studies.html

It's been thought for a long time that not everyone is able to make the conversion of EPA to DHA properly. However, a recent study compared DHA levels in various groups eating different diets (including fish-eaters, meat-eaters who didn't eat fish, vegans, etc.) and it was discovered that groups not consuming a lot of DHA in fish were still able to make the conversion, which was reflected in their blood levels of the fatty acid.[119]

This means that it's not necessary to consume fish to get DHA since the human body is capable of converting ALA into EPA and then DHA, although fish-eaters tend to have better levels of DHA than those who don't eat it.

Women are better at synthesizing DHA from EPA than men, maybe because DHA is so critical for their growing children.[120]

Aging and bad health can also affect the body's ability to properly convert EPA to DHA. Also, DHA levels in the brain are an important regulator of brain glucose uptake, which means that without proper nourishment, the brain will degenerate![121]

So, a vegan does not have to consume fish oil, or even any fat at all, to get all the DHA she needs, as long as she eats enough fruits and vegetables, generous quantities of greens, and with a more concentrated source of omega-3, such as flax or hemp, she can be sure to get enough.

119 Welch, A., Shakya-Shrestha, S., Lentjes, M., Wareham, N., &Khaw, K. (2010). Dietary intake and status of n-3 polyunsaturated fatty acids in a population of fish-eating and non-fish-eating meat-eaters, vegetarians, and vegans and the precursor-product ratio of [alpha]-linolenic acid to long-chain n- 3 polyunsaturated fatty acids: results from the EPIC-Norfolk cohort. *American Journal of Clinical Nutrition, 92*(5), 1040-1051.

120 Burdge, G., &Wootton, S. (2002). Conversion of alpha-linolenic acid to eicosapentaenoic, docosapentaenoic and docosahexaenoic acids in young women.*British journal of nutrition, 88*(4), 411-420.

121 Freemantle, E., Vandal, M., Tremblay-Mercier, J., Tremblay, S., Blachère, J., Bégin, M., et al. (2006). Omega-3 fatty acids, energy substrates, and brain function during aging.*Prostaglandins, Leukotrienes, And Essential Fatty Acids, 75*(3), 213-220.

However, to be on the safe side, it would be wise to get your essential fatty acid profile done and check your DHA levels. If there's any doubt or deficiency you could consider supplementing with vegan DHA. Vegan DHA is derived from algae, and therefore, it is completely free of fish oil, but with a similar DHA content.

Superfood or Kryptonite?

In my book *The Raw Vegan Coach*, I answer all the questions I have received over the years about specific superfoods that are popular in the raw food movement.

So I will not try to cover everything here, but instead, I will give you my opinion and experience with some of these superfoods, in a nutshell.

Raw cacao — Fortunately, raw cacao was not popular when I first started on the raw food path. Cacao may be rich in antioxidants and magnesium, but so are other raw fruits and vegetables. On the other hand, cacao contains a generous amount of theobromine, a substance that acts like caffeine in the body. Cacao is a stimulant and not a health food. It can be used occasionally as a treat, although I prefer the caffeine-free carob powder as a substitute, which is also lower in fat and alkaline-forming. Many raw foodists have reported problems like insomnia, cravings, depression and adrenal fatigue from consuming cacao regularly.

Green juice — Vegetable juices have their value. Vegetable juice is in a sense easier to digest than raw vegetables, and it can be a valuable source of alkaline minerals in an easily absorbable form. The fiber is gone, but lack of fiber is generally not a problem in the raw food diet. The best juices come from mild green vegetables (such as celery, lettuce, spinach, cucumber and kale), which can be flavored with some carrot or apple juice. Celery juice can be a useful source of natural sodium as well.

The problem is that the proponents of vegetable juicing have been taking a good thing to an extreme, transforming these vegetable juices into miracle cures. I see many people drowning their bodies in green juices, thinking it's going to offset the negative effects of the rest of their bad diet. I recommend some vegetable juice if you have the time to make it, although there is nothing you find in vegetable juice than you cannot find in whole vegetables. It may just be easier to assimilate. One or two

8-ounce glasses of green juice per day is enough and beneficial. More is just a waste, and the body will reject what it doesn't need anyway.

Raw Honey — Honey is a rich and sweet food that has been used by humans for at least 10,000 years. It's a mixture of fructose (38.5%) and glucose (31%), as well as other simple and complex sugars. Contrary to popular belief, honey contains only trace amounts of vitamins or minerals. Honey has certain antiseptic and antibacterial properties, and certain types of honey are full of antioxidants.[122] For these reasons, it's traditionally been used as a folk remedy, mostly with topical applications. The pH of honey is quite low, and this high acidity is part of the reason why it is believed to be antibacterial.

Honey is a refined sugar, and it should never be an important source of calories in any diet. It does have certain beneficial properties, especially in topical use (on the skin). I occasionally use honey in certain recipes, and my wife uses raw honey on her skin for health benefits and wound treatment.

Green Powder — Green powders, often made with barley grass or wheatgrass and other vegetables, used to be very popular. The hype is not justified because there's nothing you find in green powders that you cannot find in fresh greens. The cost-per-nutrient ratio is often very high. The only advantage is the convenience factor for traveling. I have used some barley grass powder when I traveled to places where vegetables were not available. I find that it's better to have some barley grass powder than no vegetables at all, but if I have access to organic greens, then I don't use green powders at all.

Coconut Oil — Coconut oil is a refined fat and a concentrated source of saturated fats. The claims regarding the "healing" powers of coconut oil are largely exaggerated. It remains a highly concentrated source of saturated fat, as one tablespoon of coconut oil contains more saturated fat than a Big Mac. Eat fresh coconuts in moderation and you will

---

122 Blasa, M., Albertini, M., Piatti, E., Piacentini, M., Candiracci, M., &Accorsi, A. (2006). Raw Millefiori honey is packed full of antioxidants. *Food chemistry*, *97*(2), 217-222.

enjoy any possible benefit of coconut oil. Most coconut oils are also not actually raw: they are spun in a huge centrifuge at high speeds that heat up the coconut meat well past 118°F to separate the oil from the meat. Also, any raw fresh oil would go rancid at room temperature and when exposed to light. If you believe there are health benefits to consuming raw coconut oil, I suggest you contact the manufacturer and find out exactly how it is "pressed" and at what temperature, because very few are actually raw. Personally I do not consume coconut oil but I am not opposed to the topical use of coconut oil, as it is a wonderful oil for the skin to moisturize and cleanse the face.

Agave Nectar — This is a popular sweetener used as a vegan alternative to honey. The problem with this sweetener is the same as with all other refined sugars. Agave is composed of mostly fructose (56%) and glucose (20%) and there is no evidence to prove that it is significantly better than refined sugar. Agave is generally often touted as raw, but any product that is shelf-stable and in a clear refined liquid form is rarely minimally processed, or truly raw either.

Açaí — Açaí (pronounced "ah-sigh-ee") is a Brazilian fruit from a particular palm tree mainly found in that country. It's a little fatty and not very sweet, but it has a strong taste and a very high antioxidant content.[123]

In Brazil, they sell it in big frozen blocks, and they blend in a sweetener with it and serve it in a bowl with granola. It's quite popular in the South of Brazil, where I tried it in my visit of 2003. Now, this popularity has spread to the Western world, where açaí products are a new craze. Ridiculous claims were made about açaí when it started to be sold as a nutritional supplement (including increased libido, which is usually the cheapest argument supplement companies like to use to sell their product). I have nothing against açaí as a food, but I object to it as a nutritional supplement. Açaí may be rich in antioxidants, but so are

---

123 Kang, J., Li, Z., Wu, T., Jensen, G., Schauss, A., & Wu, X. (2010). Anti-oxidant capacities of flavonoid compounds isolated from acai pulp (Euterpeoleracea Mart.). *Food Chemistry, 122*(3), 610-617.

plenty of other foods that are cheaper, such as pomegranate, concord grapes and blueberries. Frozen açaí served as a sorbet, mixed with a sweetener and fruit, is a great recipe and probably the best way to enjoy this fruit, but don't kid yourself that it has magical healing powers.

Spirulina — Spirulina is a common superfood. It's a microscopic blue-green algae that was used by some American pre-colonial civilizations, such as the Aztecs. It's rich in protein, essential fatty acids, vitamins, minerals and antioxidants. Spirulina is often recommended as a source of Vitamin B12. However, current research shows that the Vitamin B12 in spirulina is not bioavailable. True Vitamin B12 (cobalamin) is similar in structure to other compounds, such as that contained in spirulina, that cannot be utilized by the human body. In other words, this B12 analog competes with B12 and increases the requirement.[124] Some raw foodists I know, such as author Wayne Gendel, recommend spirulina over other types of blue-green algae, which can be contaminated. If you take spirulina, make sure it's from a reputable company.

Maca — Maca is a Peruvian root vegetable that is often sold dried and powdered as a supplement and superfood. The dried root is mostly carbohydrates and contains 10% protein and only 2.2% fat. Maca is rich in minerals and contains other substances that have been reputed to enhance sexual function. Some people use maca to help with hormonal function, skin tone and sex drive. These claims have not been documented through many reputable studies. Although I included maca in my smoothies a long time ago, I never noticed any benefits, so I eventually discarded it. Some people find it to be really valuable. My mind is open, but I think the benefits have been largely overrated.

Goji Berries — There was a time when goji berries sold for $30 a pound in some online raw stores, when you could go to any Asian market and buy the same quantity for only $6. Goji berries are rich in nutrients and

---

124 Watanabe, F., Katsura, H., Takenaka, S., Fujita, T., Abe, K., Tamura, Y., et al. (1999). PseudovitaminB(12) is the predominant cobamide of an algal health food, spirulina tablets. *Journal Of Agricultural And Food Chemistry*, 47(11), 4736-4741.

antioxidants, so I'm not opposed to them as long as you can get a good price on them.

Seaweed — Over the years, I have consumed some seaweed on and off. It's always been a sort of replacement for salt, as I find many salads absolutely unappealing without some sort of salty condiment. Seaweeds are a part of many Asian diets, and they have been consumed for thousands of years. Sea vegetables, such as kelp, contain some useful minerals and trace elements (such as iodine) that can be hard to find on an unsupplemented raw vegan diet (or any diet, for that matter). The sodium content of both kelp and dulse powder is low, so for that reason, and as another way to obtain extra nutrients, I encourage the moderate, but regular, consumption of some sea vegetables. My favorites are kelp powder and dulse flakes, available from Maine Coast Sea Vegetables.[125] I don't eat them every day, but I consume them usually once or twice a week.

Sprouts — For a long time, sprouting was synonymous with the raw food diet. A raw or "living foods" diet was a diet that included a lot of sprouts.

The arguments used to promote sprouts were a bit more philosophical than scientific. For example, it's often been said that sprouts are very rich in vitamins and are true "living foods," because the enzymes are converting complex substances into simple ones that are easy to assimilate.

This is all true. Sprouts are very rich in vitamins, compared to the seeds that they come from. They are also full of enzymes, because the sprouts are producing them to grow from a simple seed to a full-grown plant.

When we look at the nutritional content of sprouts, we can be impressed. However, let's remember that fresh greens are often more nutritious than sprouts.

---

125 www.seaveg.com

For example, here's the comparison between 100 grams of spinach and 100 grams of alfalfa sprouts:

Nutrient	Alfalfa	Spinach
Vitamin A	155 IU	9376 IU
Vitamin C	8.2 mg	28.1 mg
Folate	36 mcg	194 mcg
Calcium	32 mg	99 mg
Iron	2.7 mg	1 mg
Magnesium	79 mg	27 mg
Zinc	0.9 mg	0.5 mg
Manganese	0.2 mg	0.9 mg

As you can see, spinach beats alfalfa hands-down in most key nutrients, except for iron, magnesium and zinc.

I could go down the list comparing various greens with various sprouts, and we'd quickly come to the conclusion that greens are more nutritious as a food category.

Plus, it's not very easy to eat a lot of sprouts. One can easily eat half a pound of spinach in a salad, but it would be more difficult to do the same with sprouts, due to their strong taste.

Also, certain sprouts have known toxins in them that can injure health when consumed in large quantities.

A few years ago, a man from Quebec named Gilles Arbour contacted me, because he had found out that buckwheat greens contained a toxin that caused his skin to be ultra-sensitive to sunlight.

This man had visited the *Hippocrates Health Institute* and had decided to follow the program recommended by the institute very strictly upon his return to Quebec.

The health program recommended the consumption of generous quantities of green juice made with various vegetables (including buckwheat sprouts).

After a few weeks of this regimen, he noticed that his skin became very sensitive to sunlight. Montreal in the winter is certainly not known as a sunny place, but even a bit of sunshine through windows was enough to burn his skin!

He couldn't figure out what caused it, but after a lot of research, he identified the culprit: buckwheat greens.

On his website, he writes:

"The basic problem with buckwheat greens is that they contain fagopyrin, a naturally occurring substance in the buckwheat plant. When ingested in sufficient quantity, fagopyrin is known to cause the skin of animals and people to become phototoxic, which is to say hypersensitive to sunlight. This condition, specifically known as fagopyrism, occurs when the ingested fagopyrin accumulates under the skin and is subsequently activated by sunlight, resulting in a toxic reaction within the skin. Typically, exposed areas of skin turn pink or red within minutes, and a strong burning sensation accompanies the reaction. Within a few hours, the exposed areas usually appear to return to normal, however continue to remain ultra-sensitive to cold water, hot water, and to friction. This sensitivity can last for days."

After this event, he contacted the Hippocrates Health Institute to inform them of the results of his research and his bad experience with buckwheat greens. The institute reviewed the scientific literature on the subject and *decided to stop serving and recommending buckwheat greens at their institute!*

Sprouts have not been used in human foods for a long period of time and, therefore, have not been cultivated to be toxin-free. There are possibly more toxins in sprouts that haven't been identified yet, but that could pose problems for raw foodists eating large quantities of them.

For all those reasons, I do not recommend eating sprouts on a regular basis. Certainly, some sprouts, such as alfalfa, clover, sunflower, or even buckwheat, can be added to salads occasionally. There's nothing wrong with that. But it makes more sense to focus on consuming plenty of greens rather than sprouts.

CHAPTER 26

Fat: The Good, the Bad and the Ugly

The biggest question I receive about the raw food diet is this: "Why so much fruit? Can't eating that much fruit be bad for you?"

Another common question relating to the low-fat diet is this: "But... don't we need to eat some fat to be healthy? What about essential fatty acids? What about Good Fats?"

In the 1990s, the Mediterranean Diet became trendy, and nutrition experts worldwide advised us to put olive oil on everything.

In recent years, all kinds of oils, from fish to flax, have been used as supplements, and even as medicines, and gained tremendous popularity.

Although the vast majority of diets are no longer low-fat, most nutritionists advise against eating too much fat in the diet, even though they often promote diets containing around 30% fat.

What is the true story?

As mentioned previously, essential fatty acids (EFA's) are very important for many metabolic functions. Contrary to popular belief, a low-fat diet will not cause an EFA deficiency, because these fats are found in all leafy vegetables, whole fruits and vegetables, and of course nuts, seeds and avocados.

On the diet that I advocate, which contains from 7 to 15% fat, you will be way above the minimum requirement of 2-4% of calories from essential fats.

Fish contains a siginificant amount of EFA's because like humans, fish consume plant foods such as algae, which made the EFA's in the first place.

But EFAs are best obtained in natural whole foods, such as vegetables, green vegetables, nuts, and seeds. And, yes, even fruits contain a certain percentage of fat. By eating enough fruits and vegetables to meet your needs, as well as the equivalent of about one ounce of nuts or seeds per day, you can get all the EFAs you need.

The Problems with Fat

It's common knowledge that too much saturated fat from animal foods (eggs, beef, etc.) causes heart disease and other health problems.

When I first went raw, I was told that the problem is not *fat* per se, but the *cooked* and *denatured* fats that most people eat in the typical Standard American Diet. I was told that as long as I ate the raw, natural fats found in nuts, seeds and avocado, I would be okay. I could eat as much of those fats as I wanted and still be healthy.

My experience over the past 14 years, not only with myself, but also with the thousands of raw foodists I have met, shows that this way of thinking is wrong.

Cooked fats are less healthy than raw fats because heat denatures the fat and often renders it toxic. When oils begin to smoke, they become carcinogenic. The smoke point of different oils is reached at different temperatures. When oils are reused (such as in deep frying), their smoke point is reached at an even lower temperature.

Cooked fats could be very bad for you because they are *denatured*. However, they are still fat. Eating fats raw, in their "natural" state, doesn't change their basic chemical composition as a fat.

All fats, when consumed in excess, have their problems, including the so-called "healthy" fats found in olive oil, avocado, nuts and seeds.

Dr. John McDougall writes:

"Most people have assumed olive oil to be protective against heart disease because of the low incidence of heart disease in Mediterranean countries and that EFA also prevent heart disease. However, research indicates otherwise. A study on humans conducted by David Blankenhorn, M.D., and his associates compared the effects of different types of fats on the growth of atherosclerotic lesions inside the coronary arteries of people by studying the results of angiograms taken one year apart (JAMA 263:1646, 1990).

The study demonstrated that all three types of fat--saturated animal fat, monounsaturated (olive oil), and polyunsaturated (EFA)--were associated with a significant increase in new atherosclerotic lesions. Most importantly, the growth of these lesions did not stop when polyunsaturated fats of the w-6 type (linoleic acid) and monounsaturated fats (olive oil) were substituted for saturated fats. Only by decreasing all fat intake--including poly- and monounsaturated fats--did the lesions stop growing.

Dietary polyunsaturated fats (EFA), both the w-3 and w-6 types, are incorporated into human atherosclerotic plaques; thereby promoting damage to the arteries and the progression of atherosclerosis (Lancet 344:1195, 1994). In part, this is because these oils are easily oxidized, forming free radicals that damage the arteries. Most research indicates w-6 type EFA are much more damaging to the arteries than w-3 type EFA (Am J Clin Nutr 49:301, 1989).

Furthermore, high-fat meals, in contrast to low-fat meals, can cause considerable increases in plasma triglycerides and plasma levels of blood coagulation factors, which lead to a blood clot or thrombosis in the heart artery. One of the most important clotting factors predicting the risk of a heart attack is factor VII.

The five fats tested--rapeseed oil (canola), olive oil, sunflower oil, palm oil, and butter--showed similar increases in triglycerides and clotting factor VII after eating. According to the authors, "These findings indicate that high-fat meals may be prothrombotic (causing a blood clot leading to a heart attack), irrespective of their fatty acid composition." (Aterioscler Thromb Vasc Biol 17:2904, 1997).

Since w-3 EFA cause a variety of changes that both decrease and increase the risk of a heart attack, the overall impact of consuming these as free oils will have to be determined by future experiments. Undoubtedly, the w-6 varieties are artery damaging. Most likely, the heart benefits of a Mediterranean diet are due to it being a nearly vegetarian diet. The Mediterranean diet is good in spite of the olive oil (Am J Clin Nutr 61:1321S, 1995).[126]"

In the same article I'm quoting above, McDougall continues to bring even more evidence from scientific research indicting vegetable or fish oils for:

- Increased risk of cholesterol and diabetes

- Increased risk of bleeding

- Nutritional imbalances

- Immune system repression

- Obesity

- Cancer

A vegetable oil — even if cold pressed with the most natural methods — is still a refined product. It is 100% fat by calorie, and contains no fiber.

But even without consuming refined oils, it's still possible to consume too much fat in whole foods such as avocado, nuts and seeds.

Fat and Blood Sugar

The main problem caused by the overconsumption of fat is decreased insulin sensitivity. In his book *Breaking the Food Seduction*, Dr. Neal Barnard, M.D., describes an experiment that shows how a high-fat diet affects blood sugar.

"Marjorie was one of our research volunteers. In a laboratory test, we asked her to drink a syrup containing 75 grams of pure sugar. Taking blood samples over the next two hours, we saw what happened to her blood sugar. As you can see in the graph below, it peaked at about thirty minutes, then quickly cascaded downwards. That's a pretty

126 SOURCE: http://www.drmcdougall.com/res_vegetable_fat_med.html

typical pattern. If your blood sugar falls too precipitously, you may be set up for another binge, which is your body's way of bringing your blood sugar back up again.

Here's the problem: Insulin is the hormone that escorts sugar from your bloodstream into the cells of the body. It is like a doorman who turns the knob on the door to each cell, helps sugar go inside, and then closes the door. Now, while insulin is busily storing sugar in cells, it slows down fat-burning. Biologically, this makes sense, because if you've just taken in food there's no need to be burning off fat for energy. If your insulin is working efficiently, it quickly stores the sugars coming from whatever foods you've eaten and then goes away, so fat-burning can resume.

But everything changes when you eat fatty foods, or when you gain a significant amount of weight. Insulin can't work in an oil slick. When there's too much fat in the bloodstream, insulin's hand slips on the knob. Unable to open the door to the cells, insulin lets sugar build up in the blood. Your body responds by making more and more insulin, and eventually, it will get the sugar into the cells. But meanwhile, that large amount of insulin traveling in the bloodstream has been slowing down your fat-burning.

The answer is to get that grease out of the diet. Research shows that reducing fat, especially the saturated fat that is common in chicken, beef, fish (yes, anywhere from 15 to 30 percent of fish "oil" is nothing but saturated fat), dairy products, eggs, tropical oils, like palm or coconut oil, has a tremendous effect on your body's ability to handle sugar. Cutting fat from your meals improves what is called insulin sensitivity, meaning that insulin efficiently escorts sugar into the cells of the body. It does its job and gets out of the way. Boosting fiber helps, too.

With our guidance, Marjorie adjusted her diet to scrupulously cut fat and boost fiber. A few weeks later, we repeated the test. She again drank exactly the same sugar solution, but the changes in her blood sugar were very different. Because the low-fat diet had tuned up her insulin, the blood-sugar rise was more muted, the peak was lower, and the fall was gentler than before. In the ensuing weeks, not only was her blood sugar stabilized, but she found that cravings were much less insistent. With a simple diet adjustment, you can do precisely the same thing — dramatically changing your body's blood sugar response to any food. In our clinical studies, we have found that simple diet changes alone boost insulin sensitivity by an average of 24 percent, and it can increase even more if you also exercise."

The same author I quoted above also has another book, *Dr. Neal Barnard's Program for Reversing Diabetes*, which presents more research on the role of diet in insulin resistance and type-2 diabetes.

In this book, Dr. Barnard presents the results of two studies, one done on 13 patients and published in *Preventive Medicine* in 1999, and another with 59 patients, published in the *American Journal of Medicine* in 2005.

His researched showed that dietary changes alone are enough to improve insulin sensitivity and bring blood sugar back to healthy levels. The core of Dr. Barnard's program is this:

-Follow a vegan diet (no meat, dairy products, eggs or fish)

-Avoid oils and keep all fats to a very minimum. (He recommends avoiding avocados, nuts and seeds for those on the program.)

-Favor foods with a low glycemic index.

On the last point, raw foodists should be happy to hear that nearly all fruits have a low glycemic index. The glycemic index shows how certain foods affect blood sugar levels in most people. The higher the GI, the more these foods tend to raise blood sugar fast. Most fruits are rather low on the glycemic index, and the only ones that make it to the "high" category are watermelon and pineapple.

Traditional "diabetes" diets tend to deal with the problem of type-2 diabetes rather than offering a solution. They tend to control blood sugar by limiting carbohydrates and spacing meals throughout the day to avoiding spikes and drops in blood sugar.

The low-fat approach to type 2 diabetes looks at the problem from another angle: high-carbohydrate foods do not cause type-2 diabetes. In fact, before the advent of western civilization, most populations in the world lived on a very high-carb diet and were free of diabetes. The solution is to improve insulin sensitivity (which measures how efficiently insulin works at escorting sugar to your cells), which is usually done with a combination of:

- Low-fat diet
- Exercise
- Achieving optimal weight

If you'd like to gain a better understanding of the mechanisms behind blood sugar and diet, and how a high-fat diet can create insulin resistance, I recommend that you read the two books by Dr. Neal Barnard that I mentioned. It is beyond the scope of this book to fully explain how it works.

Even Low-Carb Pundits Get It

Most of the natural health movement is essentially divided between two camps:

- Those who recommend a low-carb, high-protein diet.
- Those who recommend a low-fat, high-carbohydrate diet.

Loren Cordain belongs to the first category. He's the author of *The Paleo Diet*, a popular book that promotes a return to Stone Age nutrition (a diet of lean meat, fruits and vegetables). Although he promotes a high-protein diet, he's also aware of the damage caused by excessive quantities of saturated fats in the diet. In his book, he made an interesting remark:

"Some scientists believe that high-saturated-fat diets make insulin metabolism less efficient. Others, including Dr. Gerald Reaven at Stanford University, believe that high-carbohydrate diets — both low- and high-glycemic foods — are to blame. Still others single out high-glycemic carbohydrates. However, the obvious has been ignored: Most people who develop obesity and diseases of insulin resistance do it with mixtures of high-fat and high-glycemic carbohydrates. Some examples of these bad food combinations: Baked potato and sour cream. Bread with butter. Eggs with toast and hash browns.

Pizza with cheese. Ice cream, candies, cookies, pizza, chips. These and all of the other processed foods we eat have both high fat and high-glycemic carbohydrates.[127]

If carbohydrates were truly the cause of type-2 diabetes, then nobody would get better on the type of diet promoted by Dr. Barnard, which limits fat but encourages high-carb foods.

The problem is the fat. Even worse than a high-fat diet is a diet that is both high in fat and high in sugar. This is the type of diet that I followed for many years, with disastrous results. Although I never stopped to check my blood sugar at the time, I could feel it going out of control.

Author Steve Pavlina is a well-known personal development guru (**www.stevepavlina.com**), who enjoys using himself as a human laboratory for all kinds of experiments and sharing the results with his readers.

One of his experiments was to try going for 30 days on a raw food diet. However, the most interesting part of his trial was the fact that he decided to go on a low-fat, high-fruit diet. After completing the trial, he wrote:

"I monitored my blood sugar using a blood sugar testing device, the same kind diabetics may use. It showed no discernible spikes in blood sugar throughout the trial whatsoever — absolutely none. In fact, my blood sugar remained incredibly steady throughout the trial. My highest blood sugar reading of the trial was 94, which is still medium-low. All that sweet fruit in my diet simply did not have any adverse effect on my blood sugar.

Eating this way gave my blood sugar more consistency than ever. I couldn't spike my blood sugar on this diet if I tried. Even eating 19 bananas in one day made no difference.[128]"

---

127 The Paleo Diet, Loren Cordain, Ph.D.
128 **www.stevepavlina.com/blog/2008/02/raw-food-diet/**

Saturated Fat

Of all categories of fat, saturated fat is the type that has been most consistently linked to heart disease, high cholesterol levels and cancer.

One would think that saturated fat is only found in animal foods, but it can also be found in high levels in certain plant foods. In general, most raw foods that are higher in fat are relatively low in saturated fats, but there are some exceptions. Coconut products are the richest source of saturated fat, containing even more than beef. Of all nuts, cashews contain the most saturated fat. Durian is also an appreciable source of saturated fat, but at the time of this printing I was unable to find out how much. (Durian is not a common food item in American nutritional databases!)

Food	Total Fat Content	Saturated Fat Content
100 grams of lean ground beef	16.3 g	5.7 g
McDonald's Big Mac	29 g	10 g
1 large egg (boiled)	5.3 g	1.6 g
Almonds, 3 ounces	42 g	3.3 g
Cashews, 3 ounces	37.2 g	6.6 g
Avocado, 3 ounces	13.8 g	1.8 g
Durian flesh, 1 cup	13 g	
Coconut milk (canned), 1/2 cup	28.6 g	25.3 g
Coconut oil, extra virgin, 1 Tbsp.	14 g	14 g

Too Much Fat is Too Much Fat

Everybody knows that eating cheesecake is not healthy for you. It's probably the most indulgent dessert, combining lots of fat and sugar together. In recent years, "raw vegan" cheesecake has been widely popular. I now see it sold in many health food grocery stores, and I've even found it on display in health restaurants in Bali and Thailand!

Raw vegan cheesecake is often made using coconut oil, cashews, seeds and dried fruit. Is it healthy and low in fat?

I compared a *New York Style Deli Cheesecake* recipe containing graham crackers, butter, four packages of cream cheese, white sugar, milk, eggs, sour cream and flour - to a raw vegan cheesecake. The results are astonishing.

Although the raw vegan cheesecake is slightly lower in calories per serving, it contains more fat.

As with the regular cheesecake recipe, the portions are quite conservative. They divide a 9-inch cake into 12 portions, which is a tiny slice. Most people would eat a slice twice as big, which means a whopping 1000 calories (but very few nutrients) from your raw vegan cheesecake!

Type of "Cheesecake"	Calories per entire recipe	Calories per serving	Total Fat per serving	Saturated Fat per serving
Regular New York Style Cheesecake*	6368	530 calories	35 g	21.24 g
Raw Vegan Cheesecake**	6068	505 calories	41.5 g	16.74 g

* The regular cheesecake recipe comes from: **http://allrecipes.com// Recipe/chantals-new-york-cheesecake/Detail.aspx**

** The raw vegan cheesecake recipe comes from: **http://blissfullyvegan. wordpress.com/2010/07/27/raw-cheesecakes/**

Can Fruit Sugar Make You Fat?

One of the reasons people are afraid of fruit sugar and tend to go for high-fat diets instead is the fear that eating all this fruit sugar will cause elevated blood sugar levels. We've already seen that this is not the case at all. However, there is still a concern that all this sugar may cause weight gain, as it may be converted into fat.

Fat gain is easier on a high-fat diet because the fat consumed can be stored directly as body fat.

Joel Fuhrman, M.D., writes in his book *Eat to Live*:

> "Fat, such as olive oil, can be stored in your body within minutes without costing the body any caloric price; it is just packed away (unchanged) on your hips and waist. If we biopsied your waist fat and looked at it under an electron microscope, we could actually see where the fat came from. It is stored there as pig fat, dairy fat, and olive fat — just as it was in the original food. It goes from your lips right to your hips. Actually, more fat from your last meal is deposited around your waist than on your hips, for both men and women. Analyzing these body-fat deposits is an accurate way for research scientists to discern food intake over time."

As a second resort, if one consumes calories in excess of the daily needs, a small percentage of the sugar consumed can be transformed into fat by the liver through a process known as *de novo lipogenesis*. This tends to reduce sugar in the blood but raise triglyceride levels (blood fat). However, studies that have looked at the role of sugar in *de novo lipogenesis* have used refined sugar as a model.

They have found, although not conclusively, that the sugar itself causes *de novo lipogenesis*, not the total carbohydrate content of the diet.[129]

Other studies have shown that fructose consumption is more likely to lead to *de novo lipogenesis* than other types of sugar. Because fruit usually contains about 50% of its sugar content as fructose, it is possible one may gain some body fat eating too much of it.

My theory on this is that a combination of fat intake and increased caloric intake is necessary for significant weight gain to occur.

It is possible to gain body fat from a high-fruit, low-fat raw diet, but it is often difficult to do, as many people undereat on calories. One would have to consume more calories than one burned, in order to gain body

---

129 Chong, M., Frayn, K., & Fielding, B. (2007).Metabolic interaction of dietary sugars and plasma lipids with a focus on mechanisms and de novo lipogenesis [electronic resource].*Proceedings of the Nutrition Society*, 66(1), 52-59.

fat; but because fruit is not dense in calories, it's not something that's easy to do.

Some people (especially women) sometimes have trouble losing those last 10 pounds. Other long-term raw foodists complain of weight gain years after they started eating raw. This is probably due to the fact that they are not exercising enough to burn the excess fruit sugar they are eating, and they are also able to eat larger quantities of fruit than they used to when they first started.

If that happens while eating a lot of fruit, you should look at cutting down some of the sweeter fruits in your diet (like bananas and mangoes) and replacing them with low-calorie fruits, like berries and papaya. Increase the vegetable content of your diet, and decrease the fruit content. If you miss all that fruit, then earn it by exercising more!

Too Much Fruit Sugar?

I have found that although the low-fat raw vegan diet is best, in some cases, some people transitioning to this diet have true problems with the high quantity of fruit sugar in the diet. This is usually the case when they start off the diet with severe candida or other major health problems.

For those cases, I recommend a gentle approach that doesn't brutally introduce large amounts of fruit into the diet all at once. It's best to transition gradually, using low-glycemic index, cooked complex carbohydrates as a temporary replacement for some of the fruit intake.[130]

---

130 Examples of low-glycemic carbohydrates include all beans, brown rice, sweet potato, most vegetables and pasta. High-glycemic index carbs to avoid are: bread, white rice, white potato.

There are also other protocols that can be incorporated to improve digestion and eliminate candida that are beyond the scope of this book. But the most important thing is a gradual approach with an emphasis on overcoming the root issues of your health problems.

CHAPTER 27

Conclusion: The Ideal Diet

When I first discovered the raw food diet, I had an image of paradise in my head. To me, raw foodism represented the key to a lost ideal. I conjured images of Adam and Eve and ancient human tribes living in harmony with Nature. Lacking in references from popular Hollywood movies with an anti-civilization agenda (the movie Avatar hadn't been made yet), I relied on my knowledge of philosophy and the myth of the "noble savage" that I got from reading the French philosopher Jean-Jacques Rousseau.

Armed with a new vision of ideal human society, I envisioned the "noble raw foodist," the perfect version of optimal human accomplishment, who lived in a state of "Paradise Health" (a term used by raw food diet author Arnold Ehret). For a number of years, I thought that most of humanity's problems were mainly caused by eating cooked foods! It was the fall from grace. Even worse than eating the fruits from the tree of knowledge, we cooked them!

When I first went raw, I thought that this diet would make everything better. I thought that anybody eating raw would automatically become a better person in almost every way. Then I met real-life raw foodists, and I realized that they had their problems and shortcomings just like everybody else. Each of them had a different idea of what the raw food diet represented. Some smoked pot, and they didn't see a contradiction there. Others went to different extremes, such as living on one type of fruit alone, trying to eat nothing but green juices for weeks at a time, or, even worse, trying to practice 100% breatharianism.

Raw foodism often carries this idea that modern civilization has corrupted everything. Through our bad diet, our health has declined, and all other problems of society followed. It's the belief that sometime, somewhere, in the past, humans lived in perfect harmony with nature, eating fruit off the tree and probably nothing else. Then, one day, they lost their way and started eating cooked foods, a process which eventually got out of hand with the invention of the Big Mac.

I now realize how naive and misguided this idea was. Not only is it false to say that civilization has corrupted everything (after all, aren't raw foodists using their computers to distribute their ideas?), but raw foodism itself is a product of civilization!

All the scientific evidence shows that in all of our history as human beings, we've eaten some form of cooked foods or animal foods. There is also a good reason to think that this change in our diet enabled us to get more concentrated calories in less time, which enabled the development of the human brain.

Our brain is three times larger in volume than those of the apes that are the most closely related to us genetically. Our brain uses about 25% of the calories we get in food and 20% of the total oxygen we breathe.

It is quite possible that the evolution of the human being would not have been possible without cooked foods or animal foods. Yet, at the core of our being, we are fundamentally fruitarian creatures. Some research has shown that pre-human ancestors were probably living on a fruitarian diet (see sidebar at the end of the chapter).

This particular ability that the human being has to function on almost any diet, up to a point, has enabled us to establish human cultures everywhere on the planet, and even send people to the moon and back (unless you're like some raw foodists I know and believe that's a conspiracy too).

Although we can survive on almost anything, it is not without consequences. The modern Western diet has been a disaster for our health, and it is with good reason that we seek alternatives.

Going back to "Nature" is a little bit misleading, since at no point in our history as humans proper have we lived solely on raw fruits and vegetables. Throughout our history, human cultures have always relied on one main source of calories. For the Polynesians, it was taro root and breadfruit. For the Peruvians, it was potatoes. For much of Asia, it was rice. For the Eskimos, it was animal fat. At no time in recorded history did humans live on fruits and vegetables alone.

As I heard Dr. John McDougall say in a debate between himself and Dr. Fuhrman on the role of starches in the human diet,

> "All successful populations that have lived on a plant-based diet have lived on a starch-based diet. There's no exception. (...) Basically, if a society, a village, decided to go on a raw diet or a high green/yellow vegetable diet, their caloric intake would be so sparse that what would happen is they would become too weak to fight their battles, and the next-door tribe would come and kill all the men, rape the women, and they'd be gone. So it would never happen! To live successfully, you must understand the importance of starches, as the Asians have with rice, as the Peruvians have with potatoes, as the Native Americans have with corn, as the Hawaiians have with Poi. Every single society that's ever existed on a plant-based diet always ate a starch-based diet. You need the calories. You can't do otherwise. You won't win the battles. You won't survive."

No human society has ever lived on fruits and vegetables, because in pre-modern days, they were not reliable sources of calories for entire societies to live on. Fruits cannot be stored for long periods of time, and unless one grows tropical varieties, they are generally too low in calories for primitive societies to use as a staple. Even modern raw foodists, with their access to blenders and imported fruits from all over the world, still often struggle to get enough calories eating only fruits and vegetables.

Can you imagine how much more difficult it would have been throughout the rest of human history? The fact is that as long as we've been humans, we have not subsisted on a fruit-based diet. However, our basic physiological design is still that of the fruitarian, but with a curious ability to adapt to a wide range of diets (often with negative consequences).

Monkeys can afford to spend eight hours a day eating, but their digestive tract is also much different from ours, and they can handle tough, fibrous and astringent fruits that even the most motivated raw foodist would find hard to swallow.

Could Humans Live on a Chimpanzee Diet?

The idea is appealing: chimpanzees live on fruit. Therefore, we can also live on fruit. However, we should ask ourselves: what kinds of fruit do chimpanzees live on?

"Evolutionary adaptation to cooking might likewise explain why humans seem less prepared to tolerate toxins than do other apes. In my experience of sampling many wild foods eaten by primates, items eaten by chimpanzees in the wild taste better than foods eaten by monkeys. Even so, some of the fruits, seeds, and leaves that chimpanzees select taste so foul that I can barely swallow them. The tastes are strong and rich, excellent indicators of the presence of non-nutritional compounds, many of which are likely to be toxic to humans — but presumably much less so to chimpanzees. Consider the plum-size fruit of Warburgia ugandensis, a tree famous for its medicinal bark. Warburgia fruits contain a spicy compound reminiscent of a mustard oil. The hot taste renders even a single fruit impossibly unpleasant for humans to ingest. But chimpanzees can eat a pile of these fruits and then look eagerly for more. Many other fruits in the chimpanzee diet are almost equally unpleasant to the human palate. Astringency, the drying sensation produced by tannins and a few other compounds, is common in fruits eaten by chimpanzees.

(. . .) Astringency is caused by the presence of tannins, which bind to proteins and cause them to precipitate. Our mouths are normally lubricated by mucoproteins in our saliva, but because a high density of tannins precipitates those proteins, it leaves our tongues and mouths dry: hence the "furry" sensation in our mouths after eating an unripe apple or drinking a tannin-rich wine. One has the same experience when tasting chimpanzee fruits, such as Mimusops bagshawei or the widespread Pseudospondias microcarpa. Though chimpanzees can eat more than 1 kilogram (2.2 pounds) of such fruits during an hour or more of continuous chewing, we cannot.

(…) The shifts in food preference between chimpanzees and humans suggest that our species has a reduced physiological tolerance for foods high in toxins or tannins. Since cooking predictably destroys many toxins, we may have evolved a relatively sensitive palate."

~ Catching Fire, by Richard Wrangham

Even Raw Foodists "Cook" Their Foods

Let's take a look at the way raw foodists prepare their foods. Even smart raw foodists, like low-fat raw vegans, do the equivalent of "cooking" without using any heat. Let me explain:

- We get more calories from our raw foods by making smoothies and other blended foods.

- We assimilate more from our greens by blending them into soups, or even juicing them.

- We favor high-calorie fruits such as bananas, dates, mangoes, and other tropical fruits, which have been bred to be high in sugar and low in fiber.

- We make rich dressings by blending nuts, seeds and avocados.

- Some raw foodists also ferment certain tough vegetables like cabbage for easier digestion.

Why do you think that blending is so popular in the raw food world? Why do you think that green smoothies are such a craze? Why do you think vegetable juicing has so many fans? These are all techniques we use to get the most out of our raw foods! In other words, most people inherently understand that eating just carrot sticks doesn't work. They know that raw foods are lower in calories and, therefore, have discovered all kinds of ingenious ways to make them more digestible.

The raw food diet CAN work when we use some of these tools. On the other hand, it would be almost impossible to live off wild foods. Anyone who eats a significant quantity of wild food in their diet gets the bulk of their calories from cultivated fruits, cooked rice or grains, potatoes or avocados, or eats animal products.

It's not that cooking food is one of the defining aspects of civilization. It's the "processing" of foods that makes the difference. This includes: blending, cultivating, hybridizing, juicing, etc. Raw foodists may just be a lot smarter because they use methods that don't create toxins that are harmful to the body when processing their raw foods.

We are civilized by nature. Even the modern raw food diet is completely "unnatural."

Now, for the first time in history, it is possible to attempt to live on a raw food diet. Modern agricultural techniques developed over the last hundreds of years enable us to grow fruits that are sweet enough to use as a staple, and modern trade and globalization brings us a variety of high-quality fruits and vegetables from all over the world. Combined with a little knowledge of human nutrition, a good blender, and a few recipes, the average person can now live on the cleanest and healthiest diet in the world, and yet, they can still get enough calories to get through the day. This is, in effect, a return to our pre-human roots, because our digestive tract and physiology is still mostly adapted to a fruitarian diet (with greens), even though no human tribe has ever lived on fruit for reasons of survival and practicality.

This raw food diet, when done properly, is the healthiest diet one could conceive of because of its extremely high nutrient density, low level of toxicity, ease of digestibility, and high antioxidant level.

Let's not fool ourselves into thinking that the raw food diet is "natural." Eating cooked food is as natural for a human being as grazing on grass is for a cow, but so is grabbing a bunch of bananas and blending them into a smoothie. A chimpanzee wouldn't do it, but for us humans, processing food is the only natural way to live. Without easy access to calories, no human society can thrive. (Why do you think populations all over the world have skyrocketed in the past 100 years? The advent of the industrial era and mass production of food with a long shelf life.)

The fundamental flaw of the raw food diet is falling for the trap of primitivism (everything in nature is better, reject modernity!), and this false idea that going raw can somehow defy the laws of nature.

Most raw foodists imagine that over time, they'll be able to live on less and less as their bodies will more "efficiently process the food they eat." We also have certain gurus who claim that they only need to eat a few peaches a day, or that they could live on air if they wanted. They say the great sin of raw foodists is eating too much. Nonsense! If there's a sin that raw foodists commit, it is quite the opposite: not eating enough, or grazing like a cow on low-calorie vegetables, flavored with fat and salt.

Have you ever seen a monkey eat fruit? A chimpanzee can literally engulf banana after banana after banana. Monkeys in the wild are on a constant search for calories, as is the rest of the animal kingdom. Can we humans escape the laws of nature that the same deluded raw foodists pretend to wholeheartedly embrace?

Teeth Show Fruit Was the Staple, No Exception Found

By Boyce Rensberger

May 15, 1979 issue of the New York Times

BALTIMORE - Preliminary studies of fossil teeth have led an anthropologist to the startling suggestion that early human ancestors were not predominantly meat eaters or even eaters of seeds, shoots, leaves or grasses. Nor were they omnivorous. Instead, they appear to have subsisted chiefly on a diet of fruit.

Not until the advent of Homo erectus, the species immediately ancestral to Homo sapiens, is there evidence of the omnivorous diet that is typical of human beings today.

If confirmed, the findings would upset several widely held assumptions about the diet of early hominids, or human-like creatures. It is generally held, for example, that the large, flat-topped molars of the robust forms of Australopithecus were used to grind tough nuts and roots. The smaller form of Australopithecus and a similarly gracile form of true human being called Homo habilis were thought to have been omnivorous, mixing meat with roots, nuts, eggs, shoots and fruit.

"I don't want to make too much of this yet", said Dr. Alan Walker, a Johns Hopkins University anthropologist, who discovered the dental evidence. "But it is quite a surprise."

No Exceptions Found

The sample of teeth studied so far is small - fewer than two dozen representing four major types of hominids. But, while the sample is small, no exceptions have been found.

Every tooth examined from the hominids of the 12-million-year period leading up to Homo erectus appeared to be that of a fruit-eater.

Every Homo erectus tooth was that of an omnivore. Homo erectus was the first form of human being known to have migrated out of Africa. Specimens have been found in many parts of Africa and Asia.

The findings are based on extremely detailed analysis of the microscopic wear patterns on the chewing surfaces of the teeth. The method, which Dr. Walker invented, uses a scanning electronic microscope to see scratches and pits that are invisible to the naked eye.

Dr. Walker has found that different kinds of food contain materials that mar the enamel surface of a tooth in characteristic ways. It is possible even to distinguish between a grass-eater and a leaf-eater because each food contains characteristic types and quantities of silica crystals that form naturally within plant cells. These crystals, called phytoliths, are harder than tooth enamel and scratch it slightly as the animal chews its food.

Grasses contain a much higher proportion of phytoliths than do leaves of bushes and trees. Fruits contain almost none at all. As a result, fruit eaters' teeth are highly polished, lacking any of the wear patterns characteristic of other food sources. Meats contain no phytoliths but the teeth of carnivores show scratches caused by crunching into bone.

Consistent Patterns of Wear

Using the teeth of various living mammals whose diets are known, Dr. Walker has established that the basic pattern of microwear on teeth is fairly consistent from one species to another. This is largely because tooth enamel is essentially the same substance throughout the animal kingdom.

To prove his method, Dr. Walker has compared the microwear patterns on closely related species of animals that are known to have different feeding habits. For example, of two closely related species of hyrax (rodent-sized hooved mammals sometimes called conies), one feeds predominantly on grass while the other is a browser, eating leaves of bushes and trees. Their teeth can be told apart easily using a scanning electronic microscope.

Dr. Walker has established similar patterns in the various types of wild pig, such as warthog, and among a number of monkeys and apes. It is against these patterns that the hominid teeth are checked.

If it is true that the earliest hominids were all predominantly fruit eaters, the fact would suggest a way of life more like that of chimpanzees living in forests than most anthropologists had suspected.

There are many stories and interesting episodes that I didn't include in the book simply through lack of space or time. I could have told you about a raw foodist whose nickname was *Skeletor* because he was so thin, who almost burned down his house on a one-time cooked food binge.

I could have talked about the guy in Costa Rica I knew who lived for 6 months on just coconut water, who ended up losing his mind walking around buck naked at a bus stop. He was sent back to his home country, Germany, after being taken to the hospital and pumped up with Vitamin B12 that he was apparently deficient in.

The moral of all these stories is that some people tend to follow an ideal a little too religiously, without paying attention to good common sense.

When I first went raw, I thought that people's personalities would change on the raw food diet. Shy people would become socially confident, and angry people would calm down.

I was wrong.

The raw food diet may not change who you are fundamentally, but it can have a profound effect on your health, which in turn can affect other aspects of your life.

Do you want that change to be positive or negative?

In spite of the crazy stories I told you, there's countless more stories of incredible recoveries and renewed health that represent the other side of the coin. Most raw foodists experience amazing, positive results in the first few years on the diet, but are unable to succeed in the long run for the reasons I outlined in this book.

The traditional raw food diet, the one I tried to follow for my first few years as a raw foodist, and the one that is generally promoted in most books on the subject, simply does not work.

In all the years I have been following this movement, I can honestly say that I have never seen anyone eat this way for a long time without eventually crashing. Almost every person I featured in this book is no longer eating this way, because it does not work. Eventually, they all did one of the following:

- Gave up entirely

- Continued eating mostly raw, but introduced some cooked foods in the diet

- Cut down the fat and dramatically increased the amount of fruit they ate

- Started eating animal foods (because they got deficient on a low-calorie diet)

Most raw food chefs eventually stop eating the food they prepare, as they prefer eating more simply (read: fruits and vegetables). Yet, they continue to serve their high-fat, gourmet raw food as an "excellent transition" for new would-be raw foodists.

I don't know a single vegan chef who doesn't eat what he makes... except for raw foodists! This is a covert admission that their diet simply does not work, and they cannot eat these meals day after day themselves.

In the introduction to this book, I promised to try to answer the question: "what is the ideal diet?"

I will answer it now.

The ideal diet is a raw food diet of fruits and vegetables, with plenty of fruits to meet your caloric needs and plenty of green vegetables to cover the rest. Nuts and seeds, as well as other fatty foods, can be eaten, but only in small quantities. Vitamin B12 is a concern, so supplementation in that area is recommended.

Although, in my experience, this diet is ideal, no human population has ever eaten this way, and very few people have done it for a long period of time. Because no long-term studies of raw food nutrition have ever been done, we don't know if the low-fat, raw vegan diet is ideal in the long-term or if children could be raised successfully on it. We're in unknown territory here, so we just have to keep an open mind.

In spite of my more moderate approach to the raw food diet and my own personal consumption of cooked foods on occasion, I still feel the best when I eat raw. As much as I've made mistakes eating this way over the years, and as costly as these mistakes have been, it would have been foolish to toss the baby out with the bath water, as they say in America. The raw food diet can work if you make it work, and if you keep your mind open to new information and research.

Is it necessary to eat 100% raw to be healthy?

No. Besides the rigorous and ascetic discipline of 100% raw and (by comparison) the debauchery of eating whatever pleases our senses, there exists a third way of eating.

I call this way the *Mostly Raw Plan.*

This way is for people who, for whatever reason, find it easier to be able to eat some cooked foods. Some people just don't like the pressure of eating all raw. Some people (like myself) get bored eating only raw and actually enjoy the taste of plain steamed vegetables. Some places have poor quality fruit during the winter, and there isn't enough variety for some people to stay raw and get enough calories. Others want more flexibility in social situations. Others still might be worried they are not getting everything they need from just raw food (a fair concern, especially if you undereat) or even just get tired of so much fruit sugar.

Contrary to what is commonly believed by some raw food gurus, it is possible to make this *third way* work in practice. There is a big trap there of letting this *Mostly Raw Plan* turn into a *Mostly Cooked Plan,* and thereby forego the benefits of eating raw altogether. However, there's also a way to make it work.

I intend to publish another program called the *Mostly Raw Plan* sometime in 2011, with a more detailed explanation of this particular way of eating, full of new tips and ideas that have never been explained before. I believe that some people really want to eat just mostly raw, and feel that the pressure of 100% plans is too great for emotional health. So my program will be for them.

In the beginning of this book, I said I would tell my story, present all the evidence, and let you decide for yourself. I promised you it was not an "all-or-nothing" proposition.

Some people — the perfectionists — will not be happy unless they have the very best. I belonged to that category for a long time. If they can afford it, they would rather have the Lexus with all the advanced features, than a simple Toyota Corolla to get from point A to point B. In diet, they will opt for 100% raw, and then find a way to make it even better, like removing all sources of fat from the diet or even living on fruit or juice exclusively.

After so many experiments, I realized that I didn't *have* to be perfect to get the results I wanted. I just needed to follow the 80-20 rule and mainly focus on the 20% that gave me 80% of the results, without trying to worry about every single little thing that I could be doing better.

I once heard an expert on investing saying that the biggest mistake people make is not starting to invest soon enough. They seek the perfect investment, and because of their confusion, they procrastinate taking any action at all. Don't let this confusion about nutrition delay you from taking action.

Now that you know the mistakes to avoid, and have a good understanding of what to do instead, you should be able to decide how you're going to make it work in practice. No matter how you choose to do it, you're going to get positive results.

If you'd like more information on the practical side of the raw food diet, make sure to check out the companion DVD to this program, called *Raw Food Nutrition Explained.*

If you didn't grab this DVD when you bought this book, make sure to get it with a special discount for readers of this book by going to

www.rawcontroversies.com/dvds

I hope that you've enjoyed my story and have learned something from my experience. As I like to say in my email newsletter, I wish you great health and success, in all areas of your life.

Frederic Patenaude

November 2010

Chiang Mai, Thailand

CHAPTER 28

A Little Update

In this book, I wrote the most thorough "diet autobiography" I could, focusing on the part of my journey that seemed the most relevant to my readers, starting with my discovery of the raw food diet in 1996. I took you through all of my diet experiments over the years, all the way up until my fast in 2005, with a brief overview of what happened after.

A lot of things happened in my life since 2005 — enough to fill another book of the same size! I've decided to keep things simple and focus on what would be the most relevant to any aspiring raw vegan.

Some people might be curious about what happened "after," and wish for a few more details about the person behind this book.

I was barely 20 when I discovered the raw food diet. I am 34 at the time of publication, quickly going on 35.

My passion for the raw food diet and health has led me to publish over 50 different books, eBooks, DVDs and other information products on the subject. Although I have no formal training in nutrition, I have an unquenchable thirst for knowledge and a natural skepticism that leads me to question everything.

Every year I read dozens and dozens of books and information on health and nutrition from authors of every kind of program and diet plan.

Over the years, I have earned a reputation for my common-sense approach to the raw food diet, in a field where many are often led astray by the latest scam. Although I do believe it's valuable to question established knowledge, it's also wise to not fall for any particular health philosophy as the "ultimate and indisputable truth."

405

My publishing career in this field really began after 2005, when I became more involved in the Internet community of raw food enthusiasts by building an e-zine readership of over 30,000 people worldwide, sharing my insights and ideas about raw foods and health. (You can check out my main website at **www.fredericpatenaude.com**).

In spite of my interest in health and nutrition, a bigger part of my work consists of teaching aspiring writers and health-food enthusiasts how to make a living in the natural health movement, through my other website www.dowhatyoulove.com

After my fast in Costa Rica in 2005, I have developed a special relationship with that country, and even decided to move there more or less permanently in 2006. Since then, I have returned to Canada, while continuing to spend my winters in tropical countries.

Last year in 2009, I met my wife Veronica on a raw food discussion forum. We exchanged many emails and phone conversations for a long time before finally meeting in person, and we've been together ever since! We got married in May 2010 near the beautiful tropical waterfalls of Southern Costa Rica, where we also spent the winter. Right after our wedding, we embarked on a trip around the world that is currently still underway as I'm writing these lines, taking us to an impressive number of countries, from Iceland to New Zealand.

At some point during our trip, Veronica gave me the idea for writing this book. I've hesitated for a long time to share my story with the world, but now I'm glad I did. I hope that many people can benefit from this information and avoid the mistakes that others and I made.

In this book, I have told stories and mentioned certain public figures in the raw food movement that could represent these people in a negative way.

I want to emphasize that although everything I wrote is true and actually happened, everyone involved in the early phases of the new boom of the raw food movement was guilty of some form of magical thinking (including myself). Too often, we simply did not know what we were doing and would often "wing it".

In this book, I told you the story of my own evolution through all of my different diet experiments. It is natural to assume that the other people I have mentioned in the book that are still active in the natural health field today also went through their own personal evolutions and most likely see things quite differently today from how they did in the past.

I hope that you feel empowered by my book, somewhat demystified about the whole raw food movement, and can avoid some of the mistakes it took me a lot of years and frustration to figure out.

Thank you for coming on this journey with me, and I hope that you take something valuable away from the experience.

What Happened to the Characters in this Book?

Dominic— My great friend Dominic still lives in Montreal, works full-time publishing books and information products on energy medicine and self-improvement, and tries to eat as healthy as he can, paying attention to his body. He never went back to raw foods after his first experiences being 100%, but he regularly makes green smoothies, and he studies various health philosophies, including the low-fat vegan diet of Dr. John McDougall.

Mario — Mario, my mom's friend, who turned our family on to vegetarianism and natural health, continues his financially-independent, young retiree's lifestyle. We haven't been in touch for many years, so I don't know what diet he's following now. One day I saw him, and he told me that the secret to success was probably "Eat raw and make passive income!"

Albert Mosséri — Albert Mosséri is now 85, and he still lives in the same little village in France. He continues to publish his newsletter and does telephone consulting. We finally met for the first time in 2010, and I did an interview with him that appeared on my website.

Sebastien — My brother, Sebastien, never went back to raw foods after his adventures eating raw for many years in Montreal. The social aspects of eating raw were too restrictive for him, and because he did not have any health problems to worry about, he decided to give up the diet and enjoy eating a normal diet, but rarely eating meat and animal products. He's working in the film-editing business, and he has created a few documentaries since, including producing my *Raw Vegan Cuisine* DVD series.

Andrew — I fell out of friendship with Andrew a few years ago. Since then, I heard he decided to make the move permanently to Guatemala. After a life-long disgust for civilization, he finally decided to escape from America for good. He's currently interested in a new concept of fasting in the dark, and he shares his thoughts on the subject at **www. andrewdurham.com**

RC Dini — At some point, RC Dini had over 57 websites, with unusual names such as **www.giggleisland.com, www.fruitmessiah. com,** and **www.rawsoldier.com.** It seems that all of these websites were not renewed, and we don't know what happened to RC since.

David Wolfe — David Wolfe still travels the world, spreading the word about the raw food diet, superfoods and optimal nutrition. His website is **www.davidwolfe.com.** Even though I may have portrayed David in a negative light in this book, all of my criticism was directed at the ideas that were part of the raw food movement that I joined in the late 90s. I know that David has changed his mind on many topics and kept evolving, just like I did, although in a different direction. I may not agree with everything he claims, but I can credit him for having been an important, mostly positive, force earlier in my life. I will always be grateful for his help in getting me involved in the raw food movement.

Stephen Arlin – Stephen changed his name to Thor Bazler, and he now lives in beautiful Northern Idaho. He sells a high-quality raw protein supplement available at **www.rawpower.com.** Over the years, Thor and I have stayed in touch and shared some ideas about diet and health, but more importantly, music, as Thor's great passion is symphonic metal music. Every few years, he'll introduce me to a new band that I'll get addicted to for a while.

Durian — The last time I spoke to Durian was over 9 years ago. He was still living in San Diego and was still a vegan, but he had given up the 100% raw food ideal.

Claudia — Every other year, I would speak to Claudia on the phone. The last time was over 5 years ago. She was still living in Switzerland and still doing her best to stay healthy, but not eating 100% raw.

Raven — Raven still lives in New York City, and promotes her "Age-Defying Solutions" for women. Her website is: **www.ravenpelan.com**

Jeremy Safron — Jeremy still lives on the island of Maui. He is still a raw foodist, but after about 15 years of high-fat raw, he decided to introduce some animal products into his diet. He claimed he didn't have as much energy and strength as before. So he started eating goat cheese and eggs, and claims that he is doing much better since. His website is **www.lovingfoods.com**

Doug Graham — Doug Graham still follows the 80/10/10 diet, which has gained tremendous popularity in the last few years. He claims that the 80/10/10 diet is the fastest-growing segment of the raw food movement, and from my point of view, I would agree. His website is **www.foodnsport.com**

David Jubb — David still seems to be active in New York City, although last time I checked, his website was no longer working.

Ready for the Next Step?

If you were to buy a car, would you just buy any model right away without even thinking about it, or would you research the subject thoroughly before making a decision? I'm sure you would spend a lot of time analyzing the different options before making the right decision.

Yet, when it comes to their health, many people are careless.

They search the Internet, looking for quick fixes, and read free articles. They try to make sense of it all by asking complete strangers for health advice on a random bulletin board. They do not take the subject seriously.

This is how they hurt their health unnecessarily, like I did when I first started on the raw food diet without knowing what I was doing.

That's why I've created the **Raw Health Starter Kit.**

For a long time, I've wanted to put together a collection of resources that would give anyone everything they would need to successfully switch to a raw food diet, include more raw food in their diet, or improve their current raw food program.

It took me over 8 years of research to put together all of the resources that are included in the Raw Health Starter Kit, and, in fact, I keep updating it all the time with new information.

When properly done, either at the 100% or the 70% level, the Raw Food Diet can bring you the following benefits and more:

- Gives you amazing energy. You wake up in the morning ready to go, and you rarely feel ups and downs in your energy during the day.
- Improved complexion. People will comment on how clear your skin is.
- Reach your ideal weight effortlessly.
- No feeling of deprivation.
- Great sleep and no insomnia problems.

- Regular bowel movements, with no constipation or indigestion.
- Looking younger than most people of your age.
- Clear and bright eyes
- Makes you happy for no reason. You don't need coffee to stimulate you or alcohol to make you laugh.
- Better focus and concentration.

If you are not experiencing all of these benefits, then it's time to revise your current program.

With **Raw Health Starter Kit**, you'll get everything you need to get started on raw foods (or improve your current program), including:
- My best-selling book, *The Raw Secrets: The Raw Vegan Diet in the Real World*
- My course, *How to End Confusion about Nutrition*
- My recipe book, *Instant Raw Sensations*
- My DVD Series, *The Low-Fat, Raw Vegan Cuisine* (three DVDs)
- My menu planner, *Best Foods on the Planet*
- My new book *The Raw Vegan Coach*
- Tons and tons of other bonuses and resources not available anywhere else. That totals over $400+ in REAL value.

Plus, as a reader of *Raw Food Controversies*, you'll save $20 on your order! (See below)

Here's what one of my readers had to say about the **Raw Health Starter Kit:**

"After having a mixed experience eating all-raw foods and reading numerous websites and cookbooks about the subject, I decided to give the Raw Health Starter Kit a try.

I was skeptical after participating in some other raw food programs, including a local delivery service. Although I felt a million times better than when I was eating cooked food, I was still getting sleepy and sluggish at times.

The Raw Health Starter Kit is honestly the best money I've spent going raw, and I wish that I had found this website first. I think Fred's observations and advice are spot-on and the way to be a healthy, supercharged raw-foodist.

His recipes are fantastic and incredibly simple; even my non-raw fiancé has taken to making some of the salads and smoothies.

Perhaps the best thing about Fred is that he is non-dogmatic about raw food, and, at the same time, his system is firmly rooted in science and practical common sense. Anyone who wants to eat more raw food would definitely benefit from this kit, not just raw-foodists. Given how poor the nutritional information is out there, I recommend this to anyone who simply wants to eat better.

Danica Radovanov

Los Angeles, California, USA

Here's another letter I recently received:

Dear Frederic,

Hi! I'm 53 years young and getting younger. I ordered the Raw Health Starter Kit about a month ago, and I am really enjoying all the great information and recipes contained therein.

4 months ago, I found out that my blood sugar was through the roof! My cholesterol, blood pressure, and triglycerides were all out of control. I had been taking pills for several years to "control" these things. I was tired of just covering it up, knowing good and well that I could do something about it.

Well, that pushed me right into getting healthy. The great thing is now that I am eating raw and exercising. It just, overall, gets easier, because I feel better than I have in years. As part of my recovery, I started reading everything that I could online about true, healthy living that I found your site and all the other free information, so I decided to get more info. I ordered the Raw Health Starter Kit to give me more specific info and more motivation.

There are so many recipes, tips, and general good health info that I am still reading, acting on, and then reading more and again. I really like having both the e-books/files, hard cover books, and CDs.

Well, I have been monitoring my blood pressure and sugar levels, went to my doctor for cholesterol and triglyceride levels, as well as A1C (long term sugar level), she has taken me off all those harmful chemical meds, because every level is in the excellent zone.

I look better and feel better. I want to get out, and exercise my body. All the fruits and veggies taste so clean and wonderful. I went out to dinner with the family and ordered just a raw veggie salad no dressings, cheese, etc.

Had a little craving for what they were eating, but seeing all the oils, salt, grease, and fat just reminded me of how poorly most people in the world eat.

Also, I knew that if I didn't cave into false desires and went to bed that I would be glad in the morning. True enough, the next morning those cravings from the night before had no emotional hold on me, and I was glad that I woke up light and healthy.

Thank you for your inspiration and easy-to-digest information programs. They are helping me stay the course and motivating me to do great things in my life.

Don Webber

Encino, California, USA

Here's another story from a reader in Australia:

Dear Frederic,

Since ordering the Raw Health Starter Kit, life has definitely changed for the better. I am 61 years old, thought that I was eating well, and was a bit dubious about such a different way of eating. However, I gritted my teeth and began to follow the eating pattern that you recommended.

In only a few weeks, I noticed that I no longer had hot flashes, my asthma had disappeared (I no longer take any medication which I was taking for 14 years), and the arthritis in my hands vanished. I have noticed too that the liver spots on my hands have faded and are now almost non- existent.

When I did the pinch test on my hands, previously, the skin stayed erect, but now it goes back down immediately. I feel as if there is a glow about my skin. Additionally, the dentist has commented that my teeth are in better condition. I highly recommend the Raw Health Starter Kit for a healthier, fitter, and longer life.

Ann

Australia

You'll find many more testimonials on the **Raw Health Starter Kit**, great success stories, and before and after stories of people who have completely transformed their life with the raw food diet on my website.

In fact, we recently completely redesigned the **Raw Health Starter Kit** to offer an even more complete package.

I won't try to convince you anymore about it.

Go to www.rawstarterkit.com and learn more. Make sure to use the coupon code RAWCONTROVERSIES to get a $20 discount (this offer expires soon).

I hope that you've found this book useful. I certainly would have benefited if someone had written it when I first got started, as this information was not available back then.

I'm looking forward to adding your story to our long list of success stories from people who have successfully applied the teachings in the **Raw Health Starter Kit!**

Wishing you health and success,

Frederic

Other Products By Frederic Patenaude

The following products are also available at **www.fredericpatenaude. com/products.html**

Some of these products are included as part of the **Raw Health Starter Kit.**

The Raw Vegan Mentor Club

This is my exclusive membership program offering monthly raw food menu planners, a "members only" newsletter that you receive by mail and online, interviews with health & success gurus, special reports, members' discussion forum, and more!

Sign up for a trial subscription and get over $1200 in gifts. Just go to **www.fredericpatenaude.com/mentorclub.html**

Low Fat Raw Vegan Cuisine DVD Set

An invaluable amount of knowledge laid out in a step-by-step format you can easily follow. This set includes two DVDs presenting my simple and easy low-fat raw cuisine, as well as a bonus DVD on how to make the diet work in practice.

This DVD set is included as part of the Raw Health Starter Kit! Get it now by going to **www.rawstarterkit.com**

The Raw Secrets

The groundbreaking book I first published in 2002. It offers a fresh perspective and research on the raw-food diet. This book was completely revised just two years ago.

This book is included as part of the Raw Health Starter Kit! Get it now by going to **www.rawstarterkit.com**

Instant Raw Sensations

The easiest, simplest, most delicious raw-food recipes ever. This recipe book shows you recipes that can be in 5-10 minutes with ingredients that are easy to find.

This book is included as part of the Raw Health Starter Kit! Get it now by going to **www.rawstarterkit.com**

Perfect Health Program

This is a complete home-study course on achieving radiant health, happiness and peak performance. Features over 13 hours of interviews with Dr. Doug Graham and complete transcripts.

Get more information on the Perfect Health Program at **www. fredericpatenaude.com/perfecthealth.html**

How to Heal and Prevent Dental Disasters in 21 Days or Less

Put an end to tooth pain, bleeding gums, gingivitis and decay. This information can save you thousands of dollars and lots of unnecessary pain.

Get more information on this dental health program, go to: **www. fredericpatenaude.com/oralhealth.html**

Toothsoap

Best selling item! This dental product has helped many with bad gums, cavities, periodontal disease, and more.

To get more information on toothsoap, go to: **www.fredericpatenaude. com/toothsoap.html**

Do What You Love Products

Do you dream of moving to a tropical paradise?

Would you like to know my complete system for making a living in the natural health movement, doing what you love?

Would you like to work from anywhere, including a beach home or an exotic country, and get regular income through your own website?

Discover my secrets at my other website! Sign up now for your special report at **www.dowhatyouloveuniversity.com**

Want the Whole Enchilada?

If you want every single program I've ever done, including all of my books, DVDs, and CDs, we have a complete package that saves you hundreds of dollars. You also get exclusive bonuses not available anywhere else.

The Whole Enchilada offers all Raw Vegan products and programs, plus bonus material not offered with any other program.

Find out more about the Whole Enchilada Package at **www. fredericpatenaude.com/enchilada.html**

Want to Keep In Touch?

Check out my main websites at:

www.fredericpatenaude.com

www.dowhatyoulove.com

Make sure to sign up for my e-zine to get regular news and updates, as well as three free special reports.

Made in the USA
Lexington, KY
11 July 2012